Advancements in Cardiovascular Research and Therapeutics: Molecular and Nutraceutical Perspectives

Edited by

V. V. Sathibabu Uddandrao

Department of Biochemistry
K.S. Rangasamy College of Arts and Science (Autonomous)
Tiruchengode-637215
Tamilnadu, India

&

Parim Brahma Naidu

ICMR-National Animal Resource Facility
for Biomedical Research (NARFBR)
Hyderabad-500078
Telangana, India

Advancements in Cardiovascular Research and Therapeutics: Molecular and Nutraceutical Perspectives

Editors: V. V. Sathibabu Uddandrao and Parim Brahma Naidu

ISBN (Online): 978-981-5050-83-7

ISBN (Print): 978-981-5050-84-4

ISBN (Paperback): 978-981-5050-85-1

© 2022, Bentham Books imprint.

Published by Bentham Science Publishers Pte. Ltd. Singapore. All Rights Reserved.

First published in 2022.

need for a court order if at any point you breach any terms of this License Agreement. In no event will any delay or failure by Bentham Science Publishers in enforcing your compliance with this License Agreement constitute a waiver of any of its rights.

3. You acknowledge that you have read this License Agreement, and agree to be bound by its terms and conditions. To the extent that any other terms and conditions presented on any website of Bentham Science Publishers conflict with, or are inconsistent with, the terms and conditions set out in this License Agreement, you acknowledge that the terms and conditions set out in this License Agreement shall prevail.

Bentham Science Publishers Pte. Ltd.
80 Robinson Road #02-00
Singapore 068898
Singapore
Email: subscriptions@benthamscience.net

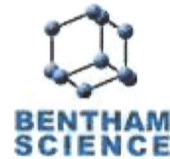

CONTENTS

FOREWORD i

PREFACE ii

LIST OF CONTRIBUTORS iv

CHAPTER 1 CARDIOVASCULAR DISEASES AND NUTRACEUTICALS: UNDERLYING MECHANISM AND THERAPEUTIC BIOMARKERS 1
Pallavi Saxena, Vinod Kumar, Noopur Khare, Neeraj Pal, Dibyabhaba Pradhan
Pradeep K Chaturvedi, Arun Kumar Jain, Manoj Kumar, V. V. Sathibabu Uddandrao
and *Umesh Kumar*

  1. INTRODUCTION 2
    1.1. Cardiovascular Disorders 2
    1.2. Cardiovascular Diseases Burden: Global and National 2
    1.3. Potential Risk Factors for CVD 4
    1.4. Therapies in Use for CVD Treatment 6
      1.4.1. ACE Inhibitors 6
      1.4.2. Angiotension II Receptor Blockers 6
      1.4.3. Antiarrhythmics 6
      1.4.4. Antiplatelet Drugs 8
      1.4.5. M. Anti-coagulants Drugs 8
      1.4.6. Diuretics 9
  2. NUTRACEUTICALS AND CARDIOVASCULAR HEALTH 10
    2.1. Nutraceuticals 10
    2.2. Potential Nutraceuticals 10
      2.2.1. Plant Sterols/ Stanols 11
      2.2.2. Cruciferous Vegetables 11
      2.2.3. Garlic 12
      2.2.4. CoQ10 12
      2.2.5. Turmeric 12
      2.2.6. Grape Skin 12
      2.2.7. Fish Oil/Olive Oil 13
      2.2.8. Vegetables 13
      2.2.9. Carnitine 13
      2.2.10. Berberine 13
      2.2.11. Flavonoids 14
      2.2.12. Prebiotics 14
      2.2.13. Probiotics 14
      2.2.14. Protein and Protein Peptides 14
      2.2.15. Vitamins 15
  3. NUTRACEUTICALS MODULATE GENETIC EXPRESSION 16
    3.1. NF-κB Regulatory Network 16
    3.2. Nrf2 Regulates Antioxidant and Detoxification Genes 16
  4. BIOINFORMATICS APPLICATION IN NUTRACEUTICALS AND CVD PREVENTION 17
    4.1. Identification of New Therapeutic Biomarkers 18
  CONCLUSION 18
  CONSENT FOR PUBLICATION 19
  CONFLICT OF INTEREST 19
  ACKNOWLEDGEMENTS 19
  REFERENCES 19

CHAPTER 2 CONGESTIVE HEART FAILURE: INSIGHT ON PHARMACOTHERAPY 25
Sri Bharathi G.S, Sakthi Sundaram S, Prabhakaran S, Lalitha V, Haja Sherief S
Duraisami R and *Sengottuvelu S*
1. INTRODUCTION 26
    1.1. Hypertrophic Cardiomyopathy (HCM) 27
    1.2. Left Ventricular Noncompaction (LVNC) 27
    1.3. Arrhythmogenic Right Ventricular Cardiomyopathy (ARVC) 27
    1.4. Restrictive Cardiomyopathy (RCM) 27
2. PREVALENCE 28
3. PATHOPHYSIOLOGY 29
4. DRUG THERAPY 29
    4.1. Diuretics 29
    4.2. Angiotensin Converting Enzyme Inhibitors (ACE Inhibitors) 29
    4.3. Beta-adrenergic Blocking Agents (Beta Blockers) 30
    4.4. Vasopressin Receptor Antagonists 30
5. MANAGEMENT OF HEART FAILURE 30
    5.1. Acute Decompensation 30
    5.2. Chronic Management 30
    5.3. Palliative Care 31
    5.4. Cardiac Glycosides 31
        5.4.1. Chemistry of Cardiac Glycosides 31
        5.4.2. Sources of Cardiac Glycosides 32
        5.4.3. Mechanism of Cardiac Glycosides 33
        5.4.4. Pharmacological Activity of Cardiac Glycosides 33
6. DIGOXIN 34
7. TOXICOKINETICS 34
CONCLUSION 35
CONSENT FOR PUBLICATION 35
CONFLICT OF INTEREST 35
ACKNOWLEDGEMENTS 35
REFERENCES 35

CHAPTER 3 DIET, INFLAMMATION AND CARDIOVASCULAR DISORDERS 38
M Kesavan and *HV Manjunathachar*
1. INTRODUCTION 38
    1.1. Diet Induced Inflammation 38
    1.2. Dietary Inflammatory Index (DII) 39
2. DIFFERENT PATTERNS OF DIET AND THEIR CHARACTERISTICS 39
    2.1. The Zone Diet 40
    2.2. Ketogenic Diet 40
    2.3. Mediterranean Diet 40
    2.4. DASH (Dietary Approaches to Stop Hypertension) Diet 41
    2.5. The Paleo Diet 41
    2.6. Vegan and Vegetarian Diet 42
3. CARDIOVASCULAR DISEASES (CVD), PRO AND ANTI-INFLAMMATORY
AGENTS 42
4. SPICES 45
CONCLUSION 47
CONSENT FOR PUBLICATION 47
CONFLICT OF INTEREST 47
ACKNOWLEDGEMENTS 47

REFERENCES 47

CHAPTER 4 RODENT AND NON-RODENT ANIMAL MODELS FOR CARDIOVASCULAR DISEASES 52
Irfan Ahmad Mir, HV Manjunathachar, R Ravindar Naik, SSYH Qadri and Taniya Saleem
   1. RODENT MODELS FOR CVD 53
   2. ATHEROSCLEROSIS AND DIABETIC MODELS 53
      2.1. LDLR−/− Mice 54
      2.2. ApoE−/− Mice 55
      2.3. SR-BI KO Mice 56
      2.4. db/db Mouse 56
      2.5. Ob/ob Mice 57
      2.6. Zucker Fatty Rat 57
      2.7. Zucker Diabetic Fatty (ZDF) Rat 58
      2.8. Otsuka Long–Evans Tokushima fatty (OLETF) Rats 58
      2.9. Goto-Kakizaki (GK) Rats 59
      2.10. WNIN/GR-Ob Rat 59
   3. HEART FAILURE MODELS 61
      3.1. Myocardial Ischemia-Induced Heart Failure 62
      3.2. Pressure Overload Models 62
      3.3. Chemical-induced Cardiomyopathy Models 62
   4. NON-RODENT MODELS OF CARDIO-VASCULAR DISEASES 63
      4.1. Overview of Advantages and Disadvantages of Non-rodent Animal Models 63
      4.2. Pigs 64
      4.3. Atherosclerotic Disease Models 66
      4.4. Pig Models for Stent Application 68
      4.5. Pig Models of Infarction and Heart Failure 68
      4.6. Dogs 70
      4.7. Sheep 71
   CONCLUSION 72
   CONSENT FOR PUBLICATION 72
   CONFLICT OF INTEREST 72
   ACKNOWLEDGEMENTS 72
   REFERENCES 73

CHAPTER 5 APPLICATION OF 21ST CENTURY GENETIC ENGINEERING TOOLS AND CRISPR-CAS9 TECHNOLOGIES TO TREAT MOST ADVANCED CARDIOVASCULAR DISEASES OF HUMANS 79
J. Venkateshwara Rao, R. Ravindar Naik, S. Venkanna and N. Ramesh Kumar
   1. INTRODUCTION 80
   2. THE CRISPR/CAS9 PROTEIN TECHNOLOGY 82
   3. APPLICATION OF CRISPR/CAS9 TECHNOLOGY AS A THERAPEUTIC TOOL FOR HUMAN DISEASES 83
      3.1. Cystic Fibrosis (CF) 83
      3.2. Sickle Cell Anemia 84
      3.3. Thalassemia 85
      3.4. Huntington's Disease 85
      3.5. Duchenne Muscular Dystrophy 86
      3.6. Hemophilia 86
      3.7. Chronic Granulomatous Disorders (CGD) 87
   4. MULTIFACTORIAL DISEASES 87

4.1. Cancer 88
4.2. Cardiovascular Diseases (CVD) 88
5. APPLICATIONS OF CRISPR/CAS9 IN CARDIAC RESEARCH 89
5.1. Gene Therapy for CVD 90
5.2. The Future of CRISPR/Cas9 Genome Editing in Cardiac Research 92
6. CHALLENGES OF APPLICATION OF CRISPR/CAS9 93
6.1. Delivery Systems of CRISPR/Cas9 93
6.2. Off-target Effects 94
6.3. Ethical Issues 94
6.4. Emerging CRISPR Technologies 95
CONCLUSION 96
CONSENT FOR PUBLICATION 96
CONFLICT OF INTEREST 96
ACKNOWLEDGEMENTS 97
REFERENCES 97

**CHAPTER 6 ROLE OF VYANA VAYU IN CARDIOVASCULAR SYSTEM,
ETIOPATHOGENESIS AND THERAPEUTIC STRATEGIES: AN AYURVEDA
PERSPECTIVE** 104
Savitri Vasudev Baikampady, C. S. Hiremath, Reeta Varyani and *Venketesh*
1. INTRODUCTION 104
2. A PREAMBLE TO VATA 106
2.1. Vyana Vayu 106
2.1.1. Role of Vyana Vayu in the Heart 107
2.1.2. Role of Vyana Vayu in Vasculature (Dhamani and Sira) 108
2.1.3. Role of Vyana Vayu in Skeletal Muscles and other Organs 108
3. ETIOLOGY 109
4. PATHOGENESES 112
4.1. Stage of Accumulation (Sanchaya) 112
4.2. Stage of Aggravation (Prakopa) 112
4.3. Stage of Dissemination (Prasar) 113
4.4. Stage of Localization (Sthanasamshraya) 113
4.5. Stage of Manifestation (Vyakta) 114
4.6. Stage of Complication (Bheda) 114
5. CONCOMITANT CONCEPT 115
6. CLINICAL IMPLICATIONS 116
7. TREATMENT STRATEGIES 117
7.1. Diet 117
7.2. Exercise 118
7.3. Pharmacological Approach 118
7.3.1. Terminalia Arjuna (TA) 118
7.3.2. Innula Recemosa 118
7.3.3. Fagonia Arabica 118
8. OMICS STUDY AND AYURVEDIC THERAPEUTIC STRATEGIES 118
CONCLUSION 119
10. HIGHLIGHTS 119
CONSENT FOR PUBLICATION 120
CONFLICT OF INTEREST 120
ACKNOWLEDGEMENTS 120
REFERENCES 120

CHAPTER 7 NUTRACEUTICALS: THE POTENTIAL AGENTS TO RESCUE HUMAN RACE FROM CARDIOVASCULAR DISEASES (CVDS) 125
Sreedevi Gandham, Ghali. EN.Hanuma Kumar and Balaji Meriga
1. INTRODUCTION 125
2. CVDS: PATHOPHYSIOLOGY 127
3. CVDS: TREATMENT OPTIONS 129
4. PLANTS AND HERBS FOR TREATMENT OF CVDS 134
  4.1. Polyphenols 136
  4.2. Flavonoids 136
  4.3. Carotenoids 136
  4.4. Other Phytochemicals 137
  4.5. Vitamins 137
5. NUTRACEUTICALS TO TREAT CVDS 137
6. SPICES AS EFFECTIVE NUTRACEUTICALS TO TREAT CVDS 138
  6.1. Ginger (Zingiber Officinale) 138
  6.2. Turmeric (Curcuma Longa) 139
  6.3. Black pepper (Piper Nigrum) 140
  6.4. Coriander (Coriandrum Sativum) 141
  6.5. Cinnamon (Cinnamomum Zeylanicum) 142
  6.6. Garlic (Allium Sativum) 143
  6.7. Cloves (Syzygium Aromaticum) 144
  6.8. Other Common Spices 145
7. NUTRACEUTICALS/SPICES: MODE OF ACTION 147
CONCLUSION 148
CONSENT FOR PUBLICATION 148
CONFLICT OF INTEREST 148
ACKNOWLEDGEMENTS 148
REFERENCES 148

CHAPTER 8 AMELIORATIVE POTENTIAL OF BIOCHANIN-A AGAINST DEXAMETHASONE INDUCED HYPERTENSION THROUGH MODULATION OF RELATIVE MRNA AND PROTEIN EXPRESSIONS IN EXPERIMENTAL RATS 156
V. V. Sathibabu Uddandrao, P. P. Sethumathi, Parim Brahma Naidu, S. Vadivukkarasi, Mustapha Sabana Begum and G. Saravanan
1. INTRODUCTION 157
2. MATERIALS AND METHODS 157
  2.1. Chemicals 157
  2.2. Animals 158
  2.3. Induction of Hypertension 158
  2.4. Experimental Design 158
  2.5. Measurement of Body Weight 158
  2.6. Indirect Measurement of Blood Pressure in Conscious Rats 158
  2.7. Hemodynamic and Vascular Responsiveness Measurements 159
  2.8. Assay of Nitric Oxide Metabolites 159
  2.9. Assay of Superoxide Production 159
  2.10. RT-PCR Analysis 159
  2.11. Western Blot Analysis 160
  2.12. Statistical Analysis 161
3. RESULTS 161
4. DISCUSSION 165
CONCLUSION 168

CONSENT FOR PUBLICATION 168
CONFLICT OF INTEREST 168
ACKNOWLEDGEMENTS 168
REFERENCES 168

CHAPTER 9 ZINGIBERENE, AN ACTIVE CONSTITUENT FROM ZINGIBER
OFFICINALE AMELIORATED HIGH-FAT DIET-INDUCED OBESITY
CARDIOMYOPATHY IN RATS 171
   S. Jaikumar, G. Somasundaram and *S. Sengottuvelu*
   1. INTRODUCTION 171
   2. MATERIALS AND METHODS 173
      2.1. Chemicals 173
      2.2. Animals 173
      2.3. HFD Composition 173
      2.4. Experimental Design 173
      2.5. Measurement of Body Weight, Anthropometrical and Morphological Parameters 174
      2.6. Estimation of Biochemical Markers 174
      2.7. Determination of Cardiac Lipid Profile 174
      2.8. Assessment of Oxidative Stress Markers in Heart 174
      2.9. Statistical Analysis 174
   3. RESULTS 175
      3.1. Effect of ZB on Anthropometrical and Morphological Parameters 175
      3.2. Influence of ZB on Diabetic Markers 176
      3.3. Effect of ZB on Cardiac Lipid Profiles 177
      3.4. ZB Ameliorated Oxidative Stress in Heart 178
   4. DISCUSSION 179
   CONCLUSION 182
   CONSENT FOR PUBLICATION 182
   CONFLICT OF INTEREST 182
   ACKNOWLEDGEMENTS 183
   REFERENCES 183

CHAPTER 10 BETAINE, A NUTRACEUTICAL AMELIORATED MYOCARDIAL
INFARCTION BY ATTENUATION OF PRO-INFLAMMATORY CYTOKINES AND MATRIX
METALLOPROTEINASE PRODUCTION IN RATS 186
   G. Somasundaram, S. Jaikumar and *S. Sengottuvelu*
   1. INTRODUCTION 187
   2. MATERIALS AND METHODS 188
      2.1. Animals 188
      2.2. Experimental Design 188
      2.3. Measurement of Heart Weight and the Ratio of Heart Weight to Body Weight 189
      2.4. Assessment of Cardiac Diagnostic Markers 189
      2.5. Estimation of Serum Inflammatory Markers 189
      2.6. Determination of Serum Matrix Metalloproteinases 189
      2.7. RT-PCR Analysis 189
      2.8. Statistical Analysis 190
   3. RESULTS 190
   4. DISCUSSION 194
   CONCLUSION 197
   CONSENT FOR PUBLICATION 197
   CONFLICT OF INTEREST 197
   ACKNOWLEDGEMENTS 197

REFERENCES 197

SUBJECT INDEX 201

FOREWORD

I was delighted when I received a request from Dr. P. Brahmanaidu and Dr. V. V. Sathibabu Uddandrao to write a brief foreword to the reprint of this book because, for many years, I have admired their incredible contribution to research especially in the field of metabolic disorders and nutraceuticals. I was excited when they started writing a book on "Advancements in Cardiovascular Research and Therapeutics: Molecular and Nutraceutical Perspectives" and I would be first in line to buy it. In fact, editors sent me a copy of the book draft and I was humbled. Not only was this a great book, but it was also a great way to write and construct chapters.

Looking through this magnificent volume, I am absolutely amazed by the way they presented this book about the pathophysiology of cardiovascular disorders and their novel treatment approaches by nutraceuticals. It is more than a book of lovely illustrations and a mine of information, demonstrating therapeutic approaches and it is a source of inspiration and information in the field of cardiovascular pharmacology. This book is unique and surely a work of treasure for anyone who is interested in cardiovascular research. So, I strongly recommend you to read it, enjoy it and learn from it.

Dr. Ramachandra Subbaraya Gudde
ICMR- National Animal Resource
Facility for Biomedical Research (NARFBR)
Hyderabad, Telangana,
India- 500078

PREFACE

Cardiovascular diseases (CVD) belong to the most severe health problems and are considered the main cause of morbidity and mortality in modern society. CVDs consist of a broad spectrum of diseases, including atherosclerosis, hypertension, myocardial ischemia, cardiomyopathy, and heart failure. Risk factors for CVDs include hypertension, hyperlipidemia, obesity, diabetes mellitus, metabolic syndrome, and a sedentary lifestyle. Therapeutic effects against CVD have been demonstrated by several medicinal plants and nutraceuticals thus presenting new possibilities for the treatment of CVD risk. Evidence suggests that this approach is very promising. So, the aim of this book is to present an update on the most recent evidence related to the use of nutraceuticals in the context of the prevention and treatment of CVD.

Chapter 1 discusses CVD and nutraceuticals and the underlying mechanism and therapeutic biomarkers. The chapter presents the beneficial effects of nutraceuticals on the heart and also gives an insight into the bioinformatics approach to identify novel therapeutic biomarkers in order to update the practitioner's awareness of the use of nutraceuticals for CVD management. Chapter 2 provides detail about congestive heart failure and insight into pharmacotherapy. This chapter explains possible pharmaceutical approaches to treat congestive heart failure. Chapter 3 provides a review of diet, inflammation, and CVDs. The chapter reveals the role of diet in the prevention of vascular inflammation and the usefulness of antioxidants in preventing CVD. Chapter 4 represents the applications, advantages and disadvantages of various rodent and non-rodent animal models in the research on CVD especially while evaluating nutraceuticals' effects against CVD. On the other hand, chapter 5 discusses the CRISPR-cas9 technologies in the 21st century and their applications in cardiovascular diseases.

Chapter 6 discloses the role of Indian Ayurvedic approaches to the cardiovascular system, etiopathogenesis, and therapeutic strategies. The chapter highlights the precipitants that attenuate Vyana Vayu and addresses curative measures to restore Vyana Vayu. Chapter 7 depicts nutraceuticals as potential agents to rescue the human race from CVD. The chapter point outs the current scenario of CVD, pathophysiology, therapeutic drugs available, the role of nutraceuticals in treating CVD, and their mode of action with a special emphasis on commonly used kitchen spices. Chapter 8 explains the therapeutic potential and mode of action of Biochanin-A, a natural compound predominantly found in soy, chickpea, peanuts, alfalfa sprouts, and red clover against hypertension in experimental rats. Chapter 9 concentrates on the ameliorative potential of Zingiberene, a monocyclic sesquiterpene that is the principal constituent of ginger (Zingiber officinale) against obesity and cardiomyopathy. Finally, chapter 10 presents the amelioration of myocardial infarction through the attenuation of pro-inflammatory cytokines and matrix metalloproteinase production by Betaine, a well-known nutraceutical widely occurring in plants, animals and rich dietary sources.

Dr. V. V. Sathibabu Uddandrao
Assistant Professor
Department of Biochemistry
K.S. Rangasamy College of Arts and Science
Tiruchengode-637215
Tamilnadu, India

Dr. Parim Brahma Naidu
DST-Inspire Faculty
ICMR-National Animal Resource Facility
for Biomedical Research (NARFBR)
Hyderabad-500078
Telangana, India

List of Contributors

Arun Kumar Jain	ICMR- National Institute of Pathology, Safdarjung Hospital Campus, New Delhi, 110029, India
Balaji Meriga	Department of Biochemistry, Sri Venkateswara University, Tirupati, Andhrapradesh, India
C. S. Hiremath	Department of Cardiology, Sri Sathya Sai Institute of Higher Medical Sciences, EPIP Area, Whitefield, Bangalore, India
Dibyabhaba Pradhan	ICMR AIIMS Computational Genomics Centre, New Delhi, 110029, India
Duraisami R	Department of Pharmacognosy, Nandha College of Pharmacy, Erode Tamilnadu, India
Ghali. EN.Hanuma Kumar	Department of Biochemistry, Sri Venkateswara University, Tirupati, Andhrapradesh, India
G. Saravanan	Department of Biochemistry, Centre for Biological Sciences, K.S. Rangasamy College of Arts and Science (Autonomous), Tiruchengode, Namakkal District, Tamilnadu, 637215-India
G. Somasundaram	Department of Pharmacology, Sri Lakshmi Narayana Institute of Medical Sciences, Puducherry, 605502-India
Haja Sherief S	Department of Pharmacology, Nandha College of Pharmacy, Erode, Tamilnadu, India
HV Manjunathachar	CMR- National Animal Resource Facility for Biomedical Research, Genome Valley, Hyderabad,Telangana-500101, India
Irfan Ahmad Mir	ICMR-National Animal Resource Facility for Biomedical Research, Genome Valley, Hyderabad,Telangana-500101, India
J. Venkateshwara Rao	Department of Zoology, Osmania University, Hyderabad, Telangana, India
Lalitha V	Department of Pharmacology, Nandha College of Pharmacy, Erode, Tamilnadu, India
M Kesavan	Division of Pharmacology and Toxicology, ICAR-Indian Veterinary Research Institute, Izatnagar, Bareilly, Uttar Pradesh-243 122, India
Manoj Kumar	Biochemistry Department Ghaziabad, Narinder Mohan Hospital and Heart Center, Uttar Pradesh, 201007, India
Mustapha Sabana Begum	Department of Biochemistry, Muthayammal College of Arts and Science, Rasipuram, Namakkal, Tamil Nadu 637408, India
Neeraj Pal	GB Pant University of Agriculture and Technology, Pantnagar, Uttarakhand-263145, India
NoopurKhare	Shri Ramswaroop Memorial University, Barabanki, Uttar Pradesh, 225001, India
Prabhakaran S	Department of Pharmacology, Nandha College of Pharmacy, Erode, Tamilnadu, India
Pallavi Saxena	ICMR- National Institute of Pathology, Safdarjung Hospital Campus, New Delhi, 110029, India

Pradeep K Chaturvedi	Department of Reproductive Biology, All India Institute of Medical Sciences, New Delhi, 110029, India
P. P. Sethumathi	Department of Pharmacology, Nandha College of Pharmacy, Erode, Tamil Nadu, 638052-India
Parim Brahma Naidu	Animal Physiology and Biochemistry Laboratory, ICMR-National Animal Resource Facility for Biomedical Research (ICMR-NARFBR), Hyderabad, 500078-India
R Ravindar Naik	ICMR-National Animal Resource Facility for Biomedical Research, Genome Valley, Shamirpet, Hyderabad, 500101-India
N. Ramesh Kumar	Department of Genetics, Osmania University, Hyderabad, Telangana, India
Reeta Varyani	Department of Cardiology, Sri Sathya Sai Institute of Higher Medical Sciences, EPIP Area, Whitefield, Bangalore, India
Sri Bharathi G.S	Department of Pharmacology, Nandha College of Pharmacy, Erode, Tamilnadu, India
Sakthi Sundaram S	Department of Pharmacology, Nandha College of Pharmacy, Erode, Tamilnadu, India
Sengottuvelu S	Department of Pharmacology, Nandha College of Pharmacy, Erode, Tamilnadu, India
SSYH Qadri	ICMR-National Institute of Nutrition, Jamai-Osmania PO, Hyderabad-500007, India
S. Venkanna	Department of Zoology, Osmania University, Hyderabad, Telangana, India
Savitri Vasudev Baikampady	Department of Cardiology, Sri Sathya Sai Institute of Higher Medical Sciences, EPIP Area, Whitefield, Bangalore, India
Sreedevi Gandham	Department of ECE, Siddhartha Educational Academy Group of Institutions, Tirupati, Andhrapradesh, India
S. Vadivukkarasi	Department of Biochemistry, Centre for Biological Sciences, K.S. Rangasamy College of Arts and Science (Autonomous), Tiruchengode, Namakkal District, Tamilnadu, 637215-India
S. Jaikumar	Department of Pharmacology, Sri Lakshmi Narayana Institute of Medical Sciences, Puducherry, 605502-India
S. Sengottuvelu	Department of Pharmacology, Nandha College of Pharmacy, Erode, Tamilnadu, India-638052
Taniya Saleem	Department of Veterinary Parasitology, SKUAST-Jammu, India
Umesh Kumar	School of Biosciences, IMS Ghaziabad, University Courses Campus, Ghaziabad, Delhi NCR, 201015, India
Vinod Kumar	Department of Reproductive Biology, All India Institute of Medical Sciences, New Delhi, 110029, India
V. V. Sathibabu Uddandrao	Department of Biochemistry, Tiruchengode, Namakkal District, Centre for Biological Sciences, K.S. Rangasamy College of Arts and Science (Autonomous), Tamilnadu, 637215, India
Venketesh	Department of Cardiology, Sri Sathya Sai Institute of Higher Medical Sciences, EPIP Area, Whitefield, Bangalore, India

V. V. Sathibabu Uddandrao   Department of Biochemistry, Centre for Biological Sciences, K.S. Rangasamy College of Arts and Science (Autonomous), Tiruchengode, Namakkal District, Tamilnadu, 637215-India

CHAPTER 1

Cardiovascular Diseases and Nutraceuticals: Underlying Mechanism and Therapeutic Biomarkers

Pallavi Saxena[1], Vinod Kumar[2], Noopur Khare[3], Neeraj Pal[4], Dibyabhaba Pradhan[5], Pradeep K Chaturvedi[2], Arun Kumar Jain[1], Manoj Kumar[6], V. V. Sathibabu Uddandrao[7] and Umesh Kumar[8,*]

[1] *ICMR- National Institute of Pathology, Safdarjung Hospital Campus, New Delhi, 110029, India*

[2] *Department of Reproductive Biology, All India Institute of Medical Sciences, New Delhi, 110029, India*

[3] *Shri Ramswaroop Memorial University, Barabanki, Uttar Pradesh, 225001, India*

[4] *GB Pant University of Agriculture and Technology,Pantnagar, Uttarakhand- 263145, India*

[5] *ICMR AIIMS Computational Genomics Centre, New Delhi, 110029, India*

[6] *Biochemistry Department, Narinder Mohan Hospital and Heart Center, Ghaziabad, Uttar Pradesh, 201007, India*

[7] *Centre for Biological Sciences, Department of Biochemistry, K.S. Rangasamy College of Arts and Science (Autonomous), Tiruchengode, Namakkal District, Tamilnadu, 637215, India*

[8] *School of Biosciences, IMS Ghaziabad, University Courses Campus, Ghaziabad, Delhi NCR, 201015, India*

Abstract: Food and nutrients are essential for the body's regular functioning. They aid in the preservation of an individual's health and the reduction of the danger of certain diseases. As a result of the widespread recognition of this fact, a link was established between "nutrition and health," and the term "nutraceuticals" was coined. Nutraceuticals are therapeutic foods that aid in maintaining well-being, enhancing health, regulating immunity, and preventing as well as curing certain diseases. Nutraceuticals might thus be thought of as one of the missing pieces in a person's overall health. More than any other illness, cardiovascular disease has numerous risk variables that are susceptible to nutraceutical treatment. It is critical to see nutraceuticals' ability to improve cardiovascular risk factors as a huge opportunity in the treatment of a disease that affects so many people. Nutraceuticals show promise in clinical treatment since they have the potential to minimize the risk of chemotherapy-related side effects while also lowering the overall cost of health care. In this study, an attempt was made to summarize some of the most recent research findings on garlic, omega-3 fatty acids, soy products, dietary fibers, vitamins, antioxidants, plant sterols,

---

[*] **Corresponding author Umesh Kumar:** School of Biosciences, IMS Ghaziabad, University Courses Campus, Ghaziabad, Delhi NCR, 201015, India; E-mail: umeshkumar82@gmail.com

flavonoids, prebiotics, and probiotics that have beneficial effects on the heart, as well as to provide insight into a bioinformatics approach to identify novel therapeutic biomarkers in order to keep practitioners up to date.

Keywords: CVD, Diet, Heart disease, Metabolic syndrome, Nutraceuticals, Nutrition.

1. INTRODUCTION

1.1. Cardiovascular Disorders

The term "cardiovascular disorders" (CVD) or "heart disease" refers to a variety of illnesses that affect the heart and blood arteries [1]. Coronary artery disease, cerebrovascular disease, angina, heart attack, heart failure, dilated and hypertrophic cardiomyopathy, peripheral arterial disease, rheumatic heart disease, heart rhythm problems (arrhythmias), congenital heart defects, deep vein thrombosis, and pulmonary embolism are all diseases that fall under the heart disease umbrella. Electrocardiogram (ECG), Holter monitoring, Echocardiogram, Stress test, cardiac catheterization, cardiac computed tomography (CT) scan, and cardiac magnetic resonance imaging are commonly used to diagnose it (MRI) [2]. CVD has surpassed cancer as the top cause of mortality worldwide, and it is a major public health issue. Obesity, metabolic syndrome, atherosclerosis, hyperlipidemia, type 2 diabetes, hypertension, and lifestyle risk factors such as smoking, physical inactivity, and dietary factors are all common and growing in popularity across the world [3]. Reducing risk variables in the population, particularly blood pressure control and cholesterol reduction can have an influence on CVD mortality [4]. Hypertension is to blame for 45% of heart attacks and 51% of strokes, as well as 9.4 million CVD-related deaths throughout the world [5]. Despite significant advancements in medical care, the prognosis for CVD remains dismal, and identifying causes and new therapeutic methods remains a high priority [6].

1.2. Cardiovascular Diseases Burden: Global and National

Cardiovascular diseases (CVDs) are the leading cause of death worldwide and a significant contributor to poor quality of life [7]. CVD claimed the lives of 17.8 million people globally in 2017, resulting in 330 million years of life lost and another 35.6 million years of disability [8]. Heart attacks and strokes account for four out of every five CVD fatalities, with one-third of these deaths occurring before the age of 70 [9]. Furthermore, case fatality due to CVD appears to be significantly greater in low-income nations than in middle- and high-income countries [10].

The burden of cardiovascular disease (CVD) in India is one of the highest in the world. Noncommunicable diseases (NCDs), including cardiovascular disease (CVD), are projected to account for 60% of all adult fatalities in India, with CVD accounting for approximately 26% of these deaths [11]. The yearly number of CVD fatalities in India is expected to increase from 2.26 million in 1990 to 4.77 million in 2050 (2020). The age-standardized CVD mortality rate in India is 272 per 100,000, which is higher than the global average of 235 per 100,000 [8]. Over the last 25 years, the incidence of CVD risk factors has been significantly increasing in India, particularly in metropolitan areas [12].

Coronary heart disease prevalence rates in India have varied from 1.6% to 7.4% in rural populations and from 1% to 13.2% in urban populations during the last several decades [13]. Ischemic heart disease (IHD) and stroke account for the bulk of CVD mortality in India (83%) [14]. The ratio of IHD to stroke mortality in India is significantly greater than the worldwide norm and equivalent to that in Western developed nations [15]. IHD and stroke account for more than a twentieth (21.1%) of all deaths and one-tenth of all years of life lost in India [16]. The Macroeconomic Commission for Health predicted that the number of IHD patients in India would increase from 36 million in 2005 to 62 million in 2015 (70% increase). In general, India's stroke incidence and stroke-related case fatality rates are greater than those of Western industrialised nations, but the rates among women are especially high. Haemorrhagic strokes are more prevalent in India than in the Western population, according to current neuroimaging research [17].

Hypertensive heart disease, among other cardiovascular diseases, is a serious problem in India, with 1.47 million fatalities in 2019, up 138%from 1990 [18]. Rheumatic heart disease (RHD) is a concern in many regions of India, with an estimated 88,674 fatalities (7 per 100,000 population) in 2010. Though, from 2000 to 2010, the Indian Council of Medical Research (ICMR) began community management and prevention of RHD using hospital-based passive monitoring and secondary prophylaxis as part of the Jai Vigyan Mission Mode Project [19]. At the national level, there is no systematic program for the prevention and control of RHD. However, following adopting an economic liberalization and globalization strategy in 2000, India's socioeconomic situation, improved living circumstances, and increased connectivity and access to health-care institutions are predicted to have resulted in a decrease in the burden of RHD [20]. According to estimates from the Global Burden of Disease research, atrial fibrillation and flutter contribute very little to the total CVD burden in India. Furthermore, other types of

CVDs, such as aortic aneurysms, peripheral vascular disease, and endocarditis, have a tiny proportionate death and morbidity impact [21].

Although CVD risk factors are widespread in India, there are significant variations across and within areas. Diabetes mellitus appears to be more frequent in India's southern states, whereas hypertension tends to be more prevalent in the north-eastern regions. This variability may be the cause of cultural variety (leading to variances in food preferences, cigarette use, and physical activity patterns) as well as differences in economic growth across and within Indian states [22]. In India, the relationship between socioeconomic position and CVD has been well investigated. CVD is no longer a wealthy man's illness, according to a recent large cohort research in Mumbai, which found that it affects the poor equally, with lower SES males having greater CVD mortality. Low SES was linked to a greater risk of having acute myocardial infarction in a case-control study. In a cross-sectional examination of cardiovascular risk factors in Jaipur, suboptimal social features such as poor educational, occupational, and SES levels were linked to a cluster of cardiovascular risk factors and a higher Framingham risk score. In most cases, social factors have a significant impact [23].

CVD diagnosis and under-reporting are more common among the poor in India. Because medical care usually involves significant out-of-pocket expenditures, economically disadvantaged CVD patients are less likely to get evidence-based therapy. Those in the low-income category face higher out-of-pocket expenditures than those in the high-income group, with higher rates of catastrophic health spending and financing for suffering [24]. As a result, households with lower SES that are affected by CVD are more likely to face financial hardship or catastrophic health costs. Out-of-pocket expenditures are not just a feature of acute care, but they are also present in chronic care. For example, diabetes treatment costs 34% (27%) of a low-income family's yearly income in urban (rural) India. As a result, poor and marginalized populations are pushed deeper into the poverty and CVD cycle [25].

1.3. Potential Risk Factors for CVD

Over the years, the main risk factors for these disorders have been identified as high levels of low-density lipoprotein (LDL) cholesterol, smoking, hypertension, diabetes, abdominal obesity, psychosocial factors, inadequate intake of fruits and vegetables, excessive alcohol consumption, and lack of adequate physical activity (Fig. **1**). Diabetes mellitus is a documented epidemiological factor linked to the rising prevalence of CVD. Atherosclerosis, which is predominantly seen in the intima of medium and wide arteries, is the leading cause of myocardial infarction, heart failure, and stroke. Dyslipidemia in the vascular endothelium and cholesterol deposition is the major causes of atherosclerosis. When oxidized, low density lipoprotein (LDL) cholesterol is pro-inflammatory and immunogenic, and it acts as a standalone CVD risk factor [26]. The increase in oxidized LDL cholesterol adds to endothelial dysfunction and has a direct impact on the progression of atherosclerosis. Although more research is being conducted to better identify a person's cardiovascular risk in terms of genetic factors, more nuanced lipid traits, and inflammatory markers, the INTERHEART study confirmed that traditional risk factors accounted for over 90% of the population's risk of myocardial infarction [27].

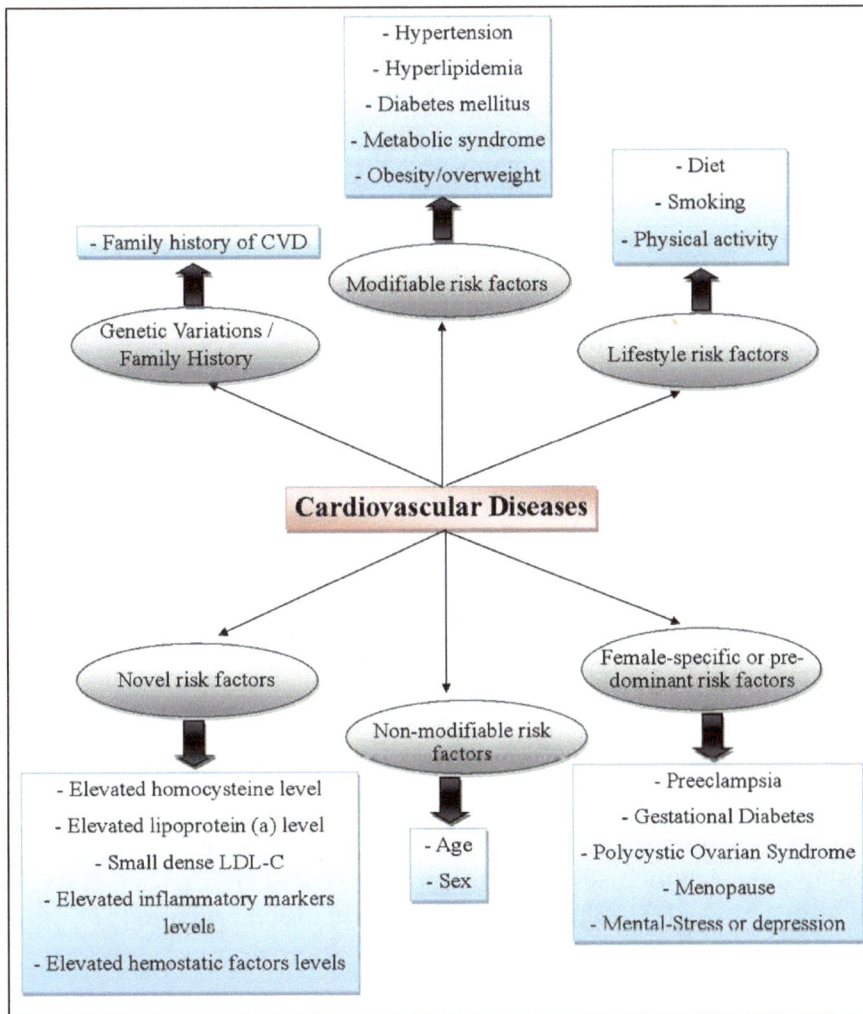

Fig. (1). Risk factors for cardiovascular diseases.

1.4. Therapies in Use for CVD Treatment

1.4.1. ACE Inhibitors

ACE inhibitors are medicines that expand, or dilate your blood arteries to increase the quantity of blood your heart pumps and reduce your blood pressure. ACE inhibitors also improve blood flow, which helps your heart work less and protects your kidneys from the consequences of hypertension and diabetes [28]. Medications include trandolapril, ramipril, benazepril and captopril.

• **Mechanism of Action of Trandolapril:** The glycoprotein ACE inhibitor is made up of a single polypeptide chain of 1277 amino acids with two functionally active domains, N and C, that result from tandem gene duplication. Despite their considerable sequence similarity, the two domains have different physiological functions. The C-domain is primarily engaged in blood pressure control, whereas the N-domain is important in stem cell differentiation and proliferation. ACE inhibitors bind to both domains and reduce their function, but the C-domain has a far higher affinity and inhibitory effect.Trandolaprilat, a metabolite of trandolapril, competes with ATI for ACE binding and inhibits ATI enzymatic proteolysis to ATII. By blocking the pressor effects of ATII, lowering ATII levels in the body lowers blood pressure [29].

1.4.2. Angiotension II Receptor Blockers

Angiotensin-converting enzyme inhibitors (ARBs) inhibit the activity of the hormone angiotensin II. This hormone causes blood vessels to constrict, causing blood pressure to rise. Angiotensin II also causes the body to retain salt and water, which raises blood pressure even further. ARBs operate by inhibiting the hormone's receptors, particularly AT1 receptors located in the heart, blood vessels, and kidneys. Blocking the activity of angiotensin II lowers blood pressure and protects the heart and kidneys from harm. These medicines help reduce substances that induce the accumulation of salt and fluid in the body [30]. Medications include candesartan, irbesartan, losartan, telmisartan.

• **Mechanism of Action of Candesartan:** Candesartan inhibits angiotensin II binding to AT1 in a variety of tissues, including vascular smooth muscle and the adrenal glands. Angiotensin II's vasoconstrictive and aldosterone-secreting actions are inhibited by AT1, resulting in a reduction in blood pressure [31].

1.4.3. Antiarrhythmics

Antiarrhythmic medication therapy's ultimate objective is to restore normal rhythm and conduction. Antiarrhythmic medications are used to modify the excitability of cardiac cells by altering the duration of the effective refractory period, and inhibit aberrant automaticity [32].

Antiarrhythmic medicines are split into four categories:

Class I: Sodium-channel blockers, which slow electrical conduction in the heart [33]. Medicines include Quinidine, Procainamide, Disopyramide and Ajmaline.

• **Mechanism of Action of Procainamide:** Procainamide is a drug used to make local or regional anesthetic and to treat ventricular tachycardia that can develop during cardiac procedures like surgery or catheterization, as well as after acute myocardial infarction, digitalis poisoning, or other cardiac conditions [34]. It is a sodium channel blocker that acts as a local anaesthetic by blocking the ionic fluxes necessary for the initiation and conduction of impulses, stabilizing the neuronal membrane.

Class II: Beta-blockers, can reduce excessive blood pressure and heart rate by inhibiting impulses that may induce an irregular heart rhythm and interfering with hormonal effects (such as adrenaline) on the heart's cells [35]. Medicines include Lidocaine, Mexiletine and Phenytoin.

• **Mechanism of Action of Lidocaine:** The main impact that lidocaine has when it binds and blocks sodium channels, reducing the ionic fluxes essential for the initiation and conduction of electrical action potential impulses necessary for muscle contraction, is believed to be related with cardiac consequences. Lidocaine has substantial effects on the central nervous system and cardiovascular system in addition to inhibiting conduction in nerve axons in the peripheral nervous system.Lidocaine may generate stimulation of the CNS followed by depression after absorption, and it works predominantly on the myocardium in the cardiovascular system, causing reductions in electrical excitability, conduction rate, and force of contraction [36].

Class III: Potassium channel blockers, By inhibiting potassium channels in the heart, it slows electrical impulses in the heart. Amiodarone, Droncdarone, Sotalol, and Bretylium are some of the medications available.

• **Mechanism of Action of Amiodarone:** It is classified as an anti-arrhythmic medication of class III. It prevents the heart muscle from repolarizing during the third phase of the cardiac action potential by blocking potassium currents. As a result, amiodarone prolongs the action potential and increases the effective refractory period of cardiac cells (myocytes). As a result, the excitability of cardiac muscle cells is decreased, avoiding and treating aberrant heart rhythms [37].

Class IV: Calcium channel blockers, It binds to calcium channels found in vascular smooth muscle, cardiac myocytes, and cardiac nodal tissue (L-type calcium channels) (sinoatrial and atrioventricular nodes). These channels are in charge of controlling calcium input into muscle cells, which drives smooth muscle contraction and cardiac myocyte contraction [38]. Medicines include amlodipine, felodipine, nifedipine, nimodipine, nitrendipine.

• **Mechanism of Action of Amlodipine:** Amlodipine is a calcium antagonist (calcium ion antagonist or slow-channel blocker) that prevents calcium ions from entering vascular smooth muscle and cardiac muscle. The transport of extracellular calcium ions into cardiac muscle and vascular smooth muscle by particular ion channels is required for contraction. Amlodipine selectively inhibits calcium ion influx across cell membranes. Amlodipine has a larger effect on vascular smooth muscle cells than it does on cardiac muscle cells Label. Amlodipine reduces blood pressure by acting directly on vascular smooth muscle [39].

1.4.4. Antiplatelet Drugs

Platelets, by virtue of their ability to cling to the damaged blood vessel wall and attract new platelets to the site of injury, are essential components of normal hemostasis and crucial actors in atherothrombosis. Although platelet adhesion, activation, and aggregation can be viewed as a physiologic repair response to an atherosclerotic plaque's sudden fissuring or rupture, uncontrolled progression of such a process through a series of self-sustaining amplification loops can result in intraluminal thrombus formation, vascular occlusion, and subsequent ischemia or infarction [40]. Aspirin is the most widely studied antiplatelet drug.

• **Mechanism of Action of Aspirin:** This medication also prevents blood clots, strokes, and myocardial infarction by inhibiting platelet aggregation (MI). Acetylsalicylic acid (ASA) inhibits the production of prostaglandins. It doesn't discriminate between COX-1 and COX-2 enzymes. Platelet aggregation is inhibited for around 7-10 days when COX-1 is inhibited (average platelet lifespan). Acetylsalicylic acid's acetyl group binds to a serine residue in the cyclooxygenase-1 (COX-1) enzyme, causing permanent inhibition. This stops pain-inducing prostaglandins from being produced [41].

1.4.5. M. Anti-coagulants Drugs

Clot buster medicines, also known as thrombolytic treatment, are a type of cardiac medication used intravenously in the hospital to dissolve blood clots. Clot busters are most commonly used to treat heart attacks and ischemic strokes.

These strong heart disease medicines are used to stop heart attacks from becoming worse, stop ischemic stroke from getting worse, and break up blood clots in other parts of the body [42]. Medication include Tenecteplase, Urokinase, Streptokinase and Reteplase

• **Mechanism of Action of Urokinase:** It is a serine protease; cleaves plasminogen to form the active fibrinolytic protease, plasmin [41].

1.4.6. Diuretics

These are sometimes referred to as "water pills." They assist your body in eliminating excess water and salt through urine. Your heart will have an easier time pumping as a result of this. It also aids in blood pressure management [43]. Medication includes Lasix, Bumex and Esidrix.

• **Mechanism of Action of Lasix:** Furosemide has direct vasodilatory actions, which explains why it is particularly successful in treating acute pulmonary edema. Vasodilation causes a decrease in the response to vasoconstrictors such angiotensin II and noradrenaline, as well as a decrease in the synthesis of endogenous natriuretic hormones having vasoconstricting characteristics. Increased synthesis of prostaglandins with vasodilating characteristics is also a result. In resistant arteries, furosemide may also open potassium channels [43].

There is strong evidence that pharmacological treatment can reduce cardiovascular events when conventional risk factors are taken into account. Several large clinical trials using HMG CoA reductase inhibitors (statins) have demonstrated that lowering LDL cholesterol with medicines lowers the risk of coronary and cerebrovascular events [44]. A reduction in high density lipoprotein (HDL) cholesterol raises the risk of atherosclerosis, whereas an increase in HDL cholesterol lowers the risk of coronary heart disease (CHD) and cardiovascular disease (CVD). Maintaining the quantity of HDL cholesterol can also induce the release of nitric oxide, which inhibits vascular bed atherogenesis [45]. Because atherosclerosis lesions take a long time to form, beginning cholesterol control early can help prevent atherosclerotic vascular disorders. Alternative therapies for lipid levels in individuals with dyslipidemia have been developed in recent years [46]. In addition to pharmacological therapy of CVD risk and the use of antithrombotic medicines, lifestyle changes are advised as a preventative strategy for controlling cardiovascular risk. The importance of dietary variables and herbal medications in the prevention and treatment of CVD is becoming more wellrecognized. Natural foods derived from medicinal plants have been shown to be beneficial to certain patients. More study, including clinical studies with extended follow-up data, is needed to determine their effectiveness against CVD disorders [47].

2. NUTRACEUTICALS AND CARDIOVASCULAR HEALTH

2.1. Nutraceuticals

CVDs are caused by a variety of interconnected variables, including age, poor eating habits, a sedentary and unhealthy lifestyle, and excessive job stress. In today's world, the traditional high fiber and carbohydrate diet has given way to a processed and packaged total fat diet. The term "nutraceutical" was coined by Dr. Stephen DeFelice in 1989, when he combined the words "nutrition" and "pharmaceutical." According to DeFelice, a nutraceutical is "a food or portion of a food that delivers medical and health advantages, including the prevention and/or treatment of disease." Isolated nutrient diets, herbal products, and genetically engineered designer meals are all examples of nutraceutical goods. "Let food be your medicine, and medicine be your nourishment," Hippocrates said over 2500 years ago. The goal of human nutrition science has shifted from preventing nutritional insufficiency to preserving human health and lowering the risk of chronic illnesses [48]. Historically, food products have been designed with the consumer's flavor, appearance, value, and convenience in mind. The creation of items to prove health advantages is a relatively new trend, reflecting the growing understanding of the importance of nutrition in illness prevention and treatment. Japan presently has eleven different categories of functional ingredients or nutraceuticals as part of FOSHU (Foods for Specified Health Use). ß Fibres in the diet ß Oligosaccharides Cardiovascular diseases are illnesses that primarily affect the heart or blood vessels (CVDs) [49].

2.2. Potential Nutraceuticals

Nutraceuticals have been proven to be helpful in the prevention and risk control of CVDs, and can be broadly described as those utilized in the prevention or treatment of congestive heart failure, arrhythmias, hypertension, angina, and hyperlipidemia. The following section discusses a variety of nutraceuticals that have been proven to be effective in the prevention and treatment of cardiovascular disease [50]. Consumer demand has risen as a result of the link between the nutritional value of food ingredients and the prevention of a number of chronic illnesses. However, in order to stay on the market, these foods must be nutritional, organic, and delicious. They may be made up of a single physiologically active molecule or may require the inclusion of additional dietary components such as omega fatty acids, prebiotics, phytochemicals, and bioactive peptides in order to be consumed [51] (Fig. **2**).

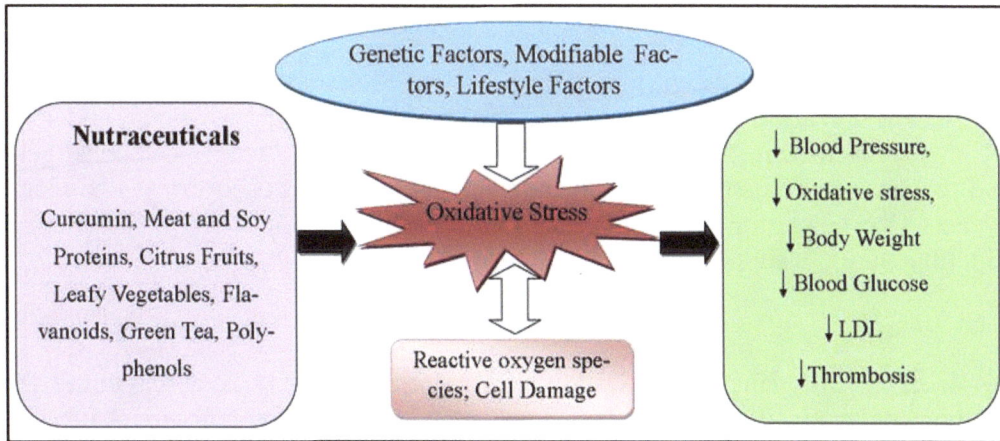

Fig. (2). Effect on nutraceuticals on cardiovascular health.

2.2.1. Plant Sterols/ Stanols

Plant sterols, also known as phytosterols, are naturally found in a range of plant sources, including vegetable oils, nuts, cereals, seeds, wood pulp, and leaves. Because they are physically similar to cholesterol, they compete with ingested cholesterol for absorption into the small intestine. This reduction in cholesterol absorption boosts LDL hepatic uptake and lowers LDL levels in the blood. Plant sterols have been demonstrated in studies to lower LDL cholesterol by 8-15%. Plant sterols are used to make natural grains like corn, maize, and sunflower. Studies have shown that plant sterols can reduce the risk of coronary heart disease [52].

2.2.2. Cruciferous Vegetables

DIM (3,3'-diin dolyl methane) and I3C (indole-3 carbinol) phytochemicals found in broccoli and kale suppress cytokine production and protect against inflammation, causing cell cycle arrest and death. Broccoli protects the myocardium from ischemia reperfusion injury through sulforaphane redox signaling. Upregulation of phase II detoxification enzymes involved in the clearance of reactive oxygen species (ROS). Sulforaphane is an anti-inflammatory agent. The antioxidant effects of phenolic substances, such as Brassica vegetables, are dependent on the amount and position of hydroxyl groups in the molecule. Quercetin, an important flavonol, inhibits cancer by chelating transition metal ions and trapping free radicals [53].

2.2.3. Garlic

As a source of flavonoids, garlic (Allium sativum) lowers the risk of hypertension and ischemic heart disease [54]. It also reduces the formation of plaque. It alters the platelet membrane's composition while also preventing superoxide leakage. It also reduces atheromatous deposition on the deepest layer of artery walls. Garlic extracts also have antihypertensive and anti-apoptotic properties [55]. Its ACE-inhibiting action also lowers blood pressure [56].

2.2.4. CoQ10

CoQ10 is an endogenous molecule, antioxidant, and free radical scavenger that functions as an electron transporter in the mitochondrial production of ATP. As a vascular superoxide antagonist, it lowers blood pressure, raises ventricular ejection fraction, and lowers arrhythmias. CoQ10 also improves mitochondrial energy generation, reduces peroxynitrite inactivation by NO, and reduces oxidative damage to LDL. In cardiac illness, there is a shortage of CoQ10. CoQ10 is found in the highest levels in meat, fish, and nuts, with considerably lower amounts in dairy products and fruits and vegetables. CoQ10 can help improve the ejection fraction in people with congestive heart failure [57].

2.2.5. Turmeric

Curcumin, an active component of turmeric, a tropical plant in the ginger family, is a polyphenolic antioxidant that reduces intracellular ROS. The primary ingredient is anti-inflammatory, and it also lowers LDL, triglycerides, and lipid peroxides. It inhibits hypertrophy and alters gene expression in cardiomyocytes. It suppresses nuclear acetylation and avoids the development of HF in hypertensive heart disease. Curcumin also suppresses platelet-derived growth factor (PDGF), which is necessary for vascular remodeling. Curcumin also causes epigenetic changes, which affect miRNAs, through food [58].

2.2.6. Grape Skin

Grape seed proanthocyanidin extract (GSPE) is a cardioprotective and antioxidant that helps to prevent cardiovascular disease. GSPE reduces infarct size and improves ventricular postischemic function. The oxidation of polyunsaturated LDL damages the arteries, resulting in atherosclerosis. Grape extracts prevent LDL from being oxidized. The efficacy of the GSPE material is dependent on the region of origin, as there is a wide range, and some estimations suggest that red wine is 20 times more active than white wine. The nuclear factor-kappa, which is implicated in the development of atherosclerotic plaques, is not activated by red wine.Resveratrol is an antioxidant and anti-inflammatory polyphenol present in grapes, red wine, and a variety of berries, but in low amounts [59].

2.2.7. Fish Oil/Olive Oil

Triglycerides reduction process is carried out by eicosapentaenoic acid (EPA) and docosahexaenoic acid (DHA) omega-3 fatty acids, and is also recommended for CHD and hypertriglyceridemia. Being, antiarrhythmic,EPA and DHA resist calcium overload in cardiac myocytes. Omega-3 and omega-6 alter the protein activity of the cell membrane and regulate gene expression. Omega-3 facilitates the release of prostaglandins that are anti-inflammatory, while omega-6 develops mediators that are inflammatory in nature. Omega-3-PUFA is antiarrhythmic and decreases the risk of cardiac arrset. It is also used for dyslipidemia treatment. It decreases blood pressure, and also has a beneficial effect on endothelial function. A third fatty acid, derived from vegetable oils, soybeans, canola oil,flaxseed, and sunflower, is alpha-linolenic acid (ALA). ALA decreases atherogenesis-related CRP values and inflammatory markers. Carotid artery plaques and intima-media thickness are decreased by ALA. Olive oil's phenol portion helps to limit platelet aggregation and inhibit an inflammatory enzyme COX-2 and MMP-9, that have an antioxidant effect [60].

2.2.8. Vegetables

Lycopene is closely related to beta-carotene, found in tomato juice, red fruits, and watermelons. It is one of the best dietary antioxidants for significantly reducing oxidation of LDL. Its antioxidant property leads to blood pressure reduction. The oxidised LDL is used by macrophages within the arterial wall to initiate plaque formation, thereby significantly lowering the LDL level. In cholesterol synthesis, lycopene prevents the function of an enzyme and helps in the CHD prevention. The aid of tomato extract leads to the improvement of hypertension [61].

2.2.9. Carnitine

Carnitine in the muscle of the heart prevents the production of lactic acid that destroys the myocardium in failed hearts. 40% carnitine content reductionis observed during myocardial infarction (MI). Thus for arrhythmias, supplementation of red meat, nuts and vegetables is recommended [62].

2.2.10. Berberine

Berberine (BBR) is an isoquinoline alkaloid that was first isolated from the Chinese plant Coptischinensis extracts (Huang lian). Berberine has a wide range of pharmacological characteristics, including anti-diarrheal, anti-arrhythmia, antihypertension, glucose and cholesterol reducing, anti-tumor, and immune-modulatory capabilities. BBR's ability to improve cardiac function may be linked to an increase in calcium concentration in heart muscle cells.Increased an inward current carried by calcium ions in the intracellular of cardiac muscle is generated by gradually raising the concentration of cyclic adenosine monophosphate (cAMP) in cardiac muscle cells [63].

2.2.11. Flavonoids

The largest group of naturally occurring phenols is the flavonoids that exist in the free-state and as glycosides. isoflavones, flavonoid glycosides, catechins, and anthocyanins are polyphenolic compounds that have been proposed to play a dominant role in the prevention of heart disease. The influence of flavonoids on the metabolism of arachidonic acid has been linked to these effects. Antioxidants present in tea, wine, fruits and vegetables are flavonoids. An epidemiological analysis found that dietary flavonoid intake and CHD were inversely associated. Due to their antioxidant properties, a lower risk of fatal and non-fatal CHD is associated with the consumption of flavanoids [64].

2.2.12. Prebiotics

A prebiotic has a non-digestible food ingredient that selectively stimulates the activity of colon and provides benefit to the host.The improvement in the composition of the colonic microflora by prebiotics contributes to the predominance of a few potentially health-promoting bacteria. Microbial food supplements enhance the immunity of the host and thus have the ability to resist major diseases such as cancer and lower serum cholesterol [65].

2.2.13. Probiotics

Probiotics are live micro-organisms administered in appropriate quantity, have a beneficial effect on the host's health. Classically, a probiotic is described as a viable microbial dietary supplement that affects the host beneficially through its effects on the intestinal tract. Probiotic bacteria favourably alter the balance of intestinal microflora, inhibit harmful bacteria growth, promote good digestion, improve immune function and increase infection resistance [66].

2.2.14. Protein and Protein Peptides

The beneficial benefits of soy and lupin proteins on the lipid profile are supported by preclinical and clinical data. Bioactive peptides found in soy and lupin (such as conglutin-gamma) are thought to be responsible for the lipid-lowering action of these legumes. Isoflavones, on the other hand, may have a role in this impact. The cholesterol-lowering mechanisms proposed for soy and lupin seem to be numerous but are still unclear, including the down-regulation of the expression of the hepatic transcription factor of sterol regulatory element binding protein (SREBP-1; *via* PI3K/Akt/GSK3β pathways, with decreased hepatic lipoprotein secretion and cholesterol content), the regulation of SREBP-2 (with increased clearance of cholesterol from the blood), the reduction of cholesterol synthesis, the increase of ApoB receptor activity, and the increase of the fecal excretion of bile salts [67].

2.2.15. Vitamins

Antioxidant vitamins are one of the main defense mechanisms of the body's non-enzymatic anti-oxidant systems. Ascorbic acid, alpha-tocopherol, and beta-carotene are the most common natural antioxidants.Vitamin D has a wide spectrum of effects in the body, varying from the role on calcium/phosphate homeostasis and muscle strength, to the action on cardiovascular, nervous, and immune systems. Vitamin D deficiency has been referred to raise the incidence of multiple chronic diseases such as CVD, cancer, multiple sclerosis, and diabetes [68].

The role of Nutraceuticals in cardiovascular health is summarised in Table **1**.

Table 1. Nutraceuticals with therapeutic potential for improvement of cardiovascular diseases.

S.No.	Nutraceutical	Bioactive Compounds	Potential Mechanism/ Effect	Reference
1.	Turmeric	Curcumin/piperine	Anti-inflammatory, Blocks NF-κB,VCAM-1, Anti-oxidative	[69]
2.	Soy proteins	Genistein and daidzein	Lowering blood cholesterol	[70]
3.	Green leafy vegetables, fruits	Carotenoids, Fiber (pectin)	Inhibition of LDL-C Oxidation. Lowering blood cholesterol	[71]
4.	Dark Chocolate	Flavanoids	Endothelial function, lowering blood pressure	[72]
5.	Citrus fruits and vegetables	Vitamin C, folate, phytochemicals	Antioxidant action, Lowering blood homocysteine	[73]
6.	Green tea	Catechin, Polyphenols	Inhibition of LDL-C Oxidation, Curtails inflammation	[72]
7.	Fish/Fish Oil	Omega-3 fatty acids	Inhibition of LDL-C Oxidation, Lowering blood triglycerides, Decreasing blood pressure	[74]
8.	Quercetin	Polyphenols, Flavanoids	Reduces blood lipids, Inhibit NF-κB regulation, Anti-oxidative	[75]

(Table 1) cont.....

S.No.	Nutraceutical	Bioactive Compounds	Potential Mechanism/ Effect	Reference
9.	Resveratrol	Phytoalexin	Deacetylates histones, Anti-oxidative	[76]
10	Carotenoids	Lycopene	Antioxidant, Curtails free radical	[77]
11	Red wine	Anthocyanins, catechins, cyanidins, and flavonols, myricetin and quercetin	Platelets aggregation, Endothelial function, Anti-inflammatory action, Decreasing blood pressure	[78]
12	Olive oil	Polyphenolics and oleic acid	Inhibition of LDL-C Oxidation	[79]
13.	Onion and garlic	Quercetin	Decreasing blood pressure	[80]

3. NUTRACEUTICALS MODULATE GENETIC EXPRESSION

By decreasing lipid adhesion and oxidative stress, nutraceuticals have endothelial effects and can predict unfavorable cardiac outcomes. When consumed, nutraceuticals activate various signaling pathways, including the transcription factors NF-B and Nrf2, and exert anti-inflammatory and anti-oxidative control by inhibiting these pathways [81].

3.1. NF-κB Regulatory Network

Although NF-kappaB is necessary for the establishment of late preconditioning against myocardial infarction, it is also important in mediating cell death following ischemia/reperfusion damage. NF-kappaB is found in the cytosol in an inactive state, complexed with the inhibitory protein 1B. This compound prevent it from binding to DNA. It also protects against hypoxia and inflammation by regulating a range of genomic processes, including hypertrophy. In the sick heart, NF-kappaB expression is elevated [82].

3.2. Nrf2 Regulates Antioxidant and Detoxification Genes

NRF2 is a master regulator of the antioxidant response, which helps the body fight oxidative stress. Unrestricted Nrf2 activity, produced by deletion of Kelch-like ECH-associated protein 1 (KEAP1) in the mouse, causes postnatal mortality, whereas Nrf2 knockouts are alive but susceptible to oxidative stresses. It operates on cytoprotective genes in response to oxidative stress. It activates antioxidant enzymes that protect against oxidative damage by attaching to antioxidant response elements (ARE) [83].

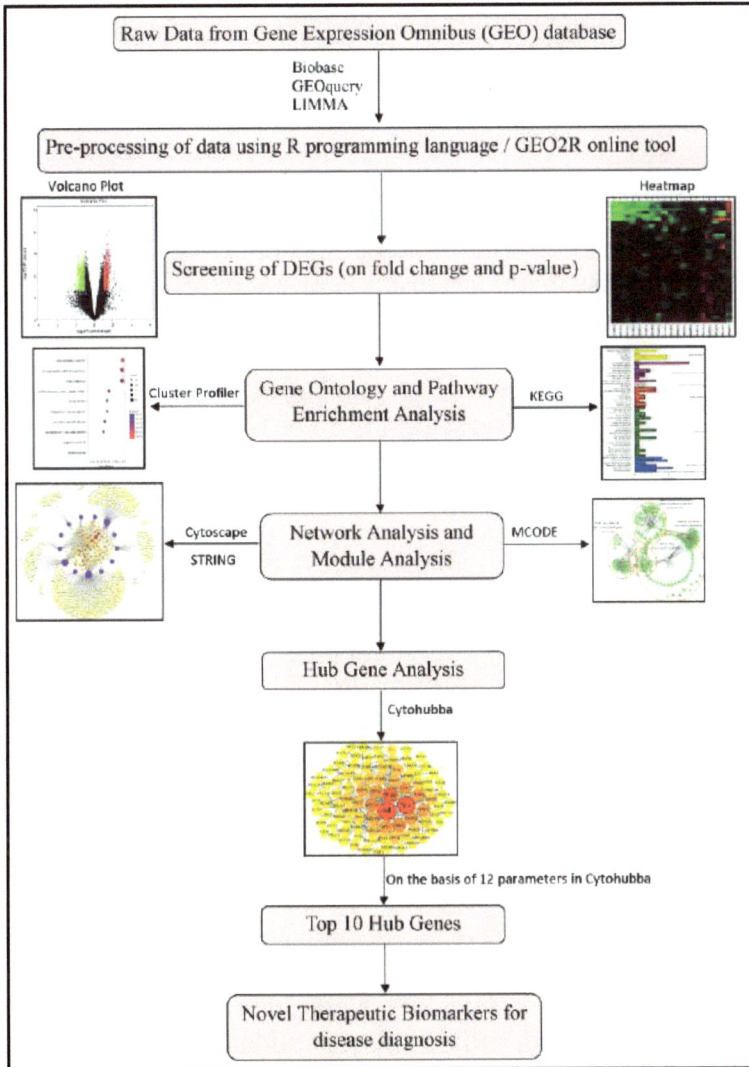

Fig. (3). Workflow for Identification of new therapeutic biomarkers using Transcriptomics approach.

4. BIOINFORMATICS APPLICATION IN NUTRACEUTICALS AND CVD PREVENTION

Researchers use a reductionist method to understand the mechanism of action of nutrients, bringing the illness to proteins and genes. The underlying metabolic process, as well as other related regulatory mechanisms and pathways, are studied at the molecular level. Arachidonate 5-lipoxygenase (ALOX5), fatty acid synthase (FASN), apolipoprotein E (APOE), and lipoprotein lipase are genes involved in metabolism and lipid production (LPL). Peroxisome-proliferator-activated receptors (PPARs) are transcription factors that detect a range of metabolites at the cellular level, including fatty acids and fatty acid derivatives, and then present a specific metabolic program by regulating the expression of a number of target genes [84].

4.1. Identification of New Therapeutic Biomarkers

The utilization of genome-wide, microarray, or RNA sequencing data to give fresh insights into disease mechanisms and uncover novel, often unexpected, therapeutic targets is one of the most promising uses for functional genomics [85]. The transcriptome study to discover differentially expressed genes (DEGs) follows a procedure to reduce a large number of DEGs down to the top 10 hub genes that would cause the disease (Fig. **3**). For CVD prevention and therapy, the proposed biomarker or therapeutic might be adjusted by pharmaceutical, lifestyle, or food changes.

CONCLUSION

Cardiovascular diseases are the consequence of the interaction of numerous complex early-life events rather than a single discrete risk factor. These include behavioral risk factors, the environment, socioeconomic risk, and hereditary risk. Rather than treating patients with cardiovascular illness, the pharmaceutical sector should instead focus on guaranteeing optimal heart health. There are several ways to address heart health, including taking supplements that directly affect heart health or supplements that aid in weight loss, general fitness, and the achievement of long-term heart objectives. Some functional foods include elements that assist intrinsic heart health; others have added such constituents, while the third group includes those that share ingredients that are harmful to heart health. Garlic, plant and marine polyunsaturated fatty acids, soy products, dietary fibers in oats, psyllium husk and flaxseed, milk protein peptides, food-containing antioxidant vitamins, certain grapes, and a variety of other foods are among them. Improved electrical stability of heart cells, reduced LDL oxidation, scavenging free radicals, lowering blood lipids, lowering blood pressure, preventing platelet aggregation, and minimizing plaque formation are only some of the processes that can help minimize the risk of cardiovascular disease. As physicians get a better understanding of natural items that improve cardiovascular health, they may include them in their treatment options. New therapeutic biomarkers might be used in the prevention and treatment of cardiovascular illnesses by medicine or diet.

CONSENT FOR PUBLICATION

Not applicable.

CONFLICT OF INTEREST

The author declares no conflict of interest, financial or otherwise.

ACKNOWLEDGEMENTS

Declared none.

REFERENCES

[1]   Bernstein AM, Sun Q, Hu FB, Stampfer MJ, Manson JE, Willett WC. Major dietary protein sources and risk of coronary heart disease in women. Circulation 2010; 122(9): 876-83.
[http://dx.doi.org/10.1161/CIRCULATIONAHA.109.915165] [PMID: 20713902]

[2]   Alissa EM, Ferns GA. Functional foods and nutraceuticals in the primary prevention of cardiovascular diseases. J Nutr Metab 2012; 2012: 1-16.
[http://dx.doi.org/10.1155/2012/569486] [PMID: 22570771]

[3]   Parim B, Sathibabu Uddandrao VV, Saravanan G. Diabetic cardiomyopathy: molecular mechanisms, detrimental effects of conventional treatment, and beneficial effects of natural therapy. Heart Fail Rev 2019; 24(2): 279-99.
[http://dx.doi.org/10.1007/s10741-018-9749-1] [PMID: 30349977]

[4]   Clark AM, DesMeules M, Luo W, Duncan AS, Wielgosz A. Socioeconomic status and cardiovascular disease: risks and implications for care. Nat Rev Cardiol 2009; 6(11): 712-22.
[http://dx.doi.org/10.1038/nrcardio.2009.163] [PMID: 19770848]

[5]   Gersh BJ, Sliwa K, Mayosi BM, Yusuf S. Novel therapeutic concepts * The epidemic of cardiovascular disease in the developing world: global implications. Eur Heart J 2010; 31(6): 642-8.
[http://dx.doi.org/10.1093/eurheartj/ehq030] [PMID: 20176800]

[6]   Roth GA, Huffman MD, Moran AE, *et al.* Global and regional patterns in cardiovascular mortality from 1990 to 2013. Circulation 2015; 132(17): 1667-78.
[http://dx.doi.org/10.1161/CIRCULATIONAHA.114.008720] [PMID: 26503749]

[7]   Goldberg RB, Mellies MJ, Sacks FM, *et al.* Cardiovascular events and their reduction with pravastatin in diabetic and glucose-intolerant myocardial infarction survivors with average cholesterol levels: subgroup analyses in the cholesterol and recurrent events (CARE) trial. Circulation 1998; 98(23): 2513-9.
[http://dx.doi.org/10.1161/01.CIR.98.23.2513] [PMID: 9843456]

[8]   Parihar A, Parihar MS. Bioactive Food Components in the Prevention of Cardiovascular Diseases. In: Mérillon JM, Ramawat K, Eds. Bioactive Molecules in Food Reference Series in Phytochemistry. Cham: Springer 2018; p. 1.
[http://dx.doi.org/10.1007/978-3-319-54528-8_55-1]

[9]   Chow C, Cardona M, Raju PK, *et al.* Cardiovascular disease and risk factors among 345 adults in rural India—the Andhra Pradesh Rural Health Initiative. Int J Cardiol 2007; 116(2): 180-5.
[http://dx.doi.org/10.1016/j.ijcard.2006.03.043] [PMID: 16839628]

[10]   Egert S, Bosy-Westphal A, Seiberl J, *et al.* Quercetin reduces systolic blood pressure and plasma oxidised low-density lipoprotein concentrations in overweight subjects with a high-cardiovascular disease risk phenotype: a double-blinded, placebo-controlled cross-over study. Br J Nutr 2009; 102(7): 1065-74.

[http://dx.doi.org/10.1017/S0007114509359127] [PMID: 19402938]

[11]   Frishman WH, Beravol P, Carosella C. Alternative and complementary medicine for preventing and treating cardiovascular disease. Dis Mon 2009; 55(3): 121-92.
[http://dx.doi.org/10.1016/j.disamonth.2008.12.002] [PMID: 19215737]

[12]   Kris-Etherton PM, Hecker KD, Bonanome A, *et al.* Bioactive compounds in foods: their role in the prevention of cardiovascular disease and cancer. Am J Med 2002; 113(9) (Suppl. 9B): 71-88.
[http://dx.doi.org/10.1016/S0002-9343(01)00995-0] [PMID: 12566142]

[13]   Taylor F, Huffman MD, Macedo AF, *et al.* Statins for the primary prevention of cardiovascular disease. Cochrane Database Syst Rev 2013; 2013(1): CD004816.
[PMID: 23440795]

[14]   Jeemon P, Reddy KS. Social determinants of cardiovascular disease outcomes in Indians. Indian J Med Res 2010; 132(5): 617-22.
[PMID: 21150014]

[15]   Gupta R, Sharma KK, Gupta A, *et al.* Persistent high prevalence of cardiovascular risk factors in the urban middle class in India: Jaipur Heart Watch-5. J Assoc Physicians India 2012; 60(3): 11-6.
[PMID: 22799108]

[16]   Gupta R, Sharma K, Guptha S, Achari V, Bhansali A, Deedwania P. Hypercholesterolemia Awareness, Treatment And Control In High Cardiovascular Risk Subjects In India: A Population-Based Study. J Am Coll Cardiol 2013; 61(10): E1405.
[http://dx.doi.org/10.1016/S0735-1097(13)61405-9]

[17]   Gupta R, Kaul V, Agrawal A, Guptha S, Gupta VP. Cardiovascular risk according to educational status in India. Prev Med 2010; 51(5): 408-11.
[http://dx.doi.org/10.1016/j.ypmed.2010.08.014] [PMID: 20817021]

[18]   Hasler CM. The cardiovascular effects of soy products. J Cardiovasc Nurs 2002; 16(4): 50-63.
[http://dx.doi.org/10.1097/00005082-200207000-00006] [PMID: 12597262]

[19]   Anjana RM, Pradeepa R, Deepa M, *et al.* Prevalence of diabetes and prediabetes (impaired fasting glucose and/or impaired glucose tolerance) in urban and rural India: Phase I results of the Indian Council of Medical Research–INdia DIABetes (ICMR–INDIAB) study. Diabetologia 2011; 54(12): 3022-7.
[http://dx.doi.org/10.1007/s00125-011-2291-5] [PMID: 21959957]

[20]   Prabhakaran D, Yusuf S, Mehta S, *et al.* Two-year outcomes in patients admitted with non-ST elevation acute coronary syndrome: results of the OASIS registry 1 and 2. Indian Heart J 2005; 57(3): 217-25.
[PMID: 16196178]

[21]   Patel V, Chatterji S, Chisholm D, *et al.* Chronic diseases and injuries in India. Lancet 2011; 377(9763): 413-28.
[http://dx.doi.org/10.1016/S0140-6736(10)61188-9] [PMID: 21227486]

[22]   Subramanian SV, Subramanyam MA, Corsi DJ, Davey Smith G. Rejoinder: Need for a data-driven discussion on the socioeconomic patterning of cardiovascular health in India. Int J Epidemiol 2013; 42(5): 1438-43.
[http://dx.doi.org/10.1093/ije/dyt181] [PMID: 24019422]

[23]   Pais P, Pogue J, Gerstein H, *et al.* Risk factors for acute myocardial infarction in Indians: a case-control study. Lancet 1996; 348(9024): 358-63.
[http://dx.doi.org/10.1016/S0140-6736(96)02507-X] [PMID: 8709733]

[24]   Karan A, Engelgau M, Mahal A. The household-level economic burden of heart disease in I ndia. Trop Med Int Health 2014; 19(5): 581-91.
[http://dx.doi.org/10.1111/tmi.12281] [PMID: 24612174]

[25]   Fathima FN, Joshi R, Agrawal T, *et al.* Rationale and design of the Primary pREvention strategies at

the community level to Promote Adherence of treatments to pREvent cardiovascular diseases trial number (CTRI/2012/09/002981). Am Heart J 2013; 166(1): 4-12.
[http://dx.doi.org/10.1016/j.ahj.2013.03.024] [PMID: 23816015]

[26]   Bandosz P, O'Flaherty M, Drygas W, *et al.* Decline in mortality from coronary heart disease in Poland after socioeconomic transformation: modelling study. BMJ 2012; 344(jan25 2): d8136.
[http://dx.doi.org/10.1136/bmj.d8136] [PMID: 22279114]

[27]   Miczke A, Szulińska M, Hansdorfer-Korzon R, *et al.* Effects of spirulina consumption on body weight, blood pressure, and endothelial function in overweight hypertensive Caucasians: a double-blind, placebo-controlled, randomized trial. Eur Rev Med Pharmacol Sci 2016; 20(1): 150-6.
[PMID: 26813468]

[28]   Nasution SA. The use of ACE inhibitor in cardiovascular disease. Acta Med Indones 2006; 38(1): 60-4.
[PMID: 16479034]

[29]   Diaz A, Ducharme A. Update on the use of trandolapril in the management of cardiovascular disorders. Vasc Health Risk Manag 2008; 4(6): 1147-58.
[PMID: 19337528]

[30]   Munger MA. Use of Angiotensin receptor blockers in cardiovascular protection: current evidence and future directions. P&T 2011; 36(1): 22-40.
[PMID: 21386934]

[31]   Meredith PA. Candesartan cilexetil – a review of effects on cardiovascular complications in hypertension and chronic heart failure. Curr Med Res Opin 2007; 23(7): 1693-705.
[http://dx.doi.org/10.1185/030079907X210723] [PMID: 17588300]

[32]   Dan GA, Martinez-Rubio A, Agewall S, *et al.* Antiarrhythmic drugs–clinical use and clinical decision making: a consensus document from the European Heart Rhythm Association (EHRA) and European Society of Cardiology (ESC) Working Group on Cardiovascular Pharmacology, endorsed by the Heart Rhythm Society (HRS), Asia-Pacific Heart Rhythm Society (APHRS) and International Society of Cardiovascular Pharmacotherapy (ISCP). Europace 2018; 20(5): 731-732, 732an.
[http://dx.doi.org/10.1093/europace/eux373] [PMID: 29438514]

[33]   Bhagatwala J, Harris RA, Parikh SJ, *et al.* Epithelial sodium channel inhibition by amiloride on blood pressure and cardiovascular disease risk in young prehypertensives. J Clin Hypertens (Greenwich) 2014; 16(1): 47-53.
[http://dx.doi.org/10.1111/jch.12218] [PMID: 24410943]

[34]   Gottlieb SS, Kukin ML, Medina N, Yushak M, Packer M. Comparative hemodynamic effects of procainamide, tocainide, and encainide in severe chronic heart failure. Circulation 1990; 81(3): 860-4.
[http://dx.doi.org/10.1161/01.CIR.81.3.860] [PMID: 2106401]

[35]   Weber M. The role of the new β-blockers in treating cardiovascular disease. Am J Hypertens 2005; 18(12): 169-76.
[http://dx.doi.org/10.1016/j.amjhyper.2005.09.009] [PMID: 16373195]

[36]   Collinsworth KA, Kalman SM, Harrison DC. The clinical pharmacology of lidocaine as an antiarrhythmic drug. Circulation 1974; 50(6): 1217-30.
[http://dx.doi.org/10.1161/01.CIR.50.6.1217] [PMID: 4609637]

[37]   Dick GM, Tune JD. Role of potassium channels in coronary vasodilation. Exp Biol Med (Maywood) 2010; 235(1): 10 22.
[http://dx.doi.org/10.1258/ebm.2009.009201] [PMID: 20404014]

[38]   Alcocer L, Bendersky M, Acosta J, Urina-Triana M. Use of calcium channel blockers in cardiovascular risk reduction: issues in Latin America. Am J Cardiovasc Drugs 2010; 10(3): 143-54.
[http://dx.doi.org/10.2165/11536120-000000000-00000] [PMID: 20524716]

[39]   Fares H, DiNicolantonio JJ, O'Keefe JH, Lavie CJ. Amlodipine in hypertension: a first-line agent with

efficacy for improving blood pressure and patient outcomes. Open Heart 2016; 3(2): e000473.
[http://dx.doi.org/10.1136/openhrt-2016-000473] [PMID: 27752334]

[40]   Lopes RD. Antiplatelet agents in cardiovascular disease. J Thromb Thrombolysis 2011; 31(3): 306-9.
[http://dx.doi.org/10.1007/s11239-011-0558-9] [PMID: 21327512]

[41]   Ittaman SV, VanWormer JJ, Rezkalla SH. The role of aspirin in the prevention of cardiovascular
disease. Clin Med Res 2014; 12(3-4): 147-54.
[http://dx.doi.org/10.3121/cmr.2013.1197] [PMID: 24573704]

[42]   Shah SU, Anjum S, Littler WA. Use of diuretics in cardiovascular diseases: (1) heart failure. Postgrad
Med J 2004; 80(942): 201-5.
[http://dx.doi.org/10.1136/pgmj.2003.010835] [PMID: 15082840]

[43]   Stroes E. Statins and LDL-cholesterol lowering: an overview. Curr Med Res Opin 2005; 21(sup6)
(Suppl. 6): S9-S16.
[http://dx.doi.org/10.1185/030079905X59102] [PMID: 16138936]

[44]   Ali KM, Wonnerth A, Huber K, Wojta J. Cardiovascular disease risk reduction by raising HDL
cholesterol - current therapies and future opportunities. Br J Pharmacol 2012; 167(6): 1177-94.
[http://dx.doi.org/10.1111/j.1476-5381.2012.02081.x] [PMID: 22725625]

[45]   Linton MF, Yancey PG, Davies SS, Jerome WG, Linton EF, Song WL, *et al.* The role of lipids and
lipoproteins in atherosclerosis 2019.

[46]   Shaito A, Thuan DTB, Phu HT, *et al.* Herbal Medicine for Cardiovascular Diseases: Efficacy,
Mechanisms, and Safety. Front Pharmacol 2020; 11: 422.
[http://dx.doi.org/10.3389/fphar.2020.00422] [PMID: 32317975]

[47]   Mehrinfar R, Frishman WH. Flavanol-Rich Cocoa. Cardiol Rev 2008; 16(3): 109-15.
[http://dx.doi.org/10.1097/CRD.0b013e31815d95e2] [PMID: 18414181]

[48]   Ohr LM. Wellness for Women-Nutraceuticals and Functional Foods. Food Technology-Chicago 2003;
57(10): 71-7.

[49]   Scicchitano P, Cameli M, Maiello M, *et al.* Nutraceuticals and dyslipidaemia: Beyond the common
therapeutics. J Funct Foods 2014; 6: 11-32.
[http://dx.doi.org/10.1016/j.jff.2013.12.006]

[50]   Massaro M, Scoditti E, Carluccio MA, De Caterina R. Nutraceuticals and prevention of
atherosclerosis: focus on ω-3 polyunsaturated fatty acids and Mediterranean diet polyphenols.
Cardiovasc Ther 2010; 28(4): e13-9.
[http://dx.doi.org/10.1111/j.1755-5922.2010.00211.x] [PMID: 20633019]

[51]   Moreau RA, Whitaker BD, Hicks KB. Phytosterols, phytostanols, and their conjugates in foods:
structural diversity, quantitative analysis, and health-promoting uses. Prog Lipid Res 2002; 41(6): 457-
500.
[http://dx.doi.org/10.1016/S0163-7827(02)00006-1] [PMID: 12169300]

[52]   Jeffery EH, Araya M. Physiological effects of broccoli consumption. Phytochem Rev 2009; 8(1): 283-
98.
[http://dx.doi.org/10.1007/s11101-008-9106-4]

[53]   Slavin JL, Lloyd B. Health benefits of fruits and vegetables. Adv Nutr 2012; 3(4): 506-16.
[http://dx.doi.org/10.3945/an.112.002154] [PMID: 22797986]

[54]   Reddy KS, Perry CL, Stigler MH, Arora M. Differences in tobacco use among young people in urban
India by sex, socioeconomic status, age, and school grade: assessment of baseline survey data. Lancet
2006; 367(9510): 589-94.
[http://dx.doi.org/10.1016/S0140-6736(06)68225-1] [PMID: 16488802]

[55]   Stevinson C, Pittler MH, Ernst E. Garlic for treating hypercholesterolemia. A meta-analysis of
randomized clinical trials. Ann Intern Med 2000; 133(6): 420-9.

[http://dx.doi.org/10.7326/0003-4819-133-6-200009190-00009] [PMID: 10975959]

[56]   Belardinelli R, Tiano L, Littarru GP. Oxidative stress, endothelial function and coenzyme Q $_{10}$. Biofactors 2008; 32(1-4): 129-33.
[http://dx.doi.org/10.1002/biof.5520320115] [PMID: 19096108]

[57]   Khurana S, Venkataraman K, Hollingsworth A, Piche M, Tai T. Polyphenols: benefits to the cardiovascular system in health and in aging. Nutrients 2013; 5(10): 3779-827.
[http://dx.doi.org/10.3390/nu5103779] [PMID: 24077237]

[58]   Dohadwala MM, Vita JA. Grapes and cardiovascular disease. J Nutr 2009; 139(9): 1788S-93S.
[http://dx.doi.org/10.3945/jn.109.107474] [PMID: 19625699]

[59]   Denruijter H, Berecki G, Opthof T, Verkerk A, Zock P, Coronel R. Pro- and antiarrhythmic properties of a diet rich in fish oil. Cardiovasc Res 2007; 73(2): 316-25.
[http://dx.doi.org/10.1016/j.cardiores.2006.06.014] [PMID: 16859661]

[60]   Micha R, Peñalvo JL, Cudhea F, Imamura F, Rehm CD, Mozaffarian D. Association between dietary factors and mortality from heart disease, stroke, and type 2 diabetes in the United States. JAMA 2017; 317(9): 912-24.
[http://dx.doi.org/10.1001/jama.2017.0947] [PMID: 28267855]

[61]   Singh RB, Niaz MA, Agarwal P, Beegum R, Rastogi SS, Sachan DS. A randomised, double-blind, placebo-controlled trial of L-carnitine in suspected acute myocardial infarction. Postgrad Med J 1996; 72(843): 45-50.
[http://dx.doi.org/10.1136/pgmj.72.843.45] [PMID: 8746285]

[62]   Kunamneni A, Ravuri B, Saisha V, Ellaiah P, Prabhakhar T. Urokinase-a very popular cardiovascular agent. Recent Adv Cardiovasc Drug Discov 2008; 3(1): 45-58.
[http://dx.doi.org/10.2174/157489008783331670] [PMID: 18221128]

[63]   Geleijnse JM, Launer LJ, van der Kuip DAM, Hofman A, Witteman JCM. Inverse association of tea and flavonoid intakes with incident myocardial infarction: the Rotterdam Study. Am J Clin Nutr 2002; 75(5): 880-6.
[http://dx.doi.org/10.1093/ajcn/75.5.880] [PMID: 11976162]

[64]   Roberfroid MB, Van Loo JAE, Gibson GR. The bifidogenic nature of chicory inulin and its hydrolysis products. J Nutr 1998; 128(1): 11-9.
[http://dx.doi.org/10.1093/jn/128.1.11] [PMID: 9430596]

[65]   Khare N, Khare P. Use of Probiotics in Curing Diseases A Review. International Journal of Pharmacy. Photon 2016; 107: 502-6.

[66]   Cam A, de Mejia EG. Role of dietary proteins and peptides in cardiovascular disease. Mol Nutr Food Res 2012; 56(1): 53-66.
[http://dx.doi.org/10.1002/mnfr.201100535] [PMID: 22121103]

[67]   Debreceni B, Debreceni L. Role of vitamins in cardiovascular health and disease. Research Reports in Clinical Cardiology 2014; 5: 283-95.
[http://dx.doi.org/10.2147/RRCC.S44465]

[68]   Larson AJ, Symons JD, Jalili T. Therapeutic potential of quercetin to decrease blood pressure: review of efficacy and mechanisms. Adv Nutr 2012; 3(1): 39-46.
[http://dx.doi.org/10.3945/an.111.001271] [PMID: 22332099]

[69]   Harland JI, Haffner TA. Systematic review, meta-analysis and regression of randomised controlled trials reporting an association between an intake of circa 25g soya protein per day and blood cholesterol. Atherosclerosis 2008; 200(1): 13-27.
[http://dx.doi.org/10.1016/j.atherosclerosis.2008.04.006] [PMID: 18534601]

[70]   Chopra M, O'Neill ME, Keogh N, Wortley G, Southon S, Thurnham DI. Influence of increased fruit and vegetable intake on plasma and lipoprotein carotenoids and LDL oxidation in smokers and nonsmokers. Clin Chem 2000; 46(11): 1818-29.

[http://dx.doi.org/10.1093/clinchem/46.11.1818] [PMID: 11067818]

[71]   Grassi D, Desideri G, Di Giosia P, *et al.* Tea, flavonoids, and cardiovascular health: endothelial protection. Am J Clin Nutr 2013; 98(6) (Suppl.): 1660S-6S.
[http://dx.doi.org/10.3945/ajcn.113.058313] [PMID: 24172308]

[72]   Flint AJ, Hu FB, Glynn RJ, *et al.* Whole grains and incident hypertension in men. Am J Clin Nutr 2009; 90(3): 493-8.
[http://dx.doi.org/10.3945/ajcn.2009.27460] [PMID: 19571218]

[73]   Harris WS, Miller M, Tighe AP, Davidson MH, Schaefer EJ. Omega-3 fatty acids and coronary heart disease risk: Clinical and mechanistic perspectives. Atherosclerosis 2008; 197(1): 12-24.
[http://dx.doi.org/10.1016/j.atherosclerosis.2007.11.008] [PMID: 18160071]

[74]   Cardoso S, Pereira O, Seca A, Pinto D, Silva A. Seaweeds as preventive agents for cardiovascular diseases: From nutrients to functional foods. Mar Drugs 2015; 13(11): 6838-65.
[http://dx.doi.org/10.3390/md13116838] [PMID: 26569268]

[75]   Berman AY, Motechin RA, Wiesenfeld MY, Holz MK. The therapeutic potential of resveratrol: a review of clinical trials. NPJ Precis Oncol 2017; 1(1): 35.
[http://dx.doi.org/10.1038/s41698-017-0038-6] [PMID: 28989978]

[76]   Wang X, Lv H, Gu Y, *et al.* Protective effect of lycopene on cardiac function and myocardial fibrosis after acute myocardial infarction in rats *via* the modulation of p38 and MMP-9. J Mol Histol 2014; 45(1): 113-20.
[http://dx.doi.org/10.1007/s10735-013-9535-2] [PMID: 24213878]

[77]   Pérez-Jiménez J, Saura-Calixto F. Grape products and cardiovascular disease risk factors. Nutr Res Rev 2008; 21(2): 158-73.
[http://dx.doi.org/10.1017/S0954422408125124] [PMID: 19087369]

[78]   Broekmans WMR, Klöpping-Ketelaars IAA, Schuurman CRWC, *et al.* Fruits and vegetables increase plasma carotenoids and vitamins and decrease homocysteine in humans. J Nutr 2000; 130(6): 1578-83.
[http://dx.doi.org/10.1093/jn/130.6.1578] [PMID: 10827213]

[79]   Hooper L, Kroon PA, Rimm EB, *et al.* Flavonoids, flavonoid-rich foods, and cardiovascular risk: a meta-analysis of randomized controlled trials. Am J Clin Nutr 2008; 88(1): 38-50.
[http://dx.doi.org/10.1093/ajcn/88.1.38] [PMID: 18614722]

[80]   Mishra S, Singh RB, Dwivedi SP, *et al.* Effects of nutraceuticals on genetic expressions. Open Nutraceuticals J 2009; 2(1): 70-80.
[http://dx.doi.org/10.2174/1876396000902010070]

[81]   Brasier AR. The NF-kappaB regulatory network. Cardiovasc Toxicol 2006; 6(2): 111-30.
[http://dx.doi.org/10.1385/CT:6:2:111] [PMID: 17303919]

[82]   Ma Q. Role of nrf2 in oxidative stress and toxicity. Annu Rev Pharmacol Toxicol 2013; 53(1): 401-26.
[http://dx.doi.org/10.1146/annurev-pharmtox-011112-140320] [PMID: 23294312]

[83]   Pan Y, Yu C, Huang J, Rong Y, Chen J, Chen M. Bioinformatics analysis of vascular RNA-seq data revealed hub genes and pathways in a novel Tibetan minipig atherosclerosis model induced by a high fat/cholesterol diet. Lipids Health Dis 2020; 19(1): 54.
[http://dx.doi.org/10.1186/s12944-020-01222-w] [PMID: 32213192]

[84]   Wan GX, Ji LH, Xia WB, Cheng L, Zhang YG. Bioinformatics identification of potential candidate blood indicators for doxorubicin☐induced heart failure. Exp Ther Med 2018; 16(3): 2534-44.
[http://dx.doi.org/10.3892/etm.2018.6482] [PMID: 30186487]

CHAPTER 2

Congestive Heart Failure: Insight on Pharmacotherapy

Sri Bharathi G.S[1,*], Sakthi Sundaram S[1], Prabhakaran S[1], Lalitha V[1], Haja Sherief S[1], Duraisami R[2] and Sengottuvelu S[1]

[1] *Department of Pharmacology, Nandha College of Pharmacy, Erode, Tamilnadu, India*
[2] *Department of Pharmacognosy, Nandha College of Pharmacy, Erode Tamilnadu, India*

Abstract: Congestive Heart Failure (CHF) is the inability of the heart to supply blood to other organs and tissues to meet its need for metabolism. Over 64.3 million people around the world live with heart failure. Some of the common causes of CHF include myocardial infarction, increase in blood pressure, atrial fibrillation and cardiomyopathy. The complete etiology of CHF is complex. Patients with HF often experience fatigue, dyspnea, and pain, lack of energy, cognitive impairment and depression. Left ventricular ejection fraction (LVEF) is a measure of the amount of blood pumped from the heart's left ventricle during each contraction. It is used as a phenotypic marker in the indication of the pathophysiological mechanism and sensitivity to therapy. The pathogenesis of HF with low ejection fraction is that of a progressive state. The various classes of drugs used clinically for the treatment of congestive heart failure are diuretics, beta blockers, ACE inhibitors and vasopressin receptor antagonists. The management of Heart failure includes acute decompensation, chronic management and palliative care. Cardiac glycosides are a varied group of naturally obtained compounds used in the treatment of CHF. They exhibit their action by binding to and inhibiting Na^+/K^+-ATPase. Then, they consequently increase the force of myocardial contraction. The primary structure of these drugs is a steroidal framework, which is the pharmacophoric component that is responsible for their activity. The most familiar cardiac glycosides are digitoxin, digoxin, oleandrin, bufalin, ouabain, marinobufagenin, telocinobufagin and aerobufagenin. Among other cardiac glycosides, digoxin has been proven to improve symptom alleviation, functional capacity, quality of life and exercise tolerance in patients with mild to moderate HF in clinical trials. Early detection and prevention interventions, as well as lifestyle changes, are essential.

Keywords: Cardiac glycosides, Causes, Congestive heart failure, Digoxin, LVEF, Pathogenesis, Treatment.

---

* Corresponding author Sri Bharathi G.S: Department of Pharmacology, Nandha College of Pharmacy,Erode, Tamilnadu, 638052-India; E-mail: gsbharathisri98@gmail.com

Dr. V. V. Sathibabu Uddandrao & Dr. Parim Brahma Naidu (Eds.)

1. INTRODUCTION

Heart failure (HF) or Congestive heart failure (CHF) or cardiac failure is classically defined as "Clinical syndrome caused by the inability of the heart to supply blood to the tissues according to the metabolic needs of the tissues". Heart Failure results from ventricular dysfunction with volume or pressure overload, either separately or together. It also involves circulatory, neurohormonal, and molecular abnormalities [1]. Diastolic dysfunction is defined as a raised end-diastolic pressure in a normal-sized chamber, whereas systolic dysfunction is described as a lower ejection fraction and refers to the inability to fill and relax the left ventricle. Ischemic (Coronary artery disease [CAD]) and non-ischemic (hypertension, thyroid illness, valvular disease, myocarditis, adult congenital heart disease) diseases are the cause of HF [2]. Coronary artery disease or coronary heart disease, including a previous myocardial infarction (heart attack), high blood pressure, valvular heart disease, atrial fibrillation, excessive alcohol consumption, infection, and cardiomyopathy of unclear cause, are all common causes of HF [3]. Coronary artery disease is considered to be the cause of congestive heart failure (CHF) in nearly 65% of patients [4].

Heart failure patients often experience symptoms of fatigue and lack of energy, depression, pain, dyspnea and cognitive impairment. The etiology of heart failure symptoms is complex and is not completely understood. Although most patients suffer worsened dyspnea with episodes of volume overload, HF-related dyspnea and exertional fatigue are not directly related to pulmonary capillary wedge pressure or cardiac output, rather to broader, systemic effects of HF, including generalized myopathy. Some of the symptoms may also overlap with comorbid problems, which are particularly common in older individuals with heart failure. Symptoms reported by HF patients are significantly impacted by depression and by the patient's perceived control over their condition [5]. LVEF (left ventricular ejection fraction) is a clinically valuable phenotypic trait that indicates underlying pathophysiological processes and therapeutic sensitivity. Heart failure patients are currently classified as having heart failure with reduced (HFrEF; LVEF 40%–49%), mid-range (HFmrEF; LVEF 40–49%), or preserved ejection fraction (HFpEF; LVEF 50%) ejection fraction. Cut-off values are arbitrary and vary from one guideline to the next. The classification of LVEF has been challenged for oversimplifying a complex condition [2].

Congestive Heart Failure (CHF) with left ventricular systolic dysfunction has been the focus of research (LVSD). Heart failure with normal ejection fraction (HFnEF, also known as "preserved systolic function" and "diastolic dysfunction") has similar pathologic abnormalities in inflammatory and neuroendocrine function [4]. The severity of heart failure can be explained symptomatically. The commonly used system is the New York Heart Association (NYHA) functional classification [6].

CLASS	SYMPTOMS
I	Cardiac disease, but no symptoms and no limitation in ordinary physical activity
II	Mild symptoms and slight limitation during ordinary activity
III	Significant limitation in activity due to symptoms. Comfortable only at rest
IV	Severe limitations. Symptoms even while at rest

1.1. Hypertrophic Cardiomyopathy (HCM)

Hypertrophic cardiomyopathy (HCM) is a condition marked by left ventricular (LV) or septal hypertrophy in the presence of normal to hyperdynamic systolic function, no ventricular chamber dilation, and no other cardiac or systemic disease that would explain the hypertrophy.

1.2. Left Ventricular Noncompaction (LVNC)

LVNC (left ventricular noncompaction) is a cardiomyopathy marked by LV hypertrabeculation. Normal LV size and systolic and diastolic function can be related to left ventricular noncompaction. In other situations, however, underlying arrhythmias are present.

1.3. Arrhythmogenic Right Ventricular Cardiomyopathy (ARVC)

Arrhythmogenic Right Ventricular Cardiomyopathy (ARVC) is an uncommon cardiomyopathy with an incidence of 1 in 1000 to 1 in 5000 in the general population. ARVC is hypothesised to be caused by mutations in desmosomal genes such as desmoplakin (DSP), plakophilin-2 (PKP2), desmoglein-2 (DSG2), desmocollin-2 (DSC2), and plakoglobin(JUP), which cause problems in cellular adhesion.

1.4. Restrictive Cardiomyopathy (RCM)

According to data from the PCMR, restrictive cardiomyopathy (RCM) is extremely rare in children, affecting only about 5% of paediatric cardiomyopathy patients. The prognosis for these children is frequently poor, and heart transplantation is frequently required [1].

2. PREVALENCE

HF affects an estimated 64.3 million people worldwide. The prevalence of recognised heart failure is believed to be between 1% and 2% of the overall adult population in affluent countries. Despite differences in diagnostic standards, most studies indicate that more than half of all heart failure patients in the general population have maintained LVEF, and that this percentage is rising [6].

Based upon the data from NHANES 2013 to 2016, an estimated 6.2 million Americans ≥20 years of age experienced heart failure (Table 1). This represents an increase from an estimated 5.7 million US adults with heart failure based on NHANES 2009 to 2012 (NHLBI unpublished tabulation using NHANES20). Projections show that the prevalence of heart failure increases 46% from 2012 to 2030, resulting in >8 million people ≥18 years of age with heart failure. Additionally, the total percentage of the population with HF is predicted to increase from 2.42% in 2012 to 2.97% in 2030 [7].

Table 1. HF in United States [8].

Population Group	Prevalence 2013-2016 Age≥20y	Incidence, 2014,Age≥55y	Mortality, 2017, All Ages*	Hospital Discharges, 2016, All Ages	Cost, 2012
Both sexes	6200000(2.2%)	1000000	80480	809000	$30.7 billion
Males	3000000(2.4%)	495000	36824(45.8%)	415000	--
Females	3200000(2.1%)	505000	43656(54.2%)	394000	--
NH white males	2.2%	430000	30076	--	--
NH white females	1.9%	425000	36004	--	--
NH black males	3.5%	65000	4068	--	--
NH black females	3.9%	80000	4683	--	--
Hispanic males	2.5%	--	1820	--	--
Hispanic females	1.7%	--	1960	--	--
NH Asian males	0.7%	--	6331	--	--
NH Asian females	--	--	7521	--	--
NH American Indian or Alaska Native	--	--	339	--	--

3. PATHOPHYSIOLOGY

The pathogenesis of HF with reduced ejection fraction is that of a progressive condition: risk factors cause cardiac injury, which leads to myocardial dysfunction (which is initially asymptomatic), leading to worsening symptoms until the patient develops end-stage HF. Heart failure is caused by any condition that damages or overloads the heart muscle, reducing efficiency. These increases in workload, which are mediated by long-term activation of neurohormonal systems, including the renin-angiotensin system, cause dilatation, fibrosis, and structural changes in the left ventricle's shape from elliptical to spherical, over time [8]. In a normal heart, increasing ventricular filling causes the Frank–Starling law of the heart to increase contraction force, resulting in an increase in cardiac output. This mechanism fails in HF because the ventricle becomes overloaded with blood, making heart muscle contractions less effective. This is due to reduced ability to cross-link actin and myosin filaments in over-stretched heart muscle [9].

4. DRUG THERAPY

4.1. Diuretics

Diuretics, which comprise diuretics types such as thiazide-like diuretics, loop diuretics, and potassium-sparing diuretics, have long been used to treat symptoms of fluid accumulation. With the exception of mineralocorticoid antagonists such as spironolactone, evidence of their efficacy and safety is sparse, despite their widespread use [10, 11]. With diuretics, clinical trials have shown rapid improvements in sodium excretion, exercise tolerance, fluid overload symptoms, and heart function [5].

4.2. Angiotensin Converting Enzyme Inhibitors (ACE Inhibitors)

If the person develops a long-term cough as a side effect of the ACE-I, angiotensin-converting enzyme inhibitors (ACE-I) or angiotensin receptor blockers (ARBs) should be used as first-line therapy for people with HF due to impaired systolic function. Nony and colleagues discovered that mortality was considerably reduced only in the cohort with IHD in 17 of the early ACE inhibitor studies; mortality was not significantly reduced in the non-IHD category. In a later meta-analysis, Garg and Yusuf found that ACE inhibitors reduced mortality in both IHD (odds ratio 0.77) and nonischemic heart failure (odds ratio 0.8), but the upper confidence interval in the latter group was >1. However, in certain important studies with ACE inhibitors in heart failure, nonischemic HF was found to have a better effect on mortality than ischemic HF [12].

4.3. Beta-adrenergic Blocking Agents (Beta Blockers)

Beta-blockers, notably metoprolol, carvedilol, and bucindolol, have been proven in clinical trials to improve hemodynamics, LV function, and clinical status in patients with ischemic and nonischemic heart failure [13]. Beta-adrenergic blocking drugs (beta blockers) are also used as a first-line treatment, enhancing the benefits of ACE-I/ARB in terms of symptom relief and mortality [14, 15]. Beta blockers offer a lower mortality benefit in patients with systolic dysfunction who also have atrial fibrillation than in people who don't [16].

4.4. Vasopressin Receptor Antagonists

Antibodies targeting the vasopressin receptor can also be utilised to treat HF. Conivaptan is the first medicine licenced by the US Food and Drug Administration to treat euvolemic hyponatremia in heart failure patients. Hyponatremia can be treated with hypertonic 3%saline and diuretics in some situations [17].

5. MANAGEMENT OF HEART FAILURE

5.1. Acute Decompensation

Acute decompensated heart failure is a broad term for a collection of symptoms that include dyspnea, edema, and weariness. Despite the great prevalence of this disorder and the significant morbidity and mortality it causes, diagnosis can be difficult, and the best treatment is yet unknown. The treatment option for acute decompensated heart failure includes furosemide, ultra filtration, nitroglycerin, positive pressure ventilation, morphine, nesiritide, nitroprusside, vasodilatingionotropes, vasopressor ionotropes [18].

5.2. Chronic Management

Heart failure can be caused by a number of factors. Excluding reversible factors, such as thyroid disease, prolonged tachycardia, anaemia, alcohol use disorder, hypertension, and failure of one or more cardiac valves, is critical when considering therapeutic alternatives. The initial step in treating HF is usually to address the underlying cause. However, in the vast majority of cases, either no primary reason is discovered or the primary cause is not treated, and normal cardiac function is not restored. In certain circumstances, there are medicinal, behavioural, and technological treatment options that can lead to significant improvements in outcomes, such as symptom relief, increased exercise tolerance, and a lower risk of hospitalisation or death. Exercise training has been advocated as a basic component of breathlessness rehabilitation for chronic obstructive pulmonary disease (COPD) and heart failure. Other interventions, such as psychological and educational needs of people, as well as employment needs, must be included in rehabilitation to address shortness of breath [19].

5.3. Palliative Care

Palliative care must be integrated into comprehensive HF care throughout the course of treatment. The activation of neurohormonal and cytokine receptors, as well as the impact on skeletal and respiratory muscles, is the genesis of many heart failure symptoms. Evidence-based therapy for neurohormonal dysregulation in HF are among the palliative symptom interventions, however data on therapies that specifically ameliorate symptoms is scarce. Other therapies, such as opioids and particular exercise for dyspnea, are supported by evidence, but more data is needed to guide treatment of depression, pain, anxiety, and spiritual distress in heart failure patients and their families, among other issues. Clinical trials for HF, specifically to investigate palliative therapy in advanced heart failure, should include data on symptom relief. To address several aspects of patient and family pain, palliative treatment for congestive heart failure should include evidence-based HF therapies and interdisciplinary approaches [4].

5.4. Cardiac Glycosides

Cardiac glycosides are a group of naturally occurring chemicals that bind to and inhibit the Na+/K+ ATPase enzyme. Members of this family have been used to treat HF and atrial arrhythmia for many years, and the mechanism of their positive inotropic effect is well understood [20]. Plants have been utilised medically for thousands of years, including those now recognized to contain cardiac glycosides [21]. These chemicals, which are most typically found as secondary metabolites in plants such as foxglove plants, have a varied variety of biochemical effects on cardiac cell activity and have also been recommended for cancer treatment [22].

5.4.1. Chemistry of Cardiac Glycosides

Cardiac glycosides are a wide group of naturally occurring chemicals. They have a lot of structural variation, however all members of this family have the same structural pattern. The primary structure of these drugs is a steroidal framework, which is the pharmacophoric component responsible for their activity [23]. The structure of the ring at the R end of the molecule, in particular, permits it to be classed as either a cardenolide or a bufadienolide. The presence of a "enolide," a five-membered ring with a single double bond, at the lactone end distinguishes cardenolides from bufadienolides. Bufadienolides, on the other hand, contain a "dienolide," a six-membered ring with two double bonds, at the lactone end (Fig. 1) [24]. Cardiac glycosides, cardenolides, and bufadienolides are similar to steroid saponins in structure and have similar solubility and foaming properties. They are further distinguishable from other steroid glycosides by the presence of a 14-hydroxy group and a strange sugar in their skeleton [25].

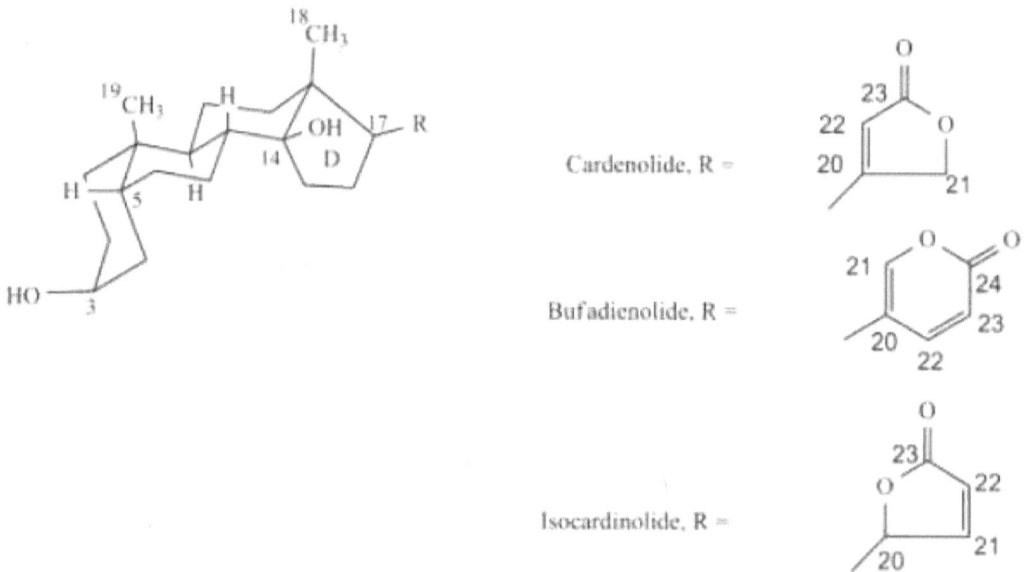

Fig. (1). Structure of cardiac glycosides [25].

5.4.2. Sources of Cardiac Glycosides

Cardiac glycosides are pharmacologically active compounds produced by several plant and toad species, and have also been found in mammalian tissues. Digoxin, digitoxin, oleandrin, ouabain, bufalin, marinobufagenin, aerobufagenin, and telocinobufagin are the most well-known. Cardiac glycosides have been found in plants in the past, and their use has been linked to cardiovascular symptoms due to the blockage of the NKA current in the heart. Ouabain is found in the Acokanthera and Strophanthus genera, digoxin is found in the Digitalis genus, such as D. lanata and D. purpurea, and oleandrin is found in the Nerium oleander plant. Another group of plants that contains cardenolides, such as caloptrin, is the Asclepias genus, also known as milkweed. These cardiac glycosides are frequently consumed by monarch butterflies, which have developed a significant ability to absorb and retain cardenolides as a result of significant NKA adaptation. Such a feature may play a crucial role in the species' defence against predators. Bufodienolide poisoning can also be used to infer heart toxicity; reports of toad poisoning encouraged research into other cardiac glycosides and associated toxicities [26].

5.4.3. Mechanism of Cardiac Glycosides

Cardiac glycosides modify the functioning of the sodium-potassium ATPase pump in cardiac muscle cells. These sodium-potassium pumps normally transport potassium ions in and sodium ions out. Cardiac glycosides, on the other hand, inhibit this pump by stabilizing it in the E2-P transition state, preventing sodium from being extruded out, resulting in an increase in intracellular sodium concentration. Because both cardiac glycosides and potassium compete for binding to the ATPase pump, variations in extracellular potassium content can possibly lead to medication efficacy being altered [27]. Such negative effects can be avoided by carefully managing the dosage. Continuing with the mechanism, increased intracellular sodium levels restrict the action of NCX, a second membrane ion exchanger that pumps calcium ions out of the cell and sodium ions in at a 3Na+/Ca2+ ratio. As a result, calcium ions are not ejected and begin to pile up inside the cell [28, 29].

Elevated calcium uptake into the sarcoplasmic reticulum (SR) *via* the SERCA2 transporter is caused by impaired calcium homeostasis and increased cytoplasmic calcium concentrations. Increased calcium reserves in the sarcoplasmic reticulum allow for more calcium release when the myocyte is stimulated, allowing for faster and more forceful contractions *via* cross-bridge cycling. Because the AV node's refractory period is lengthened, cardiac glycosides also help to lower heart rate. Digoxin, for example, causes an increase in cardiac output and a drop in heart rate without causing major changes in blood pressure; this property permits it to be widely employed in the treatment of cardiac arrhythmias [30].

5.4.4. Pharmacological Activity of Cardiac Glycosides

Because of the relevance of cardiotonic glycosides in medicine, thorough plant surveys for their existence have been conducted [31]. The effects of these cardiac glycosides in the therapy of heart failure are their most important use. In cardiac failure, also known as congestive heart failure, the heart is unable to pump enough blood to meet the body's needs. There is an input of Na+ and an outflow of K+ with each heart contraction. Na+, K+, ATPase must reestablish the concentration gradient before the next contraction by pumping Na+ into the cell against the concentration gradient. This process necessitates energy, which is obtained *via* Na+, K+, and ATPase hydrolyzing ATP to ADP. Cardiac glycosides inhibit Na+, K+, and ATPase, increasing the force of heart contraction as result. Some cardiac glycosides, on the other hand, are being studied for their anticancer properties. Furthermore, several cardiac glycosides have been shown to have antiviral effect against rhinovirus [25].

6. DIGOXIN

Digoxin has been proven to improve symptom alleviation, quality of life, functional capacity, and exercise tolerance in patients with mild to moderate HF in clinical trials. The discontinuation of digoxin medication resulted in a severe decline in clinical condition. In patients with atrial fibrillation, digoxin is suggested for ventricular response management. Digoxin can be given to ACE inhibitors, beta blockers, and diuretics to relieve clinical symptoms in patients with a normal sinus rhythm [5]. Patients with CHF who were given placebo deteriorated more frequently than would be predicted by chance compared to those who were given digoxin. Dyspnea (as judged by questionnaire) and functional exercise capacity (as measured by the 6-minute walking test) both showed small improvements with digoxin. Fatigue and emotional function were unaffected by the medication. While on digoxin, cardiac function was better as determined by ejection fraction on M-mode echocardiography and cardiothoracic ratio on chest radiograph [32].

7. TOXICOKINETICS

Due to the deadly properties of cardiac glycoside-containing plants and their crude extracts, people have employed them as arrow coatings, homicidal or suicidal aids, rat poisons, diuretics, heart tonics, and emetics since ancient times [33]. The Food and Drug Administration (FDA) has only approved digoxin for the treatment of HF and arrhythmia in humans and animals. This cardiac glycoside is available on the pharmaceutical market as an elixir, capsule, ampoule, and pill for oral and intravenous administration. The capsules have a bioavailability of close to 100%, the elixir has a bioavailability of 70 to 85% and the pills have a bioavailability of 75%. Digoxin's intestinal absorption is 50% lower than that of digitoxin, another cardiac glycoside present in medicinal formulations. The half-life of digoxin varies depending on the species. In individuals with normal renal function, the excretory half-life of ouabain is approximately 11 hours, oleandrin is 2.3 hours, and bufalin is between 0.99 and 2.47 hours in humans. Hepatic biotransformation is the primary mode of cardiac glycoside biotransformation. Dihydrodigoxin and digitoxigenin can be made from digoxin, while oleandrin can be turned into oleandrigenin. Cardiac glycosides have been found in the liver, spleen, gastrointestinal system, heart, and kidneys, indicating that tissue distribution is relatively comparable. As it crosses through the blood-brain barrier, oleandrin can build up in the central nervous system. For digoxin, urinary excretion is expected to be the primary route of elimination, but for oleandrin, faecal excretion is thought to be the primary route of elimination [26].

CONCLUSION

Congestive heart failure is a pathophysiological condition in which the heart's output is insufficient to meet the body's and lungs' needs. The main goals of CHF treatment are to alleviate symptoms and prevent the condition from progressing. Treatment involves dietary and pharmaceutical adjustments, as well as device therapy and, in rare cases, heart transplantation. Heart failure pharmacology has evolved into a combination symptomatic and preventative care strategy. Standard treatment includes ACE inhibitors, diuretics, and beta-blockers. Digoxin is given to people with atrial fibrillation to improve clinical symptoms. Early detection and prevention interventions, as well as lifestyle changes, are critical.

CONSENT FOR PUBLICATION

Not applicable.

CONFLICT OF INTEREST

The author declares no conflict of interest, financial or otherwise.

ACKNOWLEDGEMENTS

Declared none.

REFERENCES

[1]   Puggia L, Rowland TJ, Miyamoto SD, Sinagra G, Mestroni L. Molecular and cellular mechanisms in heart failure. In: Jefferies JL, Chang AC, Rossano JW, Shaddy RE, Towbin JA, Eds. Heart failure in the child and young adult. Boston. Academic Press 2018; pp. 3-19.
      [http://dx.doi.org/10.1016/B978-0-12-802393-8.00001-6]

[2]   Groenewegen A, Rutten FH, Mosterd A, Hoes AW. Epidemiology of heart failure. Eur J Heart Fail 2020; 22(8): 1342-56.
      [http://dx.doi.org/10.1002/ejhf.1858] [PMID: 32483830]

[3]   Chronic heart failure: National clinical guideline for diagnosis and management in primary and secondary care: Partial update. National Clinical Guideline Centre (UK) 2010; (August): 19-24.

[4]   Rustad JK, Stern TA, Hebert KA, Musselman DL. Diagnosis and treatment of depression in patients with congestive heart failure: a review of the literature. Prim Care Companion CNS Disord 2013; 15(4): 01511.

[http://dx.doi.org/10.4088/PCC.13r01511] [PMID: 24392265]

[5]   Goodlin SJ. Palliative care in congestive heart failure. J Am Coll Cardiol 2009; 54(5): 386-96.
       [http://dx.doi.org/10.1016/j.jacc.2009.02.078] [PMID: 19628112]

[6]   Gomberg-Maitland M, Baran DA, Fuster V. Treatment of congestive heart failure: guidelines for the
       primary care physician and the heart failure specialist. Arch Intern Med 2001; 161(3): 342-52.
       [http://dx.doi.org/10.1001/archinte.161.3.342] [PMID: 11176759]

[7]   Virani SS, Alonso A, Benjamin EJ, *et al.* Heart Disease and Stroke Statistics—2020 Update: A Report
       From the American Heart Association. Circulation 2020; 141(9): e139-596.
       [http://dx.doi.org/10.1161/CIR.0000000000000757] [PMID: 31992061]

[8]   Metra M, Teerlink JR. Heart failure. Lancet 2017; 390(10106): 1981-95.
       [http://dx.doi.org/10.1016/S0140-6736(17)31071-1] [PMID: 28460827]

[9]   Boron WF, Boulpaep EL. Medical Physiology: A Cellular and Molecular Approach (Updated ed.).
       2005; p. 533.

[10]   Pitt B, Zannad F, Remme WJ, *et al.* The effect of spironolactone on morbidity and mortality in
       patients with severe heart failure. N Engl J Med 1999; 341(10): 709-17.
       [http://dx.doi.org/10.1056/NEJM199909023411001] [PMID: 10471456]

[11]   von Lueder TG, Atar D, Krum H, Krum H. Diuretic use in heart failure and outcomes. Clin Pharmacol
       Ther 2013; 94(4): 490-8.
       [http://dx.doi.org/10.1038/clpt.2013.140] [PMID: 23852396]

[12]   Follath F, Cleland JGF, Klein W, Murphy R. Etiology and response to drug treatment in heart failure. J
       Am Coll Cardiol 1998; 32(5): 1167-72.
       [http://dx.doi.org/10.1016/S0735-1097(98)00400-8] [PMID: 9809921]

[13]   Rapid Review Pathology. 4th ed., Philadelphia, PA: Saunders/Elsevier 2014.

[14]   National Institute for Health and Clinical Excellence. Clinical guideline 108: Chronic heart failure –
       Management of chronic heart failure in adults in primary and secondary care 2010.

[15]   Kotecha D, Manzano L, Krum H, *et al.* Effect of age and sex on efficacy and tolerability of β blockers
       in patients with heart failure with reduced ejection fraction: individual patient data meta-analysis. BMJ
       2016; 353: i1855.
       [http://dx.doi.org/10.1136/bmj.i1855] [PMID: 27098105]

[16]   Kotecha D, Holmes J, Krum H, *et al.* Efficacy of β blockers in patients with heart failure plus atrial
       fibrillation: an individual-patient data meta-analysis. Lancet 2014; 384(9961): 2235-43.
       [http://dx.doi.org/10.1016/S0140-6736(14)61373-8] [PMID: 25193873]

[17]   Abraham WT. Managing hyponatremia in heart failure. US Cardiology Review 2008; 5(1): 57-60.
       [http://dx.doi.org/10.15420/usc.2008.5.1.57]

[18]   Allen LA, O'Connor CM. Management of acute decompensated heart failure. CMAJ 2007; 176(6):
       797-805.
       [http://dx.doi.org/10.1503/cmaj.051620] [PMID: 17353535]

[19]   Man WDC, Chowdhury F, Taylor RS, *et al.* Building consensus for provision of breathlessness
       rehabilitation for patients with chronic obstructive pulmonary disease and chronic heart failure. Chron
       Respir Dis 2016; 13(3): 229-39.
       [http://dx.doi.org/10.1177/1479972316642363] [PMID: 27072018]

[20]   Prassas I, Diamandis EP. Novel therapeutic applications of cardiac glycosides. Nat Rev Drug Discov
       2008; 7(11): 926-35.
       [http://dx.doi.org/10.1038/nrd2682] [PMID: 18948999]

[21]   Radford DJ, Gillies AD, Hinds JA, Duffy P. Naturally occurring cardiac glycosides. Med J Aust 1986;
       144(10): 540-4.
       [http://dx.doi.org/10.5694/j.1326-5377.1986.tb112283.x] [PMID: 3086679]

[22]   Riganti C, Campia I, Kopecka J, *et al.* Pleiotropic effects of cardioactive glycosides. Curr Med Chem 2011; 18(6): 872-85.
[http://dx.doi.org/10.2174/092986711794927685] [PMID: 21182478]

[23]   Schönfeld W, Weiland J, Lindig C, *et al.* The lead structure in cardiac glycosides is 5 beta, 14 beta-androstane-3 beta 14-diol. Naunyn Schmiedebergs Arch Pharmacol 1985; 329(4): 414-26.
[http://dx.doi.org/10.1007/BF00496377] [PMID: 4033807]

[24]   Cheeke Peter R. Toxicants of plant origin. 1989.

[25]   Nagy M. 2017. https://www.intechopen.com/books/aromatic-and-medicinal-plants-back-to-nature/cardiac-glycosides-in-medicinal-plants
[http://dx.doi.org/10.5772/65963]

[26]   Botelho AFM, Pierezan F, Soto-Blanco B, Melo MM. A review of cardiac glycosides: Structure, toxicokinetics, clinical signs, diagnosis and antineoplastic potential. Toxicon 2019; 158: 63-8.
[http://dx.doi.org/10.1016/j.toxicon.2018.11.429] [PMID: 30529380]

[27]   Fundamentals of Pharmacology. Pearson Higher Education 2013.

[28]   Babula P, Masarik M, Adam V, Provaznik I, Kizek R. From Na+/K+-ATPase and cardiac glycosides to cytotoxicity and cancer treatment. Anticancer Agents Med Chem 2013; 13(7): 1069-87.
[http://dx.doi.org/10.2174/18715206113139990304] [PMID: 23537048]

[29]   CV Pharmacology, Cardiac Glycosides. Digitalis Compounds 2017.

[30]   Patel S. Plant-derived cardiac glycosides: Role in heart ailments and cancer management. Biomed Pharmacother 2016; 84: 1036-41.
[http://dx.doi.org/10.1016/j.biopha.2016.10.030] [PMID: 27780131]

[31]   Farnsworth NR. Biological and phytochemical screening of plants. J Pharm Sci 1966; 55(3): 225-76.
[http://dx.doi.org/10.1002/jps.2600550302] [PMID: 5335471]

[32]   Guyatt GH, Sullivan MJJ, Fallen EL, *et al.* A controlled trial of digoxin in congestive heart failure. Am J Cardiol 1988; 61(4): 371-5.
[http://dx.doi.org/10.1016/0002-9149(88)90947-2] [PMID: 3277366]

[33]   Cardiac Glycoside Plant Poisoning: Practice Essentials, Pathophysiology. Etiology 2017.

CHAPTER 3

Diet, Inflammation and Cardiovascular Disorders

M Kesavan[1,*] and **HV Manjunathachar[2,*]**

[1] *Division of Pharmacology and Toxicology, ICAR-Indian Veterinary Research Institute, Izatnagar, Bareilly, Uttar Pradesh-243 122, India*

[2] *ICMR- National Animal Resource Facility for Biomedical Research, Genome Valley, Hyderabad, Telangana-500101, India*

Abstract: Diet has been implicated in cardiovascular inflammation and the development of cardiovascular disorders. Several studies have correlated the dietary pattern with cardiovascular disease incidences. Especially high carbohydrate diet consists of refined starches, sugar, and saturated and trans-fatty acids shown to cause vascular inflammation and its related CVDs. To modify or prevent CVD complications, studies have highlighted and recommended a dietary pattern rich in protein and fibers with low carbohydrates. However, the long term effects of these low carbohydrate diets have not been analysed. Further, the diet consumed in Asian countries is rich in spices and they are loaded with antioxidants. Hence, this has to be reviewed thoroughly to conclude on the role of antioxidants in preventing CVDs. Therefore, in this chapter diet-induced inflammation, the role of low carbohydrate and high fat/protein diets in preventing vascular inflammation and their long term effects on health and the usefulness of antioxidants in preventing cardiovascular diseases will be reviewed elaborately.

Keywords: Antioxidants, Atherosclerosis, Dietary interventions, High Carbohydrate diet, Metabolic syndrome, Vascular inflammation.

1. INTRODUCTION

1.1. Diet Induced Inflammation

The Sedentary lifestyle and unhealthy diets of modern society lead to the increased incidence of cardiovascular diseases. Obesity, metabolic syndrome and type-2 diabetes mellitus is on the rise and predisposing for cardiovascular diseases predisposing factors for cardiovascular diseases [1]. Meal ingestion itself causes mild oxidative stress, which leads to the raise in the levels of circulatory

---

* Corresponding authors Kesavan M & Manjunathachar HV: Division of Pharmacology and Toxicology, ICAR-Indian Veterinary Research Institute, Izatnagar, Bareilly, Uttar Pradesh-243 122, India; & ICMR- National Animal Resource Facility for Biomedical Research, Genome Valley, Hyderabad, Telangana-500101, India; E-mails: kesu.kesavan@gmail.com & drmanju.icmr@hotmail.com

inflammatory mediators [2]. It is demonstrated that glucose intake promotes reactive oxygen species generation [3] and full fat meal with saturated fats activates endothelium. It is evident that post-prandial state abnormalities are the major contributing factors for cardiovascular diseases [1]. Although several studies have examined the pro-inflammatory effects of individual macronutrients, it is pertinent to note that all the ingredients of a diet should be considered to get an insight to the overall diet related inflammation. A study by O'Neil *et al*. [4] showed the positive correlation between pro-inflammaotry diet and CVDs development in Australian men. Further, saturated fatty acid intake alone did not predict the CVD events. Therefore, dietary inflammatory index scores can be useful for recommending the best-suited diet for CVD predisposed population.

1.2. Dietary Inflammatory Index (DII)

It is a quantitative measurement for assessing diet-associated inflammation, which was first introduced in 2009 and subsequently, several modifications and additions were made. Basically, it scores the inflammatory values of dietary ingredients and classifies them as pro-inflammatory or anti-inflammatory. DII scores are comparable with the Alternative Healthy Eating Index or Mediterranean Diet (MED) score and moderately correlated with the glycemic index score. However, a moderate negative correlation was observed between DII scores and Healthy Eating Index and Mediterranean Dietary Index. Albeit, updated DII is said to be superior to the other indices as it has considered different population and their diets and the experimental evidence [5]. Including a large population and their dietary patterns and experimental evidence of individual macro/micro nutrients showing pro/ anti-inflammatory effects will provide a robust DII.

Diets consisting of a high amount of saturated and trans unsaturated fatty acids like red meats, hydrogenated fats, refined oils and high glycemic index carbohydrates, has been positively associated with dietary inflammation, while diets based on fruits, vegetables, unsaturated fatty acids, fish, yoghurt, whole grains and wine tend to reduce cardiovascular inflammation. Micronutrients such as omega-3 fatty acids, vitamins B1 (thiamine), B2 (riboflavin), B3 (niacin), folic acid, vitamin A, vitamin C, vitamin E, beta-carotene, magnesium, and zinc are proven to be anti-inflammatory [6 - 8].

2. DIFFERENT PATTERNS OF DIET AND THEIR CHARACTERISTICS

Globally several diet patterns are being practiced. Among them, a few diet patterns are practiced especially for weight reduction, weight gain and prevention of lifestyle diseases. In Ayurveda, dietary plan is one of the principles being followed for treating diseases.

2.1. The Zone Diet

This diet consists of low carbohydrates with protein and fats. This has a fixed percentage of carbohydrates (40%), protein (30%) and fat (30%) in everyday meal. This diet plan is similar to our ancestor's diet where, meat, vegetables and fruits were their dietary sources [9]. The zone diet consists of carbohydrates from unrefined cereals and fats. As the major energy source in this diet is shifted from carbohydrates to fats, a better control of blood sugar and weight loss can be achieved. The zone diet also said to be anti-inflammatory and healthy insulin to glucagon ratio can be maintained. This eventually leads to a decline in chronic disease risk, immuno-competency, better physical and mental health, longevity and lifelong weight control [10].

2.2. Ketogenic Diet

The ketogenic diet is said to cure some medical conditions like Alzheimer's disease, cancer, polycystic ovary syndrome, epilepsy, *etc.*, However, it was initially prescribed for controlling diabetes. The ketogenic diet is distinct from the zone diet with its exceptionally high-fat content (70% to 80%), Generally, ketogenic diets consist of 70-80% fat, 5-10% carbohydrate and 10-20% protein [11]. Unsaturated fatty acids or healthy fats-rich foods like avocados, coconuts, brazil nuts, oil seeds, fish and olive oil are added as a part of the diet plan. This diet artificially creates a condition called ketosis. Wherein the absence of glucose for generating energy leads to the breakdown of fats and the formation of ketone bodies [12]. This diet plan can be used for reversing metabolic syndrome such as insulin resistance, high blood pressure, dyslipidemia. Along with this, weight loss can be achieved in a very short period time. Ketogenic diet and other low carbohydrate diets are being focused on controlling type 2 diabetes [13, 14].

2.3. Mediterranean Diet

The Mediterranean diet is being followed among the people of Crete, Greece, and southern Italy, which are the populations bordering the Mediterranean Sea. Further, this pattern of diet is also consumed in Spain, southern France, and Portugal. It is primarily plant-based diet that includes whole grains, olive oil, fruits, vegetables, beans, legumes, nuts, herbs, and spices in their regular meal. In 1993, the Harvard School of Public Health, Old ways Preservation and Exchange

Trust, and the European Office of the World Health Organization introduced the "Mediterranean Diet Pyramid" for familiarizing the Mediterranean diet using commonly available foods of the region. The diet is characterized by nine dietary components according to the levels of consumption [15, 16]. It was believed that the diet with whole grains, fishes, beans, nuts, fruits and vegetables, olive oil, with a small amount of dairy foods (cheese and yoghurt) and red wine were contributed to the health benefits observed in Mediterranean Diet. Up to one-third portion of the Mediterranean diet meal consists of fat, with saturated fats not exceeding 8% of calorie intake [17]. Several studies have shown the effectiveness of the Mediterranean diet in reducing the risk of cardiovascular diseases and overall mortality [18]. A study by Ahmad *et al.* [19] conducted on nearly 26,000 women who followed this type of diet pattern over the span of 12 years showed that they had 25% less risk of developing cardiovascular diseases. Overall, the mediterranean diet is believed to be a healthy eating pattern for the prevention of cardiovascular diseases, increasing lifespan, and healthy aging. When used in conjunction with caloric restriction, the diet may also support healthy weight loss [18, 20, 21].

2.4. DASH (Dietary Approaches to Stop Hypertension) Diet

The DASH diet pattern was first introduced by American Heart Association in 1996 for the prevention of hypertension. The DASH diet meal consists of fruits, vegetables, whole grains, nuts and low-fat dairy foods with reduced amounts of saturated fat, total fat, cholesterol with restrictions on sodium, added sugars and red meat. This diet differs from other diets as it limits the fat content of the daily meal and promotes increasing the intake of potassium, magnesium, calcium, protein, and fiber, nutrients believed to help control blood pressure [22, 23]. Numerous studies show wide-ranging health benefits of the DASH diet to lower blood pressure, and preventing or reducing the risk of cardiovascular diseases, diabetes, kidney disease and gout [23, 24].

2.5. The Paleo Diet

Paleolithic diet, also called as caveman or stone-age diet, recommends eating more lean meat, fish, eggs, fats, fruits, vegetables, nuts, and seeds and does not allow to have refined carbohydrates, sugar, processed foods, potatoes and legumes. Paleo diet supporters say our genetics and anatomy haven't changed from Paleolithic hunter gatherers for adopting cereals-based diet. The diet mainly emphasizes low-glycemic fruits and vegetables. Overall, the diet is high in protein and fibre, moderate in fat (mainly from unsaturated fats) and low-moderate in carbohydrates (specifically restricting high glycemic index carbohydrates [25,

26]. The Paleo diet provides 30% of total calories from protein, 40% from fat and 30% from carbohydrates. Several clinical studies have shown that the Paleo diet produces greater benefits in a short period, such as weight reduction, reduction in waist circumference, decreased blood pressure, cholesterol and increased insulin sensitivity. Some researchers are also concerned about high protein contents, which may harm kidneys [27, 28].

2.6. Vegan and Vegetarian Diet

Vegan or plant-based diet is devoid of animal source foods and doesn't allow eggs (ovo) and dairy (lacto) products. However, in vegetarian diet, dairy products and eggs are consumed. Veganism is being followed for environmental, ethical, and compassionate reasons. Research suggests that the vegan diet can improve heart health, protect against cancer, and lower the risk of type 2 diabetes [29, 30]. Many people choose vegetarian diet for ethical reasons, as well as for maintaining good health. There are various types of vegetarianism: lacto-vegetarian, fruitarian vegetarian, ovo-vegetarian, lacto-ovo vegetarian, living food diet vegetarian, pesco-vegetarian, and semi-vegetarian. The majority of vegetarians are lacto-ovo vegetarians; in other words, they do not eat animal source foods, except for eggs, dairy, and honey. The proclaimed benefits of vegetarian diet are body weight control, less suffering from diseases and longer life expectancy. Generally, diets higher in plant foods and lower in animal foods with restricted calories were associated with a lower risk of cardiovascular morbidity and mortality in the general population [31, 32].

3. CARDIOVASCULAR DISEASES (CVD), PRO AND ANTI-INFLAMMATORY AGENTS

Cardiovascular diseases are a broad term that denotes the atherosclerotic conditions of the heart and blood vessels [33]. Atherosclerosis is the hardening of arteries due to the deposition of fat, cholesterol, calcium and other substances of blood in the tunica intima of arteries [34]. Atherosclerosis is a chronic inflammatory condition that is the underlying factor of cardiovascular diseases. Both blood vessel walls and the immune system are implicated in atherogenesis. Plasma lipoproteins, genetics and the hemodynamics of the blood flow in the artery all play important roles in the development of atherosclerosis (Fig. **1**). It is now considered a chronic inflammatory disease, with reactive oxygen species and oxidized lipoprotein particles implicated in pathogenesis and progression. It is classically believed that insults to endothelial integrity promote deposition of low density lipoprotein particles (LDL), and macrophage-dependent formation of oxidized low-density lipoprotein (oxLDL) within vascular tissues [35]. However,

CVD-promoting conditions, including obesity are associated with elevated circulating levels of oxLDL, and bioactive metabolites preformed in these particles may promote their atherogenicity [36]. Regardless, these materials trigger the activation of innate and adaptive immune responses and lead to the secretion of proatherogenic cytokines and immune cells migrations, which eventually lead to the development of atheromatous plaque [35, 37].

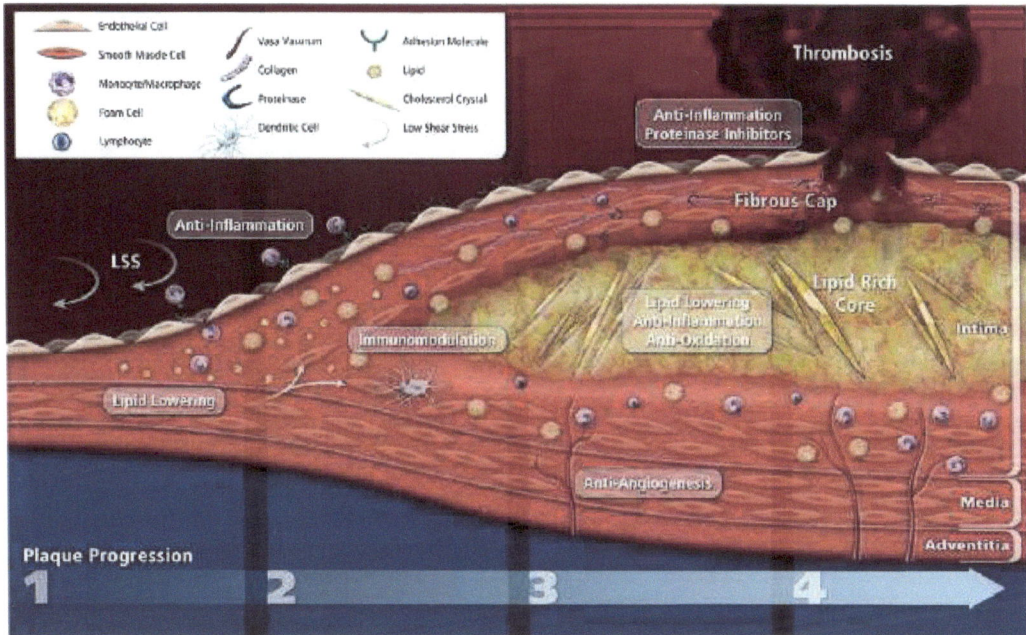

Fig. (1). Atherosclerotic plaque progression and impact of anti-inflammatory agents [39].

This disease is considered to have a multi-factorial origin, with many risk factors associated with the metabolic syndrome, including pro-atherogenic dyslipidemia, elevated blood pressure, insulin resistance with elevated blood glucose, chronic inflammation and a pro-thrombotic state. Pro-inflammatory lipoproteins are associated with arterial wall inflammation [38].

Overweight and obesity are associated with metabolic syndrome which is mediated by insulin resistance. Adipose tissue secretes several signaling molecules referred as adipokines, are involved in inflammation. In obesity, a number of mature adipocytes increase, which in turn, secrete more adipokines, inducing inflammation (Fig. **2**). Their role in inflammation can be reconfirmed by the reduction of inflammatory cytokines/markers during weight loss. Eating macronutrients with high glycemic index results in high insulinemia and ROS formation and results in inflammation. Foods containing saturated and Trans fatty acids have shown to increase inflammatory cytokines [40]. Accumulation of macrophages in matured adipose tissues secretes variety of inflammatory cytokines, which causes insulin resistance in obesity. However, acute fat overload also causes insulin resistance independent of inflammation by a process called lipotoxicity [41].

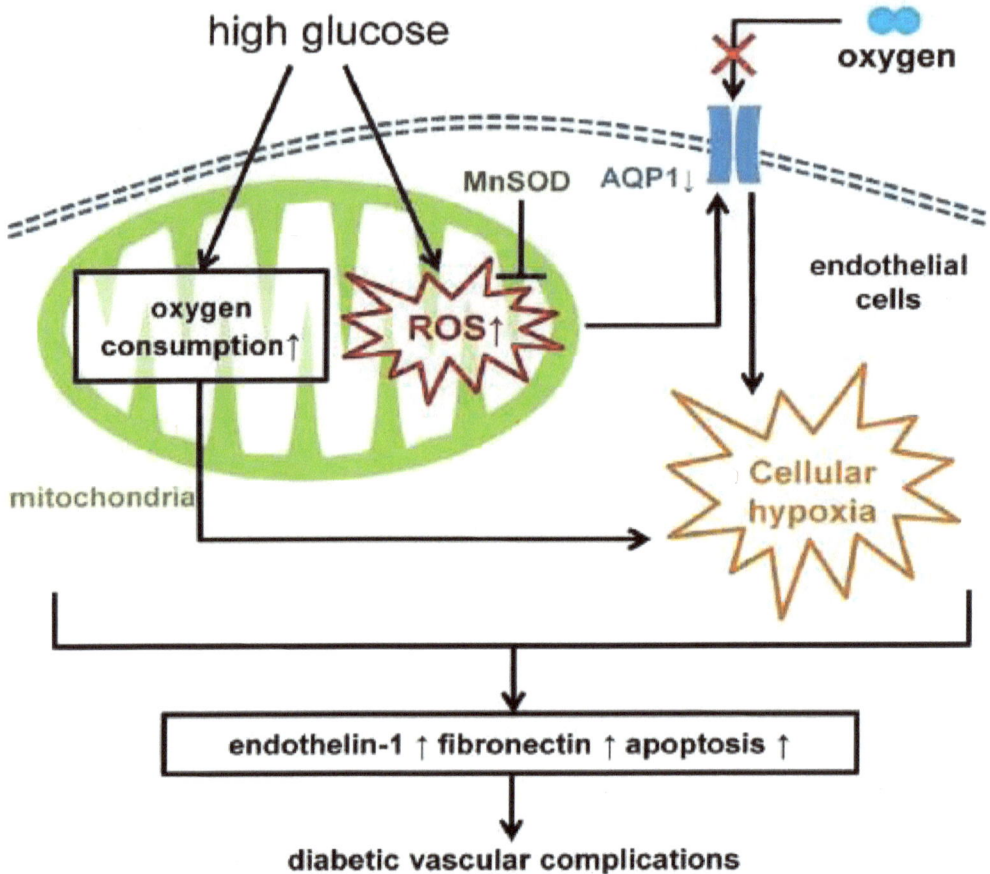

Fig. (2). Model of the diabetic pathogenesis and its complications [42].

Recently, low carbohydrate (ketogenic) diets have been prescribed for faster weight loss, Type-II diabetes mellitus, non-alcoholic fatty liver disease and autoimmune disorders. Low carb diet is said to be offering more benefits like increased insulin sensitivity, faster weight loss, increased immune function, reduced migration of pro-inflammatory macrophages in visceral adipose tissues, reduction in inflammatory mediators, correcting dyslipidemia and hypertension [43 - 46]. It is also shown to be beneficial in cancer and neurodegenerative disorders [47]. However, few studies also showed ineffectiveness of ketogenic diets in reducing inflammation and insulin resistance and correcting dyslipidemia

[48, 49]. However, low carbohydrate diets have proven effective in the short term, there is a requirement to study the long term effects of low carbohydrate diets and a large population-based clinical trials are to confirm the beneficial effects of these diets.

Inflammatory and oxidative stress can rise due to an unbalanced dietary life style and consumption of high fat and high carbohydrate meals [50]. Increase in postprandial lipopolysaccharide (LPS) and Toll-like receptor-4 (TLR4) is directly associated with the up-regulation of inflammatory cytokines levels, and they activate oxidative burst [51]. Given these premises, the importance of the diet, as inducer or preventer of inflammatory and oxidative stress, is paramount.

4. SPICES

For ages, in various cultures worldwide, spices and herbs have been considered as an integral part of the diet. The wide array of phytochemicals present in them exerts antioxidant and anti-inflammatory mechanisms. Spices and herbs were widely traded items in the ancient era between the continents. Herbalist, traditional practitioners and folk practitioners have used plant and their products as remedies for centuries. In Indian systems of medicine and Chinese medicine, herbs including spices, are being used for treating various ailments. However, only in the last few decades, scientific studies have begun to identify the active components and their role in disease prevention. The anti-proliferative, anti-diabetic, anti-inflammatory, anti-hypercholesterolemic effects of spices are of greater importance, as the key health concern of mankind nowadays is cardio-vascular diseases, diabetes, arthritis and cancer. The list of spices and herbs used against several diseases were listed along with up-regulation or down-regulation of anti-inflammatory agents (Table **1**). Several spices are loaded with antioxidants and scientific evidences suggest that antioxidants are potent inhibitors of tissue damage and inflammation caused by oxidative stress due to high levels of blood sugar and circulating lipids. Spices have very low calorie content and they are reliable sources of antioxidants and other potential bioactive compounds in the diet. Spices or their active compounds could be used as ameliorative or preventive agents for these health disorders.

Table 1. List of spices and herbs used against many diseases and their response.

Compound	Disease Condition	Markers of Oxidative Status	Markers of Inflammatory Status	References
Green tea (Beverage)	Obese	IsoP ↓	CRP and IL6 ↔	[52]
Green tea extract (capsule)	Obese, hypertensive patients	NEAC ↑	TNF-α ↓ CRP ↓	[53]
Green tea extract (capsule)	Chronic dialysis	oxLDL ↓	P22phox ↓	[54]
Green tea extract (Tablets)	Haemodialysis patients	peroxides ↓	IL-8 and TNF-α receptor↓ CRP and TNF-α ↓	[55]
Curcuminoids (capsules)	Undergoing coronary artery bypass grafting	MDA↓	CRP↓	[56]
Turmeric (capsules)	Type 2 diabetes on metformin therapy	NEAC ↑ MDA↓ GSH, GPX, CAT and carbonyls ↔	CRP↓	[57]
Turmeric (capsules)	Overweight and obese women	IsoP and oxLDL↔	CRP, IL-6, IL-8 and TNF-α ↔	[58]
Ginger (capsule)	Peritoneal dialysis	MDA↔	CRP↔	[59]
Ginger (capsules)	Type 2 diabetes	NEAC↑ MDA↓	CRP↓	[60]
Curcuminoids + piperine (capsules)	Metabolic syndrome	SOD↑ MDA↓	CRP↓	[61]
Powder containing green tea extract (1g) + vitamin C and E	Cancer patients	NEAC ↑ IsoP↔	CRP ↔	[62]

CAT: catalase; CRP: C reactive protein; GPX: glutathione peroxidase; GSH: reduced glutathione; IL: interleukin; IsoP: isoprostanes; MDA: malondialdehyde; MPO: myeloperoxidase; NEAC: non-enzymatic antioxidant capacity; oxLDL: oxidized low density lipoproteins; SOD: superoxide dismutase; TNF--α: tumor necrosis factor alfa, CRP: C reactive protein; EGCG: epigallocatechingallate; IL: interleukin; IsoP: isoprostanes; oxLDL: oxidized low density lipoproteins; TBARS: thiobarbituric acid reactive substances; GPX: glutathione peroxidase; MDA: malondialdehyde; MPO: myeloperoxidase;

Many researchers have shown the potential use of spices and herbs against diseases or conditions as antibacterial, antispasmodic, antioxidant, antiseptic, and carminative agent. Studies have also explored the role of spices in controlling the blood sugar in type 2 diabetes, cancer, cardiovascular, hypertension, and AIDS.

Spices, as a part of daily dietary ingredient can provide several beneficial effects. In addition to these, spices are bestowed with immense medicinal potential. Several clinical as well as preclinical studies reported the effectiveness of various spices as a whole for different ailments.

CONCLUSION

Immune-boosting properties, along with the excellent safety profile, are making spices as the current choice of Phytochemical-research as well as the home remedies. Hence, finding their functional ingredients of spices and understanding their mechanism of actions can provide a better therapeutics beyond their culinary uses.

CONSENT FOR PUBLICATION

Not applicable.

CONFLICT OF INTEREST

The author declares no conflict of interest, financial or otherwise.

ACKNOWLEDGEMENTS

Declared none.

REFERENCES

[1]   Esposito K, Giugliano D. Diet and inflammation: a link to metabolic and cardiovascular diseases. Eur Heart J 2006; 27(1): 15-20.
[http://dx.doi.org/10.1093/eurheartj/ehi605] [PMID: 16219650]

[2]   Bowen PE, Borthakur G. Postprandial lipid oxidation and cardiovascular disease risk. Curr Atheroscler Rep 2004; 6(6): 477-84.
[http://dx.doi.org/10.1007/s11883-004-0089-3] [PMID: 15485594]

[3]   Dandona P, Aljada A, Chaudhuri A, Mohanty P, Garg R. Metabolic Syndrome. Circulation 2005; 111(11): 1448-54.
[http://dx.doi.org/10.1161/01.CIR.0000158483.13093.9D] [PMID: 15781756]

[4]   O'Neil A, Shivappa N, Jacka FN, *et al.* Pro-inflammatory dietary intake as a risk factor for CVD in men: a 5-year longitudinal study. Br J Nutr 2015; 114(12): 2074-82.
[http://dx.doi.org/10.1017/S0007114515003815] [PMID: 26450630]

[5]   Hébert JR, Shivappa N, Wirth MD, Hussey JR, Hurley TG. Perspective: The Dietary Inflammatory Index (DII)—Lessons Learned, Improvements Made, and Future Directions. Adv Nutr 2019; 10(2): 185-95.
[http://dx.doi.org/10.1093/advances/nmy071] [PMID: 30615051]

[6]   Basu A, Devaraj S, Jialal I. Dietary factors that promote or retard inflammation. Arterioscler Thromb Vasc Biol 2006; 26(5): 995-1001.
[http://dx.doi.org/10.1161/01.ATV.0000214295.86079.d1] [PMID: 16484595]

[7]   Remig V, Franklin B, Margolis S, Kostas G, Nece T, Street JC. Trans fats in America: a review of

their use, consumption, health implications, and regulation. J Am Diet Assoc 2010; 110(4): 585-92.
[http://dx.doi.org/10.1016/j.jada.2009.12.024] [PMID: 20338284]

[8] Camargo-Ramos C, Correa-Bautista J, Correa-Rodríguez M, Ramírez-Vélez R. Dietary Inflammatory Index and Cardiometabolic Risk Parameters in Overweight and Sedentary Subjects. Int J Environ Res Public Health 2017; 14(10): 1104.
[http://dx.doi.org/10.3390/ijerph14101104] [PMID: 28984835]

[9] Gardner CD, Kiazand A, Alhassan S, *et al.* Comparison of the Atkins, Zone, Ornish, and LEARN diets for change in weight and related risk factors among overweight premenopausal women: the A TO Z Weight Loss Study: a randomized trial. JAMA 2007; 297(9): 969-77.
[http://dx.doi.org/10.1001/jama.297.9.969] [PMID: 17341711]

[10] Cheuvront SN. The Zone Diet phenomenon: a closer look at the science behind the claims. J Am Coll Nutr 2003; 22(1): 9-17.
[http://dx.doi.org/10.1080/07315724.2003.10719271] [PMID: 12569110]

[11] Schwingshackl L, Hoffmann G. Comparison of effects of long-term low-fat *vs* high-fat diets on blood lipid levels in overweight or obese patients: a systematic review and meta-analysis. J Acad Nutr Diet 2013; 113(12): 1640-61.
[http://dx.doi.org/10.1016/j.jand.2013.07.010] [PMID: 24139973]

[12] Kalra S, Gupta L, Khandelwal D, Gupta P, Dutta D, Aggarwal S. Ketogenic diet in endocrine disorders: Current perspectives. J Postgrad Med 2017; 63(4): 242-51.
[http://dx.doi.org/10.4103/jpgm.JPGM_16_17] [PMID: 29022562]

[13] Paoli A. Ketogenic diet for obesity: friend or foe? Int J Environ Res Public Health 2014; 11(2): 2092-107.
[http://dx.doi.org/10.3390/ijerph110202092] [PMID: 24557522]

[14] Abbasi J. Interest in the Ketogenic Diet Grows for Weight Loss and Type 2 Diabetes. JAMA 2018; 319(3): 215-7.
[http://dx.doi.org/10.1001/jama.2017.20639] [PMID: 29340675]

[15] Willett WC, Sacks F, Trichopoulou A, *et al.* Mediterranean diet pyramid: a cultural model for healthy eating. Am J Clin Nutr 1995; 61(6) (Suppl.): 1402S-6S.
[http://dx.doi.org/10.1093/ajcn/61.6.1402S] [PMID: 7754995]

[16] Gifford KD. Dietary fats, eating guides, and public policy: history, critique, and recommendations. Am J Med 2002; 113(9) (Suppl. 9B): 89-106.
[http://dx.doi.org/10.1016/S0002-9343(01)00996-2] [PMID: 12566143]

[17] Fung TT, Rexrode KM, Mantzoros CS, Manson JE, Willett WC, Hu FB. Mediterranean diet and incidence of and mortality from coronary heart disease and stroke in women. Circulation 2009; 119(8): 1093-100.
[http://dx.doi.org/10.1161/CIRCULATIONAHA.108.816736] [PMID: 19221219]

[18] Lopez-Garcia E, Rodriguez-Artalejo F, Li TY, *et al.* The Mediterranean-style dietary pattern and mortality among men and women with cardiovascular disease. Am J Clin Nutr 2014; 99(1): 172-80.
[http://dx.doi.org/10.3945/ajcn.113.068106] [PMID: 24172306]

[19] Ahmad S, Moorthy MV, Demler OV, *et al.* Assessment of Risk Factors and Biomarkers Associated With Risk of Cardiovascular Disease Among Women Consuming a Mediterranean Diet. JAMA Netw Open 2018; 1(8): e185708.
[http://dx.doi.org/10.1001/jamanetworkopen.2018.5708] [PMID: 30646282]

[20] Loughrey DG, Lavecchia S, Brennan S, Lawlor BA, Kelly ME. The impact of the Mediterranean diet on the cognitive functioning of healthy older adults: a systematic review and meta-analysis. Adv Nutr 2017; 8(4): 571-86.
[PMID: 28710144]

[21] Correia LCL. Primary Prevention of Cardiovascular Disease with a Mediterranean Diet Supplemented

with Extra-Virgin Olive Oil or Nuts. N Engl J Med 2018; 379(14): 1387-9.
[http://dx.doi.org/10.1056/NEJMc1809971] [PMID: 30285331]

[22]   Appel LJ, Moore TJ, Obarzanek E, *et al.* A clinical trial of the effects of dietary patterns on blood pressure. N Engl J Med 1997; 336(16): 1117-24.
[http://dx.doi.org/10.1056/NEJM199704173361601] [PMID: 9099655]

[23]   Saneei P, Salehi-Abargouei A, Esmaillzadeh A, Azadbakht L. Influence of Dietary Approaches to Stop Hypertension (DASH) diet on blood pressure: A systematic review and meta-analysis on randomized controlled trials. Nutr Metab Cardiovasc Dis 2014; 24(12): 1253-61.
[http://dx.doi.org/10.1016/j.numecd.2014.06.008] [PMID: 25149893]

[24]   Rai SK, Fung TT, Lu N, Keller SF, Curhan GC, Choi HK. The Dietary Approaches to Stop Hypertension (DASH) diet, Western diet, and risk of gout in men: prospective cohort study. BMJ 2017; 357: j1794.
[http://dx.doi.org/10.1136/bmj.j1794] [PMID: 28487277]

[25]   Chang ML, Nowell A. How to make stone soup: Is the "Paleo diet" a missed opportunity for anthropologists? Evol Anthropol 2016; 25(5): 228-31.
[http://dx.doi.org/10.1002/evan.21504] [PMID: 27753214]

[26]   Tarantino G, Citro V, Finelli C. Hype or reality: should patients with metabolic syndrome-related NAFLD be on the hunter-gatherer (Paleo) diet to decrease morbidity. J Gastrointestin Liver Dis 2015; 24(3): 359-68.
[http://dx.doi.org/10.15403/jgld.2014.1121.243.gta] [PMID: 26405708]

[27]   Masharani U, Sherchan P, Schloetter M, *et al.* Metabolic and physiologic effects from consuming a hunter-gatherer (Paleolithic)-type diet in type 2 diabetes. Eur J Clin Nutr 2015; 69(8): 944-8.
[http://dx.doi.org/10.1038/ejcn.2015.39] [PMID: 25828624]

[28]   Obert J, Pearlman M, Obert L, Chapin S. Popular weight loss strategies: a review of four weight loss techniques. Curr Gastroenterol Rep 2017; 19(12): 61.
[http://dx.doi.org/10.1007/s11894-017-0603-8] [PMID: 29124370]

[29]   Heiss S, Coffino JA, Hormes JM. Eating and health behaviors in vegans compared to omnivores: Dispelling common myths. Appetite 2017; 118: 129-35.
[http://dx.doi.org/10.1016/j.appet.2017.08.001] [PMID: 28780065]

[30]   Kim H, Caulfield LE, Garcia-Larsen V, Steffen LM, Coresh J, Rebholz CM. Plant-Based diets are associated with a lower risk of incident cardiovascular disease, cardiovascular disease mortality, and All-Cause mortality in a general population of Middle-Aged adults. J Am Heart Assoc 2019; 8(16): e012865.
[http://dx.doi.org/10.1161/JAHA.119.012865] [PMID: 31387433]

[31]   Tonstad S, Butler T, Yan R, Fraser GE. Type of vegetarian diet, body weight, and prevalence of type 2 diabetes. Diabetes Care 2009; 32(5): 791-6.
[http://dx.doi.org/10.2337/dc08-1886] [PMID: 19351712]

[32]   Dinu M, Abbate R, Gensini GF, Casini A, Sofi F. Vegetarian, vegan diets and multiple health outcomes: A systematic review with meta-analysis of observational studies. Crit Rev Food Sci Nutr 2017; 57(17): 3640-9.
[http://dx.doi.org/10.1080/10408398.2016.1138447] [PMID: 26853923]

[33]   Bibbins-Domingo K, Grossman DC, Curry SJ, *et al.* Statin use for the primary prevention of cardiovascular disease in adults. us preventive services task force recommendation. JAMA 2016; 316(19): 1997-2007.
[http://dx.doi.org/10.1001/jama.2016.15450] [PMID: 27838723]

[34]   Rafieian-Kopaei M, Setorki M, Doudi M, Baradaran A, Nasri H. Atherosclerosis: process, indicators, risk factors and new hopes. Int J Prev Med 2014; 5(8): 927-46.
[PMID: 25489440]

[35]   Kattoor AJ, Pothineni NVK, Palagiri D, Mehta JL. Oxidative Stress in Atherosclerosis. Curr Atheroscler Rep 2017; 19(11): 42.
[http://dx.doi.org/10.1007/s11883-017-0678-6] [PMID: 28921056]

[36]   Rajamani A, Borkowski K, Akre S, *et al.* Oxylipins in triglyceride-rich lipoproteins of dyslipidemic subjects promote endothelial inflammation following a high fat meal. Sci Rep 2019; 9(1): 8655.
[http://dx.doi.org/10.1038/s41598-019-45005-5] [PMID: 31209255]

[37]   Taleb S. Inflammation in atherosclerosis. Arch Cardiovasc Dis 2016; 109(12): 708-15.
[http://dx.doi.org/10.1016/j.acvd.2016.04.002] [PMID: 27595467]

[38]   MGrundy S. Genetics, obesity, and the metabolic syndrome: The Professor Donald S. Fredrickson Memorial Lecture. Int Congr Ser 2004; 1262: 19-24.

[39]   Quillard T, Libby P. Molecular imaging of atherosclerosis for improving diagnostic and therapeutic development. Circ Res 2012; 111(2): 231-44.
[http://dx.doi.org/10.1161/CIRCRESAHA.112.268144] [PMID: 22773426]

[40]   Bulló M, Casas-Agustench P, Amigó-Correig P, Aranceta J, Salas-Salvadó J. Inflammation, obesity and comorbidities: the role of diet. Public Health Nutr 2007; 10(10A): 1164-72.
[http://dx.doi.org/10.1017/S1368980007000663] [PMID: 17903326]

[41]   Lee YS, Li P, Huh JY, *et al.* Inflammation is necessary for long-term but not short-term high-fat diet-induced insulin resistance. Diabetes 2011; 60(10): 2474-83.
[http://dx.doi.org/10.2337/db11-0194] [PMID: 21911747]

[42]   Sada K, Nishikawa T, Kukidome D, *et al.* Hyperglycemia induces cellular hypoxia through production of mitochondrial ROS followed by suppression of aquaporin-1. PLoS One 2016; 11(7): e0158619.
[http://dx.doi.org/10.1371/journal.pone.0158619] [PMID: 27383386]

[43]   Kosinski C, Jornayvaz F. Effects of Ketogenic Diets on Cardiovascular Risk Factors: Evidence from Animal and Human Studies. Nutrients 2017; 9(5): 517.
[http://dx.doi.org/10.3390/nu9050517] [PMID: 28534852]

[44]   Patel S, Suleria HAR. Ethnic and paleolithic diet: Where do they stand in inflammation alleviation? A discussion. Journal of Ethnic Foods 2017; 4(4): 236-41.
[http://dx.doi.org/10.1016/j.jef.2017.10.004]

[45]   Monda V, Polito R, Lovino A, *et al.* Short-Term Physiological Effects of a Very Low-Calorie Ketogenic Diet: Effects on Adiponectin Levels and Inflammatory States. Int J Mol Sci 2020; 21(9): 3228.
[http://dx.doi.org/10.3390/ijms21093228] [PMID: 32370212]

[46]   Stubbs BJ, Newman JC. Ketogenic diet and adipose tissue inflammation—a simple story? Fat chance! Nat Metab 2020; 2(1): 3-4.
[http://dx.doi.org/10.1038/s42255-019-0164-2] [PMID: 32694682]

[47]   Ludwig DS. The Ketogenic Diet: Evidence for Optimism but High-Quality Research Needed. J Nutr 2020; 150(6): 1354-9.
[http://dx.doi.org/10.1093/jn/nxz308] [PMID: 31825066]

[48]   Coppola G, Natale F, Torino A, *et al.* The impact of the ketogenic diet on arterial morphology and endothelial function in children and young adults with epilepsy: A case–control study. Seizure 2014; 23(4): 260-5.
[http://dx.doi.org/10.1016/j.seizure.2013.12.002] [PMID: 24380692]

[49]   Rosenbaum M, Hall KD, Guo J, *et al.* Glucose and Lipid Homeostasis and Inflammation in Humans Following an Isocaloric Ketogenic Diet. Obesity (Silver Spring) 2019; 27(6): 971-81.
[http://dx.doi.org/10.1002/oby.22468] [PMID: 31067015]

[50]   Serafini M, Peluso I. Functional foods for health: the interrelated antioxidant and anti-inflammatory role of fruits, vegetables, herbs, spices and cocoa in humans. Curr Pharm Des 2017; 22(44): 6701-15.

[http://dx.doi.org/10.2174/1381612823666161123094235] [PMID: 27881064]

[51]   Deopurkar R, Ghanim H, Friedman J, *et al.* Differential effects of cream, glucose, and orange juice on inflammation, endotoxin, and the expression of Toll-like receptor-4 and suppressor of cytokine signaling-3. Diabetes Care 2010; 33(5): 991-7.
[http://dx.doi.org/10.2337/dc09-1630] [PMID: 20067961]

[52]   Stote KS, Clevidence BA, Novotny JA, Henderson T, Radecki SV, Baer DJ. Effect of cocoa and green tea on biomarkers of glucose regulation, oxidative stress, inflammation and hemostasis in obese adults at risk for insulin resistance. Eur J Clin Nutr 2012; 66(10): 1153-9.
[http://dx.doi.org/10.1038/ejcn.2012.101] [PMID: 22854880]

[53]   Bogdanski P, Suliburska J, Szulinska M, Stepien M, Pupek-Musialik D, Jablecka A. Green tea extract reduces blood pressure, inflammatory biomarkers, and oxidative stress and improves parameters associated with insulin resistance in obese, hypertensive patients. Nutr Res 2012; 32(6): 421-7.
[http://dx.doi.org/10.1016/j.nutres.2012.05.007] [PMID: 22749178]

[54]   Calo LA, Vertolli U, Davis PA, *et al.* Molecular biology based assessment of green tea effects on oxidative stress and cardiac remodelling in dialysis patients. Clin Nutr 2014; 33(3): 437-42.
[http://dx.doi.org/10.1016/j.clnu.2013.06.010] [PMID: 23845383]

[55]   Hsu SP, Wu MS, Yang CC, *et al.* Chronic green tea extract supplementation reduces hemodialysis-enhanced production of hydrogen peroxide and hypochlorous acid, atherosclerotic factors, and proinflammatory cytokines. Am J Clin Nutr 2007; 86(5): 1539-47.
[http://dx.doi.org/10.1093/ajcn/86.5.1539] [PMID: 17991670]

[56]   Wongcharoen W, Jai-aue S, Phrommintikul A, *et al.* Effects of curcuminoids on frequency of acute myocardial infarction after coronary artery bypass grafting. Am J Cardiol 2012; 110(1): 40-4.
[http://dx.doi.org/10.1016/j.amjcard.2012.02.043] [PMID: 22481014]

[57]   Maithili Karpaga Selvi N, Sridhar MG, Swaminathan RP, Sripradha R. Efficacy of turmeric as adjuvant therapy in type 2 diabetic patients. Indian J Clin Biochem 2015; 30(2): 180-6.
[http://dx.doi.org/10.1007/s12291-014-0436-2] [PMID: 25883426]

[58]   Nieman DC, Cialdella-Kam L, Knab AM, Shanely RA. Influence of red pepper spice and turmeric on inflammation and oxidative stress biomarkers in overweight females: a metabolomics approach. Plant Foods Hum Nutr 2012; 67(4): 415-21.
[http://dx.doi.org/10.1007/s11130-012-0325-x] [PMID: 23150126]

[59]   Imani H, Tabibi H, Najafi I, Atabak S, Hedayati M, Rahmani L. Effects of ginger on serum glucose, advanced glycation end products, and inflammation in peritoneal dialysis patients. Nutrition 2015; 31(5): 703-7.
[http://dx.doi.org/10.1016/j.nut.2014.11.020] [PMID: 25837216]

[60]   Shidfar F, Rajab A, Rahideh T, Khandouzi N, Hosseini S, Shidfar S. The effect of ginger (Zingiber officinale) on glycemic markers in patients with type 2 diabetes. J Complement Integr Med 2015; 12(2): 165-70.
[http://dx.doi.org/10.1515/jcim-2014-0021] [PMID: 25719344]

[61]   Panahi Y, Hosseini MS, Khalili N, Naimi E, Majeed M, Sahebkar A. Antioxidant and anti-inflammatory effects of curcuminoid-piperine combination in subjects with metabolic syndrome: A randomized controlled trial and an updated meta-analysis. Clin Nutr 2015; 34(6): 1101-8.
[http://dx.doi.org/10.1016/j.clnu.2014.12.019] [PMID: 25618800]

[62]   Braga M, Bissolati M, Rocchetti S, Beneduce A, Pecorelli N, Di Carlo V. Oral preoperative antioxidants in pancreatic surgery: A double-blind, randomized, clinical trial. Nutrition 2012; 28(2): 160-4.
[http://dx.doi.org/10.1016/j.nut.2011.05.014] [PMID: 21890323]

CHAPTER 4

Rodent and Non-Rodent Animal Models for CardioVascular Diseases

Irfan Ahmad Mir[1,*], **HV Manjunathachar**[1,*], **R Ravindar Naik**[1], **SSYH Qadri**[2] and **Taniya Saleem**[3]

[1] *ICMR-National Animal Resource Facility for Biomedical Research, Genome Valley, Shamirpet, Hyderabad, 500101, India*

[2] *ICMR-National Institute of Nutrition, Jamai-Osmania PO, Hyderabad-500007, India*

[3] *Department of Veterinary Parasitology, SKUAST-Jammu, India*

Abstract: Cardiovascular diseases (CVD) come under non-communicable disease (NCD) that are responsible for the leading cause of death, globally. They involve a range of pathologies *viz.* coronary artery disease, cerebro-vascular disease, venous thrombo-embolism, peripheral vascular disease, myocardial infarction, cardiac arrhythmias and stroke. Each pathology is the result of the complex interplay of many factors which determine the prognosis of the condition. Animal experimentation has played an important role in the fundamental understanding of pathologies of cardiac diseases and discovered improved methods of diagnosis and treatment. Researchers have used a number of lab animals that involve rodents (mice, rats, hamsters, and rabbits) and non-rodent animal models (dogs, pigs, sheep, primates) as a biological system to mimic cardiovascular diseases for translational research. An ideal animal-model system should be cheap, readily manipulable, reproducible, ethically sound and reflect the complexity of cardiovascular diseases. Rodent animal models are considered the prime model for human research. Common rodent models include mice, rats and hamsters; rabbits are used for studies on cardiac hypertrophy, heart failure, aortic constriction, pulmonary vein constriction, atherosclerosis and cholesterol regulation studies. With the advancement in genetic engineering, several transgenic/humanized rodent models are available which can mimic better human systems for translational application. Among non-rodent animal models, pigs, dogs, sheep, and non-human primates serve as an excellent model in cardiovascular research; owing to the similarity in heart structure, atrio-ventricular valves, lipid metabolism and vasculature with humans. In the current chapter, we will deal with the importance of the models and their characteristic features, advantages and limitations.

Keywords: Animal Models, Cardio-vascular Diseases, Non-Rodents, Rodents.

* **Corresponding authors Irfan Ahmad Mir & HV Manjunathachar:** ICMR-National Animal Resource Facility for Biomedical Research, Genome Valley, Shamirpet, Hyderabad, 500101, India; E-mails: mirirfan441@gmail.com & drmanju.icmr@hotmail.com
# These authors have equal contribution.

Dr. V. V. Sathibabu Uddandrao & Dr. Parim Brahma Naidu (Eds.)

1. RODENT MODELS FOR CVD

Cardiovascular diseases (CVDs) are the leading principal cause of death and morbidity, globally. CVDs are a group of disorders of the heart and blood vessels that include coronary heart disease, cerebro-vascular disease, rheumatic heart disease, and other conditions. About 17.9 million people die annually (approximately 31%) due to CVDs. More than three-quarters of deaths occuring in low- and middle-income countries are due to cardiovascular diseases, depicting a serious burden on the medical field. The etiologies for cardiac and vascular complications are very complex, in which both genetic and environmental factors are implicated along with lifestyle changes [1]. Generally overweight, increased blood pressure and blood sugar level may cause cardiovascular diseases and they are categorized under two major disorders belonging to lipid metabolism and metabolic syndromes [2].

The use of animal models has contributed immensely to increasing the knowledge about pathophysiology and focused approaches to improve the diagnostic and the early treatment of diseases [3]. The CVDs' preventative and ameliorative treatments depend on animal models that mimic human disease processes. Generally, rodents are widely accepted as the model organism for studying the diseases of humans, especially for mice, with whom they share 99% of their genes. Rodents have been regarded as a reliable research species mainly due to their small size, abbreviated (short) lifespan, reproductive affluence, known genetic background, as well as ease in handling and housing practices. With the development of biotechnologies and medico-veterinary field, various manipulations allow the establishment of rodent models which accurately mimic the human disease model of interests and accurately reflect the morphological and biochemical aspects of disease pathogenesis [4 - 6]. Experimental rodent models are widely used for cardiovascular diseases research due to the effective simulation of human cardiovascular diseases, stronger reproductive ability, and detection of physiological indicators in contrast to large animal models [7]. Henceforth, in this article, we will summarize the most common models of cardiovascular diseases, and modeling methods to provide a reference for research on cardiovascular diseases. In particular, we will briefly describe atherosclerosis and diabetic models, with models of heart failure.

2. ATHEROSCLEROSIS AND DIABETIC MODELS

Atherosclerosis is a chronic inflammatory condition and one of the underlying factors of cardiovascular diseases. Atherosclerosis is a disease in which plaque builds up inside human arteries. Both the blood vessel walls and the immune system are implicated in atherogenesis. Plasma lipoproteins, genetics and the hemodynamics of the blood flow in the artery all play important roles in the development of atherosclerosis. Animal models are valuable tools for providing insights into the etiology and pathophysiology of this disease. They can be used for testing the efficacy and safety of different pharmacological therapies. As per the extensive literature survey, mouse models particularly knockout and transgenic mouse models for atherosclerosis have proved to be useful to study the development and progression of the atherosclerotic lesion, understand the molecular and cellular mechanisms involved in atherogenesis, and evaluate the effectiveness of new and existing atherosclerotic drugs [8].

Generally, wild-type mice are resistant to atherosclerotic lesion development. The current mouse models used for atherosclerosis are based on genetic modifications of lipoprotein metabolism with additional dietary changes. Among them, low-density lipoprotein receptor-deficient mice (LDLR−/− mice) and apolipoprotein E-deficient mice (apoE−/− mice) are the most widely used mouse models for atherosclerosis research. Both LDLR and APOE are important for the removal of cholesterol and triglyceride-rich lipoprotein particles from the blood. APOE is a plasma glycoprotein constituent on the surface of most lipoproteins including very-low-density lipoprotein (VLDL), intermediate-density lipoprotein (IDL) and chylomicron lipoprotein particles. LDLR is a cell-surface receptor that recognizes the ApoE, apoprotein B 100, and apolipoprotein B (APOB) to clear the lipoprotein particles from the blood. Human mutations in LDLR and APOE are associated with several hereditary dyslipidemic disorders and increase the susceptibility to atherosclerosis for the mutation carrier.

2.1. LDLR−/− Mice

The LDLR−/− mice (low-density lipoprotein, LDL, receptor) are the models for studying familial hypocholesterolemia [3]. These models have a mutation that affects the LDLR level and resembles humans' plasma lipoprotein profile. The genetic modification in the model leads to delayed clearance of very-low-density lipoprotein (VLDL) and LDL from the plasma and therefore results in an increased plasma level of cholesterol on the normal chow diet [9]. Besides, the inclusion of high-fat and high-cholesterol content in the diet increases the severity of atherosclerotic lesions and hypercholesterolemia in LDLR−/− mice [10]. The plasma levels of LDLR−/− mice fed on a high-fat western diet were 10 times higher than those of wild type, and plaques formed on the aortic roots, showing symptoms of atherosclerosis. Pan *et al.* fed 7-week-old male LDLR−/− mice (C57BL6/J background) with a western diet containing 20% fat, 20% sugar, and 1.25% cholesterol till 16 weeks of age. The evaluation of aortic atherosclerotic lesions by hematoxylin and eosin staining proves to achieve good modeling results [11].

2.2. ApoE−/− Mice

The apolipoprotein E (ApoE) is synthesized in the liver and in macrophages, and plays an important role as an antiatherogenic agent. ApoE is a constituent of plasma lipoproteins and it serves as a ligand for the cell-surface lipoprotein receptors such as LDL receptors. It promotes the uptake of atherogenic particles from circulation. The homozygous deletion of the apoE gene in mice results in a pronounced increase in the LDL and VLDL levels in plasma. It is mainly attributed to the failure of lipoprotein receptor-mediated clearance of these lipoproteins. The most obvious phenotype of ApoE−/− mice is the spontaneous development of atherosclerotic lesions, even on a standard chow diet that is is low in fat content (< 40 g/kg) and does not contain cholesterol. The apoE−/− mouse contains the entire spectrum of lesions observed during atherogenesis and was the first mouse model to resemble its human counterparts lesions. Further, the process can be strongly accelerated by a high-fat, high-cholesterol diet [12]. The researchers analyzed the aortic plaque and the vascular lumen morphology with Sudan IV staining using imaging methods and concluded that ApoE−/− mice fed with a high-fat diet containing 18% milk fat and 0.15% cholesterol for more than 18 weeks, and 12-week-old ApoE−/− mice fed with a normal diet for more than 6 weeks can achieve good modeling effects [13, 14]. In addition, LDLR−/− and ApoE double-deficient mice (LDLR−/−ApoE−/−) have increased plasma cholesterol levels and develop atherosclerotic lesions under specific normal dietary conditions. Hence, these models facilitate the study of diseases without putting burden on feeding the mice with an atherogenic diet [15].

Currently, the ApoE−/− mice are the most widely used animal model for the study of atherosclerosis. Besides, the apoE−/− mouse model was used for (i) identifying atherosclerosis susceptibility-modifying genes, by the candidate-gene and gene-mapping methods, (ii) deciphering molecular mechanisms and cell types involved in atherogenesis, (iii) searching the drug effects on atherosclerosis, and (iv) assessing novel therapies that prevent lesion progression [16]. Both LDLR−/− and ApoE−/− mice have advantages and disadvantages depending on the goals of the study. In fact, on a chow diet, ApoE−/− mice show higher plasma total cholesterol levels compared to LDLR−/− mice, thus, developing severe atherosclerotic lesions as soon as a few weeks after birth [17]. Moreover, the deficiency of the endogenous ApoE expression causes an imbalance in cholesterol loading specifically in the macrophages, results in cytokine and protease secretion and triggers subsequent inflammation and extracellular matrix degradation [18]. These peculiar aspects of ApoE −/− mice reflect the greater adaptability for studying several other diseases associated with inflammation and extracellular matrix degradation such as Alzheimer's, erectile dysfunction, diet-induced steatohepatitis, and recently also chronic obstructive pulmonary disease [19]. Other less frequently reported mouse models of atherosclerosis involving disturbance to lipid metabolism are the mice expressing mutant forms of apoE, such as apoE3Leiden (E3L) and apoE (Arg 112 →Cys→142) transgenic mice, which are the more widely studied. These mice display a lipoprotein profile comparable to that of patients with dysbetalipoproteinemia. The E3L transgenic mice develop atherosclerotic lesions with all the characteristics of human vasculopathy, varying from fatty streak to mild, moderate, and severe plaques [20]. Furthermore, E3L transgenic mice and the more recently developed E3L/Cholesteryl ester transfer protein (CETP) transgenic mice are more sensitive to a variety of hypolipidemic drugs and PPAR agonists than apoE−/− and LDLR−/− mice (Van Der Hoorn *et al.*, 2009).

2.3. SR-BI KO Mice

These models are deficient in the HDL scavenger receptor Class B Type 1, with and without apoE deficiency. The SR-BI KO models exhibit atherogenesis lesions when fed with a high-fat/high-cholesterol diet and do not exhibit lesions on the normal chow diet type. The genetic modifications in lipid metabolism and diet change lead to advanced vascular diseases similar to that seen in rare human genetic disorders. However, it does not correspond to common disease processes seen in humans with common metabolic syndrome and type 2 diabetes [21, 22].

2.4. db/db Mouse

The db/db mouse strain carries a spontaneous mutation of the leptin ObR system that is analogous to the cp gene. Mice that are homozygous for the db mutation produce a receptor with a prematurely terminated intracellular domain and a defective binding of leptin, leading to obesity, insulin resistance, hyperinsulinemia, and hypertriglyceridemia [23]. This model was used mainly for type 2 diabetes mellitus. Kobayashi *et al.* [24] conducted a study on db/db mouse, a model for diabetic dyslipidemia. They fed the animal model with human-like 0.15% (wt/wt) cholesterol and 21% (wt/wt) fat "Western" diet. The db/db mice developed elevated plasma cholesterol, accompanied by an exaggerated apolipoprotein E (apoE) response compared with the control group. They concluded that db/db mice on a western diet have a plasma lipoprotein phenotype that shows some similarities to that in patients with type 2 diabetes mellitus, and that db/db mice are a useful model to study the pathogenesis and treatment of diabetic dyslipidemia.

2.5. Ob/ob Mice

The ob/ob or obese mouse model has mutations in the leptin gene, responsible for the production of the hormone leptin, which is important in the control of appetite. This is an animal model of type II diabetes and obesity due to their hyperphagic, hyperinsulinemic, and hyperglycemic features. Strains possess a recessive mutation in leptin, the ligand for the leptin receptor, and in the C57BL/6J, DBA2/J, and FVB strains [25]. Generally, ob/ob mice are indistinguishable from their lean littermates at birth and they become heavier and develop hyperinsulinemia after the weaning period and overt hyperglycemia is observed during the fourth week of age. The blood glucose rises to reach the peak after 3-5 months when the mice also have very high food intake and rapid growth. After that, blood glucose values decrease and eventually become nearly normal at old age. The animals remain insulin-resistant, but impaired glucose tolerance and glycosuria after a glucose load are observed mostly in the post-weaning period of rapid growth, and this usually becomes normalized when the mice get older [26].

Apart from these models for providing insights into diabetic pathophysiology, other genetically-induced models (*e.g.*, NOD mice, ZDF rats), chemically induced models (*e.g.*, STZ-induced rodent diabetic models, alloxan-induced diabetic rat models), and surgically-induced models (*e.g.*, Renal ischemia-induced DN models, oxygen-induced retinopathy mouse models), have been used for testing the efficacy and safety of different pharmacological therapies for the management of diabetic complications [27 - 29].

2.6. Zucker Fatty Rat

Zucker fatty/obese rat (ZFR) is used as a model of human obesity accompanied by hyperlipidemia and hypertension. The ZFR is outbred and multicolored, with four principal coat colors: (1) predominantly brown, (2) brown and white, (3) predominantly black, and (4) black and white. The first of the new genetically unique obesity rat strains was the fatty Zucker, which was initially described by Zucker and Zucker in 1961 [30]. The Zucker rat was developed from crosses between animals from the Sherman strain and the Merck stock 13 M strain [31]. The leptin mutation ("fa") found in this strain of rat is a recessive trait and causes obesity in rats . The mutation was determined to be a shortened leptin-receptor protein resulting from a single nucleotide substitution at position 880 of the leptin-receptor gene [32]. The outbred Zucker fatty rat (Zucker fa/fa) is probably the best-known and most widely used model of the genetic obesity trait [31]. This obese rat model is characterized by hyperlipidemia, hypercholesterolemia, and hyperinsulinemia and develops adipocyte hypertrophy and hyperplasia. It has been a valuable contributor to the study of early-onset hyperplastic hypertrophic obesity.

2.7. Zucker Diabetic Fatty (ZDF) Rat

Inbreeding of the Zucker fatty rat for hyperglycemia gives rise to the ZDF rat strain, being less obese than the Zucker fatty rat, but having more severe insulin resistance. The onset of diabetes in the ZDF model is related to the loss of GLUT-2 glucose transporters in pancreatic β cells and the concomitant loss of muscle GLUT-4 transporters [33]. It is severely insulin-resistant and males become overtly diabetic at 8–10 weeks, which is due to an inability of beta cells to compensate for insulin resistance, which is associated with changes in islet morphology. But females do not develop overt diabetes [34]. The Zucker diabetic fatty (ZDF) rat is most widely used for studying type 2 diabetes associated with obesity. The diabetic ZDF rat develops symptoms of type 2 diabetes that are characterized by (1) hyperglycemia that develops between 7 and 12 weeks of age, (2) early hyperinsulinemia that begins to diminish as the beta-cells in the pancreas are destroyed, (3) fasting hyperglycemia, (4) abnormal glucose tolerance, (5) increased plasma triglycerides, and (6) mild hypertension. The ZDF model has proven to be useful in studying type 2 diabetes as well as the influence of diabetes on wound healing, periodontal disease, and neuropathy. This rat strain possesses high reproductive efficiency and therefore should serve as a useful model for young- to middle-aged adult-onset type 2 diabetes in the studies of the pathophysiology, therapeutic interventions, and complications of the disease [35]. This model is prone to hydronephrosis, which may interfere with renal studies.

2.8. Otsuka Long–Evans Tokushima fatty (OLETF) Rats

The OLETF is a spontaneously diabetic rat strain with polyuria, polydipsia, mild obesity, hypertension, and dyslipidemia derived from the Long-Evans rat. About 90% of the male animals become diabetic by 1 year of age. Statistical tests have determined that the locus containing the cholecystokinin A receptor is responsible for about 50% of the T2DM in the OLETF rats. The receptor is disrupted in the OLETF rat because of a 165-bp deletion in exon 1. Just as in human disease, the progression of T2DM in OLETF rats can be prevented by exercise and caloric restriction [25]. Multiple recessive genes are associated with the induction of diabetes, such as the odb-1 on the X-chromosome of OLETF rats.

2.9. Goto-Kakizaki (GK) Rats

GK rats are nonobese and spontaneously diabetic models which were developed by repeated selective breeding of normal Wistar rats using glucose intolerance as a selection index [36]. The models will show glucose intolerance after 2 weeks of age and significant hyperglycemia will be developed as early as 4 weeks of age, and the animals show hyperinsulinemia and decreased pancreatic insulin stores [36]. Development of type 2 diabetes mellitus in the GK model results from the complex interaction of multiple events such as (i) the presence of several susceptibility loci containing genes responsible for some diabetic traits, (ii) gestational metabolic impairment inducing an epigenetic programming of the offspring pancreas and the major insulin target tissues, and (iii) environmentally induced loss of β cell differentiation due to chronic exposure to hyperglycemia/hyperlipidemia, inflammation, and oxidative stress [37]. GK rat appears to be a suitable model for experimental studies of chronic complications of diabetes.

2.10. WNIN/GR-Ob Rat

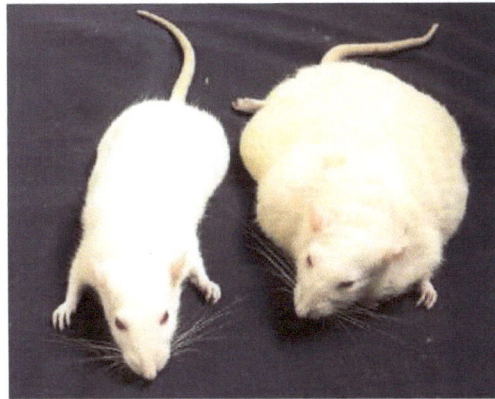

Fig. (1). WNIN/Ob Rat. Adult (left) lean (right) obese rats of the same age [40].

This is the first mutant obese rat strain with impaired glucose tolerance (IGT) developed by the ICMR- National Institute of Nutrition (NIN), Hyderabad, India, from the stock Wistar rat (WNIN) colony (Fig. **1**). The WNIN/GR-Ob mutant strain obesity is inherited as an autosomal incomplete dominant trait in this strain. The strain is characterized by high growth, polydipsia, hyperphagia, glycosuria, polyurea, and significantly lower lean body mass, and higher fat mass as compared with carrier and lean rats. At the age of 50 days, with abnormal response to a glucose load, hypertriglyceridemia, hyperinsulinemia, hypercholesterolemia and hyperleptinemia will be detected. This mutant obese model is easy to propagate, and can easily be transformed into a frank diabetes model by dietary manipulation and thus can be used for screening anti-diabetic drugs [38]. Apart from the above-mentioned strains, for a quick review of atherosclerosis and diabetic-induced or spontaneous models, basic information is summarized in Table **1** [39].

Table 1. Atherosclerosis and diabetic rodent models.

Animal Strain	Induction Type	Diet Type	Survival Rate	Remarks of the Strain
apoE/LDL-R	Stress-induced	western-type	Died after 6 months on this diet	Acute myocardial infarction, myocardial apoptosis, cardiac fibrosis, Plaque stenosis /occlusion in the proximal segment
SR-BI/apoE dKO	Spontaneous	normal chow diet	50% mortality at 6 weeks old	Extensive lipid, fibrin-rich coronary occlusion, cardiac hypertrophy, fibrosis and lipids accumulation on the myocardium
n/i/eNOS tKO	Spontaneous	normal chow diet	50% mortality after 7.5 months on this diet	Distal arteriosclerotic lesion, perivascular fibrosis and mast cell infiltration in the heart, Cardiac fibrosis and hypertrophy
SR-BI KO/HypoE	Diet-induced	PD for 4 weeks	50% mortality after 20 days on this diet	Lipid-rich occlusion, intra-plaque Hemorrhage on heart, Cardiac hypertrophy, infarction and fibrosis
SR-BI KO/HypoE	Diet-induced	PD for 1 week	50% mortality after 36 days on this diet	Multiple diffuse lipid-rich stenosis, occasional thrombus, Cardiac fibrosis, predominantly located near the endocardium
SR-BI/LDL-R dKO	Diet-induced	PD for 12 weeks	50% mortality after 3.5 weeks on this diet	Lipid-rich occlusion, platelet accumulation Cardiac hypertrophy, infarction and fibrosis
SR-BI/LDL-R dKO	Diet-induced	2% cholesterol diet for 12 weeks	50% mortality after 11.4 weeks on this diet	Lipid-rich occlusion, platelet accumulation Cardiac hypertrophy, infarction and fibrosis
SR-BI/LDL-R dKO	Diet-induced	WD with 0.5% cholesterol for 20 weeks	50% mortality after 13.9 weeks on this diet	Plaque stenosis/occlusion in the proximal Segment Cardiac hypertrophy and ischemia

(Table 1) cont.....

Animal Strain	Induction Type	Diet Type	Survival Rate	Remarks of the Strain
PDZK1/apoE dKO	Diet-induced	PD for 3 months	No mortality	Lipid-rich occlusion, perivascular fibrosis Cardiac fibrosis
eNOS/apoE dKO	Diet-induced	WD for 16 weeks	No mortality	Distal arteriosclerotic lesion with fatty streak, perivascular fibrosis, Cardiac ischemia, hypertrophy and fibrosis
WD: western-type diet; PD: paigen diet				

3. HEART FAILURE MODELS

Heart failure is characterized by reduced cardiac output and consequently. The heart is unable to meet the perfusion demands of the body. Even though the small animal models have several known advantages and disadvantages, they are widely used to explore the pathophysiology of heart failure and to develop novel therapeutic progression of this prevalent and fatal disease (Table **1**).

Table 2. Advantages and limitations of heart failure rodent models.

Model & Method	Advantage	Limitations	References
a. Surgical			
Left coronary ligation	Directly applicable to human disease, Availability of multiple modalities to assess cardiovascular function, the greater quantity of myocardial tissue for postmortem analyses	High mortality; technically demanding; relevance to other conditions?	[41, 42]
Ascending aortic constriction	Gradual onset hypertension along with the above benefits	Same as above	[43]
Cryoinjury	Technically simple	Relevance to human disease?	[44]
b. Chemical / Toxic			
Ethanol, Isoproterenol Doxorubicin, Homocysteine	Non-invasive; technically simple; reproducible	High mortality; non-cardiac effects; not generally applicable?	[44]
c. Genetic			
Muscle lim protein Knockout - Dilated cardiomyopathy	No surgery is required for heart failure stimulus, directly reproduces gene expression changes seen in disease	Non-specific effects of over expression, Developmental effects of null allele	[44]

(Table 2) cont.....

Model & Method	Advantage	Limitations	References
Inducible null/transgenic	Control of time course of induction/deletion	Control of level of trans-gene often impossible	[44]

3.1. Myocardial Ischemia-Induced Heart Failure

Surgical clipping of a coronary artery, typically the left anterior descending artery (LADL) will be done on both male and female rats weighing 200-250 grams. Briefly, a transverse incision will be made on a chest through the skin. After separating the muscles, an incision will be made in the intercostal space between the fourth and fifth ribs. Once the heart is visible, a small needle with a suture is passed through the pathway of the coronary artery and the left descending coronary artery will be ligated permanently. Later the chest incision and skin incision will be closed [45]. This murine model allows the monitoring of pathological processes occurring from coronary occlusion to late-stage heart failure at the local heart tissue and systemic levels. This model can be induced in both rats and mice, and it is the most preferred and acceptable heart failure. Coronary artery ligation offers advantages such as better reproducibility and heart failure similar to human heart failure.

3.2. Pressure Overload Models

Numerous surgical methods have been used to develop pressure overload rat models, but the ascending aortic banding is the most widely used surgical method in which a stricture is placed around the ascending aorta of weanling (3- to 4-week old) rats [46]. As these rats grow, hypertension develops gradually, during which, aortic outflow is increasingly impeded. This model shows that after 8 weeks postbanding, rats exhibit maintenance of left ventricular (LV) chamber size with evidence of LV hypertrophy, consistent with "compensated hypertrophy" though Doppler echocardiography at this stage shows evidence of increased left atrial pressure. Further, pressure overload-induced left ventricular hypertrophy and heart failure can be produced by transverse aortic banding and abdominal aortic banding in rodents. The transverse aortic constriction mice model and the ascending aortic banding rat model are the most widely used pressure overload models. Pressure overload models are valuable to study hypertrophy and the transition to heart failure.

3.3. Chemical-induced Cardiomyopathy Models

Cytotoxic drugs such as doxorubicin are known as cardiotoxins in humans and have been used to induce heart failure syndromes in rats. Doxorubicin-induced cardiac toxicity is characterized by ventricular wall thinning and dilation of the left ventricular chamber. Nakahara *et al.* [47] induced cardiomyopathy in Sprague-Dawley male rats through a single injection of high-dose doxorubicin (5-10 mg/kg) or multiple injections (2- 4 times) of low-dose doxorubicin (2.5 mg/kg) with a combined single injection of trastuzumab (10 mg/kg).

4. NON-RODENT MODELS OF CARDIO-VASCULAR DISEASES

Non-Rodent animal models used in cardiovascular research mainly involve swine, dogs and sheep. These animal models have similarities in various anatomical features of the human cardiovascular system to test various therapeutic agents for efficacy and toxicity/safety studies. The peculiar resemblances in anatomy and physiological parameters help to translate the clinically relevant protocols, imaging techniques, diagnostic procedures, and medical devices like stents, catheters, and valves for humans. Pigs, dogs and sheep are most frequently used as the animals of choice by researchers except fornon-human primates as they involve many limitations [48]. In recent years, swine models have dominated cardiovascular research in drug development, toxicology, and regulatory studies [49]. They are replacing other large animal models, particularly dogs which have high societal reasons, emotional value to humans and various anatomical and physiological differences which do not translate the result of cardiovascular research well in humans. As such we have discussed various swine models used in cardiovascular research at large in this text.

4.1. Overview of Advantages and Disadvantages of Non-rodent Animal Models

Advantages	Disadvantages
• More Relevant clinically • Heart diseases having chronic course can be studied. • Cardiac Function responses can be measured more easily in the intact animal. • All the techniques and measurements used in humans can be performed in Non-rodent models. • Anatomical and physiological parameters are more closely related than rodent models to humans.	• Housing and maintenance costs are high. • Need for trained personnel and specialized infrastructure in handling. • Gestation time and life span are longer to observe the effects in long term studies. • In the case of Dog and pig: ischemia-reperfusion induced arrhythmias occur more frequently. • Production of transgenic models is cumbersome.

4.2. Pigs

Pigs are the best animal model to study cardio-vascular diseases as they have many similarities with the human cardiovascular system. Similarity of the cardiovascular system in terms of anatomy, network of coronary arteries, and performance of ventricles, cardiac metabolism, electrophysiology and collateralization after acute myocardial infarction makes them the best suitable model for the simulation of cardio-vascular diseases in order to understand the pathophysiology, study efficacy and safety of various drugs [50]. Pigs share the heart rate at an average heart beat of 90-107 beats per minute, which is closer to humans at an average heart rate of 70-100 beats/minute. Various blood parameters, aorta size, coronary vasculature and lipid profile are more or less identical. The circulating levels of cholesterol (60%) and low density lipid level (38%) also have similarity with humans to 63% and 28% respectively [51]. Pigs and humans share the anatomical similarities of the aortic valve as both have trilayered structures and similar extracellular matrice substances, critical to simulating the aortic stenosis in humans [52]. The right dominance of the heart in both human and pigs is an added advantage in various congestive heart failure models compared to other animal models *viz.* ruminants and canines, who have left heart dominance [53].

Besides various anatomical and physiological resemblances, several hemodynamic parameters are fundamental in cardiovascular research. Haemodynamic parameters play a key role in the extrapolation of data and indicate prognosis in various haemodynamic studies, cardiac arrest and cardiac resucitation in humans [54]. However, the data is seen to vary among different species and within the same species depending on age, body weight, and type of anesthesia. These criteria should be taken into account for the research outcomes of any study. A reference set of various haemodynamic parameters which are important to cardiovascular research are provided below for various breeds of pig in Table **3** [55].

Table 3. Hemodynamic parameters in various breeds of pig used in cardiovascular research.

Parameter	Landrace–Large White	Hanford	Yucatan minipig	Yucatan micropig
Age	10–15 wk	4 mo	4 mo	4 mo
Heart rate (bpm)	116.41 ± 8.11	105 ± 7	112 ± 3	106 ± 5
Cardiac output (L/min)	5.12 ± 0.53	—	—	—
Left ventriclar systolic pressure (mm Hg)	108.97 ± 12.06	116 ± 4	58 ± 2	59 ± 3

(Table 3) cont.....

Parameter	Landrace–Large White	Hanford	Yucatan minipig	Yucatan micropig
Left ventricular diastolic pressure (mm Hg)	8.88 ± 1.81	4 ± 1	3 ± 1	6 ± 2
Right ventricular peak pressure (mm Hg)	21.24 ± 2.16	30 ± 1	24 ± 2	27 ± 2
Right ventricular diastolic pressure (mm Hg)	4.20 ± 0.72	4 ± 1	2 ± 1	5 ± 2

Several swine models which include native and altered models are available to carry out research on cardio-vascular diseases. Common breeds used as models in cardio-vascular research include large-sized pig breeds and small-sized pig breeds. Among the large sized breeds, the large Landrace pig, Yorkshire, Duroc and their crosses are commonly used. Miniature swine breeds available include the Göttingen minipig (Fig. **2**), the Yucatan miniature pig (Fig. **3**), the Troll minipig, the Hanford miniature pig, and the Sinclair minipig. Among the mentioned miniature breeds, Göttingen minipig has become very popular because of its size, easy management and docile nature of the animal. They have been developed as a result of continuous cross-breeding of the Vietnamese swine, the Hormel or Minnesota miniature swine and the German-improved Landrace at the University of Göttingen (Germany). Another advantage about the animal is that these animals reach sexual maturity at a much earlier time than other Non-rodent animal models.

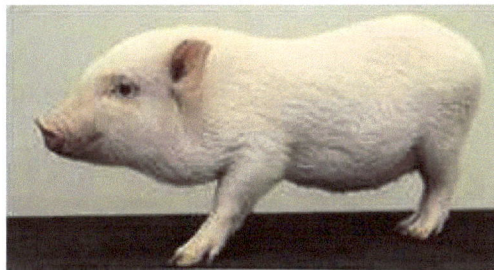

Fig. (2). A young Gottingen Miniature Pig (Source: https://en.wikipedia.org/wiki/G%C3% B6ttingen_mini-pig).

Initially, mini pigs were used as the large animal species for safety testing in the development of dermal pharmaceutical products. This was because, compared to other non-rodent species, the skin of this animal more closely resembles humans in many respects, including sparse distribution of the hair coat, overall histologic appearance, epidermal thickness, keratinocyte turnover time, xenobiotic metabolic activity, and similar dermal penetration rates for many chemicals. In addition to the dermal route of administration, mini pigs are easily dosed *via* the oral (gavage or capsule), intravenous and subcutaneous routes. Moreover, there are many cases in which mini pigs are suitable alternatives to the standard non-rodent species because of species-specific, dose-limiting toxicity to drugs. Nowadays, they have become very popular in cardio-vascular research because of several advantages particularly in long term studies.

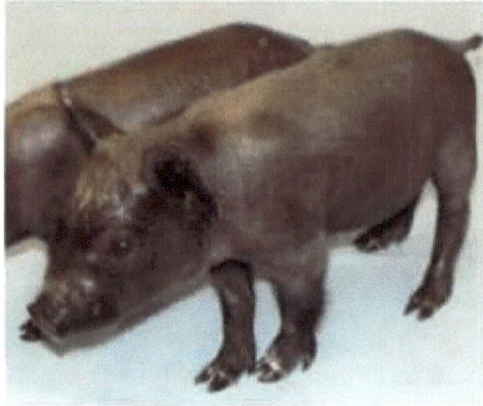

Fig. (3). Yucatan Miniature Pig (Source: https://nsrrc.missouri.edu/nsrrc0012info).

4.3. Atherosclerotic Disease Models

Porcine serves an excellent animal model for atherosclerosis as they develop lesions spontaneously when kept on high fat or high cholesterol diet [56]. Porcine models are good to examine adventitial neovascularization, on atherosclerotic plaque composition and vascular remodeling in coronary atherosclerosis. However, the lesions develop slowly and take a longer duration for the onset of atherosclerosis compared to rodent models. Importantly the atherosclerotic lesions developed in the porcine model are complex having a high degree of similarity to human lesions in terms of inflammatory mediators, extracellular matrices, calcification pattern, smooth muscle cell involvement, foam cells, fibrous cap and plaque haemorrhage [56]. Several swine models of coronary atherosclerosis which mimic advanced humanoid lesions of atherosclerosis have been developed and standardized which are critical in emerging technologies in interventional cardiology and for the study of drug-eluting stents [57, 58].

Geritty *et al.* [59] developed a pig model to simulate the atherosclerotic lesions in humans in 2001 called as Diabetic/Hypercholesterolemia pig model in Yorkshire breed. He injected streptozotocin intravenously to destroy the beta-cells of the pancreas to develop DM and kept the pigs on 5-10% lard and 0.5-1% cholesterol diet. This way the atherosclerotic lesions developed in pigs showed more severity and similarity to those human. Rapacz developed a strain of pigs with inherited hyper low-density lipoprotein (LDL) and hypercholesterolemia (IHLC pigs) and named it Rapacz-HF which developed atherosclerotic lesions having more humanoid morphology. The strain was developed by cross breeding having characteristics of six domesticated swine breeds exhibiting familial hypercholesterolemia (FHC) [60]. The strain was developed through multiple generations of breeding, while keeping them on a low-fat and low-cholesterol diets. The unique part of the model is that, it has high levels of LDL and low levels of HDL which is similar to the human subject having a predisposition to atherosclerosis. This condition is hard to achieve in other swine models through High fat/high cholesterol feeding. This unique attribute is due to the LPB-5 gene mutation and R84C-LDLR gene mutation. These two gene mutations result in low binding ability of LDL-C and LDLR, resulting in decreased clearance of LDL, leading to accumulation of LDL in the body which results in AS.

Several researchers have also induced such mutations/knock offs in genes governing the bad lipid content in blood with the help of genetic engineering. They have an added advantage in terms of size and severity of lesions of AS compared to Rapacz pig which becomes overweight and has a lot of variability in lesion severity. Scientists have developed strategies to edit the genes *viz.* LDLR-knockoff (LDLR-KO), and ApoE-knockoff (ApoE-KO) to increase the susceptibility of breeds to high cholesterol content in the blood which eventually leads to AS. One such attempt was made by Davis *et al* [61] to create an improved swine model with a genetic predisposition to hypercholesterolemia and AS was made in Yucatan miniature pigs. They used recombinant adeno-associated virus-mediated gene targeting and somatic cell nuclear transfer to produce male and female LDLR+/- pigs which were subsequently bred and selected for LDLR-/- genotype animals. These homozygotic pigs resulted in atherosclerotic lesions in the coronary arteries and abdominal aorta that resemble human atherosclerosis without any dietary changes needed. Moreover, AS was more severe and developed in a shorter time duration if the animals were fed a high fat/high cholesterol diet. This model has several advantages which include size, consistency, versatility and availability. The developed model has been used in several studies on diagnosis and treatment strategies for coronary and aortic atherosclerosis and its associated complications. The LDLR-/- homozygous animals showed extremely high LDL levels, whether at birth (490.8±19.0mg/dL *vs.* 64.2±7.0 mg/dL, compared to the normal group, same as below), fed with a normal diet (567.4±34.3 mg/dL *vs.* 67.0±6.6 mg/dL), or fed with a high cholesterol diet (960.4±46.9 mg/dL *vs.* 161.0±23.6 mg/dL). Also, the complex lesions of AS in coronary arteries and the aorta had fibrous caps, hemorrhage, calcification, and foam cells which had great similarity with advanced AS lesions.

Li *et al*. [62] attempted to make LDLR -/- from domestic pigs in to overcome the high cost and availability limitation of Yucatan miniature pigs. They successfully knocked out exon 4 of the LDLR gene-targeted deletion and generated a new LDLR knockout pig from a commonly available domestic pig. They used conventional targeting vectors for the replacement of the LDLR gene by neomycin resistance gene into fetal fibroblasts obtained from Landrace and Large White crossbred pigs using Gene Pulser II electroporation system. In the developed model, a marked resemblance of advanced human-like plaques after a relatively short time-period was observed when fed on a high fat, high cholesterol diet. This model is easily available for researchers at a very cheap rate than other LDLR knout out pigs. However, it is not suitable for studies with a longer duration of time-period as the animal becomes overweight and difficult to manage.

4.4. Pig Models for Stent Application

Pigs serve as excellent models in-stent research development for regulatory studies which involve analysis of biomechanical properties of stents, their biology and their efficacy in controlling blockage of blood vessels. Innate swine models with no alteration in vasculature or feeding schedule can be used for these studies. These animal models give us insights into toxicity studies of the naïve fabrics of stents and also drug loaded stents within normal arteries. The animal model for stent technology development also has been used for standardizing imaging tools, like optical coherence tomography, that can be used to study the effects of stenting *in vivo* [63, 64]. Several studies have supported that swine is an excellent model to study the coronary as well as peripheral stent application [65]. Researchers use generally normocholesterolemic domestic crossbred pig for relatively short term studies, as the maintenance cost is low and their availability is high. However, for studies that involve long follow-ups these pigs are not suitable as they grow very fast and become unmanageable. For longer duration of studies, researchers prefer to use mini-pigs which are smaller and easy to manage.

4.5. Pig Models of Infarction and Heart Failure

Pig models of cardiovascular disease are commonly used to study myocardial infarction and heart failure for various purposes which include surgical research, regenerative medicine, imaging studies, and other scientific purposes [66]. This is mainly due to scanty coronary collateral arteries found in swine hearts than in other animal models like dogs [67]. Several techniques are being used by the scientific community to replicate the heart failure condition. The techniques involve the open heart and closed heart surgical procedures which can either compromise or preserve the anatomical structures. Mostly closed heart procedures result in better modeling of heart failure due to several advantages:

1. The survival rate is high in the animals including a high survival rate (>90% after ischemia-reperfusion).

2. Myocardial Infarction size can be adjusted easily by varying the occlusion of the coronary artery.

3. The method is less invasive compared to open heart surgical procedures.

4. The resulting cardiac failure is highly reproducible with similar outcomes in other experiments.

The procedure for closed-chest procedure for developing Myocardial Infarction in the swine model is briefly given below;

1. The animal is placed in the dorsal spine position and restrained properly after giving pre-medication and anaesthesia. The animal is given prophylactic antibiotics and kept on maintenance anaesthesia like propofol using an endotracheal tube.

2. After the preparation of the animal, baseline echocardiography data is obtained to evaluate the pre-MI condition of the heart.

3. The onset of MI starts by puncturing a needle in the groin region of the animal and under ultrasound guidance needle is advanced into the femoral artery. The puncture of the artery is done using a modified Seldinger's technique. After that a J-tip guide wire is entered into the artery after ascertaining good pulsatile blood flow.

4. This is followed by giving a skin incision to introduce arterial vascular sheath by replacing the puncture needles.

5. A small suture is placed to secure the sheath in place.

6. Now advance a 4 OR 5 Fr size coronary catheter to the ascending aorta preceding guidance with a 0.035 inch wire. The wire is pulled back 5-10 cm and the catheter is rotated clockwise to position it in the right coronary artery. After this, the wire is removed and catheter is connected to the manifold injection.

7. Now contrast material is injected slowly after ensuring no air is in the catheter. The X-ray is taken for a test shot followed by the angiography in different views.

8. The procedure is repeated in the same way for the left coronary artery.

9. After the images of the coronary arteries are obtained, the coronary balloon for occlusion of arteries is prepared.

10. Usually, coronary balloon measuring 1.5 times that of the coronary artery segment is used to induce Myocardial infarction.

11. The coronary balloon is placed in the coronary arteries using the 6 or 7 Fr catheters with a 0.014 inch wire inside.

12. After ascertaining the perfect placement of the balloon in the coronary artery, balloons are inflated to induce MI.

13. The balloon occlusion can be permanently induced using emboli coil implantation or clot injection after reperfusion or temporarily induced for Ischaemia injury. In temporary occlusion, the balloon is deflated and reflated as per the desired time.

14. After the procedure is over, the animals should be given proper analgesics and fluid therapy till recovery.

4.6. Dogs

Dogs have played an important model in biomedical research as they share many structural and physiological similarities to humans. They are usually considered better animal models than rodent models and various large animal models. Several canine breeds have been used in cardiovascular research, particularly in understanding the aetio-pathophysiology of ischaemic heart diseases. Dogs have been modeled by several methods to produce various heart diseases. Some of the methods include chronic pacing of the dog heart at a rate of above 200 beats/minute for several weeks which results in Chronic congestive heart failure [68]; coronary artery ligation and microembolisation [69] to produce myocardial infarction/heart failure but due to extensive collateral blood circulation it is difficult to translate in humans; trans-myocardial direct-current shock to induce ventricular hypertrophy [70]; aortic constriction intervention to cause pressure overload ventricles.

Various breeds of dogs have a genetic and spontaneous predilection for various heart diseases. These breeds have given various significant leads in the research to understand the pathophysiology of various ischaemic heart diseases. Dilated cardiomyopathy is a common heart disease that occurs spontaneously in several breeds *viz.* Dobermman Pinsher, Saint Bernard, and Great Danes. These breeds have been used as clinically relevant models as the condition develops without any intervention. Researchers use different instruments to record various hemo-dynamic parameters over several weeks to monitor the changes that occur during the progression of heart failure [71].

Chronic valvular disease is another important disease that commonly develops in dog breeds like Dachshunds, miniature and toy Poodles, Chihuahuas, and Terrier breeds. This disease resembles mitral valve collapse in humans, as such, these breeds have been modeled to study the heart failure associated with mitral valve [72].

Boxer dogs with mutations associated with chromosome 17 have a predilection to develop Arrythmogenic Right Ventricular cardiomyopathy which often leads to sudden cardiac arrest. This disease is similar to humans, as boxer dogs have been modeled to study ventricular tachycardia and various abnormalities in the right ventricle to get insights into the pathological features associated with the disease [73].

Cardio-myopathic complication associated with Duchenne Muscle Dystrophy (DMD) has been modelled in Golden retriever dogs. This dog breed also develops diseases similar to humans related to a point mutation in the dystrophin gene on X chromosome. This animal is the best available model to study DMD as the clinical symptoms like progressive muscle wasting, degeneration, fibrosis, and a shortened lifespan frankly match with the disease in humans [74].

Over the years, due to high ethical concerns, animal activists, high cost factor and resources involved in housing and maintenance have limited the use of dogs in cardio-vascular research. Also, despite many similarities, differences in anatomical and physiological parameters have raised concerns in the translation of results from dogs to humans.

4.7. Sheep

Sheep is one of the large animals which have been used in cardio-vascular research owing to many similarities to human heart. Sheep are a common animal model for translational research in cardiovascular surgery particularly in heart-valve related surgeries [75]. Sheep cardiomyocytes have a similar contractile-relation functional relationship to human cardiomyocytes. The resting heart rate, systolic blood pressure and diastolic blood pressure of sheep frankly resemble to the humans. As such, sheep serve as a good pre-clinical model in cardiovascular research. Several sheep models for various heart diseases have been reported *viz*, myocardial infarction [76, 77], aortic constriction over a period of time to produce pressure overload and ventricular hypertrophy [78] and tachypacing induced degenerative dilated cardiomyopathy and heart failure [79]. A heart failure sheep model was described by Devlin *et al* [77] using the catheter-based approach to implant microemboli. The model presented stable chronic heart failure using catheter skills resulting in repetitive myocardial infarction. Emmert *et al.* [80] reported a novel fetal sheep model for intramyocardial transplantation of human mesenchymal stem cells in intra-uterine pre-immune myocardial infarction. This model has the advantage that no immune-suppressive therapy is needed to study the regenerative capacity of stem cells in myocardial infarction. This model provides a platform to study the fate of human stem cells after transmyocardial implantation without any interference from immune-suppressive drugs. Another heart failure model related to pressure afterload induced by aortic constriction was described by Moorjani *et al* [78]. In this model, they used a novel variable aortic constriction device to gradually change the after load to monitor the ventricular changes. During,experiment, they collected biopsy tissue from the ventricle to unravel the molecular changes associated with ventricular remodeling. This model can be used to study myocardial recovery by specifically targeting molecular derangements. A sheep model involving ventricular tachycardia and sudden death due to chronic myocardial infarction was reported by Killingsworth *et al* [81]. This model showed that ventricular tachycardia and myocardial infarction and bradycardia induced by AV node ablation in sheep can mimic ventricular tachycardia and sudden cardiac death in humans.

CONCLUSION

Although, sheep have been used as a good pre-clinical model for cardiac research and cardiac surgery but there are several limitations involved in their use. Most importantly, housing and management of sheep in long term studies are highly costly. It has been reported that the cost involved in sheep as a model is 80 times that of rodents. Also, anatomical and physiological differences pose challenges to complicated procedures in cardiovascular surgeries.

CONSENT FOR PUBLICATION

Not applicable.

CONFLICT OF INTEREST

The author declares no conflict of interest, financial or otherwise.

ACKNOWLEDGEMENTS

Declared none.

REFERENCES

[1]   Parim B, Sathibabu Uddandrao VV, Saravanan G. Diabetic cardiomyopathy: molecular mechanisms, detrimental effects of conventional treatment, and beneficial effects of natural therapy. Heart Fail Rev 2019; 24(2): 279-99.
[http://dx.doi.org/10.1007/s10741-018-9749-1] [PMID: 30349977]

[2]   Russell JC, Proctor SD. Small animal models of cardiovascular disease: tools for the study of the roles of metabolic syndrome, dyslipidemia, and atherosclerosis. Cardiovasc Pathol 2006; 15(6): 318-30.
[http://dx.doi.org/10.1016/j.carpath.2006.09.001] [PMID: 17113010]

[3]   Zaragoza C, Gomez-Guerrero C, Martin-Ventura JL, *et al.* Animal models of cardiovascular diseases. J Biomed Biotechnol 2011; 2011: 1-13.
[http://dx.doi.org/10.1155/2011/497841] [PMID: 21403831]

[4]   Sangeethadevi G, v v SU, Jansy Isabella RAR, *et al.* Attenuation of lipid metabolic abnormalities, proinflammatory cytokines, and matrix metalloproteinase expression by biochanin-A in isoproterenol-induced myocardial infarction in rats. Drug Chem Toxicol 2021; 1-12.
[http://dx.doi.org/10.1080/01480545.2021.1894707] [PMID: 33719799]

[5]   Brahmanaidu P, Uddandrao VVS, Sasikumar V, *et al.* Reversal of endothelial dysfunction in aorta of streptozotocin-nicotinamide-induced type-2 diabetic rats by S-Allylcysteine. Mol Cell Biochem 2017; 432(1-2): 25-32.
[http://dx.doi.org/10.1007/s11010-017-2994-0] [PMID: 28258439]

[6]   Pavithra K, Sathibabu Uddandrao VV, Chandrasekaran P, *et al.* Phenolic fraction extracted from *Kedrostis foetidissima* leaves ameliorated isoproterenol-induced cardiotoxicity in rats through restoration of cardiac antioxidant status. J Food Biochem 2020; 44(11): e13450.
[http://dx.doi.org/10.1111/jfbc.13450] [PMID: 32839989]

[7]   Jia T, Wang C, Han Z, Wang X, Ding M, Wang Q. Experimental Rodent Models of Cardiovascular Diseases. Front Cardiovasc Med 2020; 7: 588075.
[http://dx.doi.org/10.3389/fcvm.2020.588075] [PMID: 33365329]

[8]   Zadelaar S, Kleemann R, Verschuren L, *et al.* Mouse models for atherosclerosis and pharmaceutical modifiers. Arterioscler Thromb Vasc Biol 2007; 27(8): 1706-21.
[http://dx.doi.org/10.1161/ATVBAHA.107.142570]

[9]   Bentzon JF, Falk E. Atherosclerotic lesions in mouse and man: is it the same disease? Curr Opin Lipidol 2010; 21(5): 434-40.
[http://dx.doi.org/10.1097/MOL.0b013e32833ded6a]

[10]   Knowles JW, Maeda N. Genetic modifiers of atherosclerosis in mice. Arterioscler Thromb Vasc Biol 2000; 20(11): 2336-45.
[http://dx.doi.org/10.1161/01.ATV.20.11.2336] [PMID: 11073835]

[11]   Pan S, Liu H, Gao F, *et al.* Folic acid delays development of atherosclerosis in low-density lipoprotein receptor-deficient mice. J Cell Mol Med 2018; 22(6): 3183-91.
[http://dx.doi.org/10.1111/jcmm.13599] [PMID: 29571225]

[12]   Nakashima Y, Plump AS, Raines EW, Breslow JL, Ross R. ApoE-deficient mice develop lesions of all phases of atherosclerosis throughout the arterial tree. Arterioscler Thromb 1994; 14(1): 133-40.
[http://dx.doi.org/10.1161/01.ATV.14.1.133] [PMID: 8274468]

[13]   Gomez D, Baylis RA, Durgin BG, *et al.* Interleukin-1β has atheroprotective effects in advanced atherosclerotic lesions of mice. Nat Med 2018; 24(9): 1418-29.
[http://dx.doi.org/10.1038/s41591-018-0124-5] [PMID: 30038218]

[14]   Seijkens TTP, van Tiel CM, Kusters PJH, *et al.* Targeting CD40-induced TRAF6 signaling in macrophages reduces atherosclerosis. J Am Coll Cardiol 2018; 71(5): 527-42.
[http://dx.doi.org/10.1016/j.jacc.2017.11.055] [PMID: 29406859]

[15] Jawień J, Nastałek P, Korbut R. Mouse models of experimental atherosclerosis. J Physiol Pharmacol 2004; 55(3): 503-17.
[PMID: 15381823]

[16] Wang YXJ, Martin-McNulty B, Huw LY, *et al.* Anti-atherosclerotic effect of simvastatin depends on the presence of apolipoprotein E. Atherosclerosis 2002; 162(1): 23-31.
[http://dx.doi.org/10.1016/S0021-9150(01)00678-5] [PMID: 11947894]

[17] Ishibashi S, Brown MS, Goldstein JL, Gerard RD, Hammer RE, Herz J. Hypercholesterolemia in low density lipoprotein receptor knockout mice and its reversal by adenovirus-mediated gene delivery. J Clin Invest 1993; 92(2): 883-93.
[http://dx.doi.org/10.1172/JCI116663] [PMID: 8349823]

[18] Shaw PX. Rethinking oxidized low-density lipoprotein, its role in atherogenesis and the immune responses associated with it. Archivum Immunologiae Et Therapiae Experimentalis-English Edition. 2004; 52: pp. (4)225-39.

[19] Lo Sasso G, Schlage WK, Boué S, Veljkovic E, Peitsch MC, Hoeng J. The Apoe−/− mouse model: a suitable model to study cardiovascular and respiratory diseases in the context of cigarette smoke exposure and harm reduction. J Transl Med 2016; 14(1): 146.
[http://dx.doi.org/10.1186/s12967-016-0901-1] [PMID: 27207171]

[20] Leppänen P, Luoma JS, Hofker MH, Havekes LM, Ylä-Herttuala S. Characterization of atherosclerotic lesions in apo E3-leiden transgenic mice. Atherosclerosis 1998; 136(1): 147-52.
[http://dx.doi.org/10.1016/S0021-9150(97)00196-2] [PMID: 9544741]

[21] Braun A, Zhang S, Miettinen HE, *et al.* Probucol prevents early coronary heart disease and death in the high-density lipoprotein receptor SR-BI/apolipoprotein E double knockout mouse. Proc Natl Acad Sci USA 2003; 100(12): 7283-8.
[http://dx.doi.org/10.1073/pnas.1237725100] [PMID: 12771386]

[22] Zhang S, Picard MH, Vasile E, *et al.* Diet-induced occlusive coronary atherosclerosis, myocardial infarction, cardiac dysfunction, and premature death in scavenger receptor class B type I-deficient, hypomorphic apolipoprotein ER61 mice. Circulation 2005; 111(25): 3457-64.
[http://dx.doi.org/10.1161/CIRCULATIONAHA.104.523563] [PMID: 15967843]

[23] Lee GH, Proenca R, Montez JM, *et al.* Abnormal splicing of the leptin receptor in diabetic mice. Nature 1996; 379(6566): 632-5.
[http://dx.doi.org/10.1038/379632a0] [PMID: 8628397]

[24] Kobayashi K, Forte TM, Taniguchi S, Ishida BY, Oka K, Chan L. The db/db mouse, a model for diabetic dyslipidemia: Molecular characterization and effects of western diet feeding. Metabolism 2000; 49(1): 22-31.
[http://dx.doi.org/10.1016/S0026-0495(00)90588-2] [PMID: 10647060]

[25] Kong L, Wu H, Cui W, *et al.* Advances in murine models of diabetic nephropathy. J Diabetes Res 2013; 2013: 1-10.
[http://dx.doi.org/10.1155/2013/797548] [PMID: 23844375]

[26] Lindström P. The physiology of obese-hyperglycemic mice [ob/ob mice]. ScientificWorldJournal 2007; 7: 666-85.
[http://dx.doi.org/10.1100/tsw.2007.117] [PMID: 17619751]

[27] Sathibabu Uddandrao VV, Brahmanaidu P, Ravindarnaik R, Suresh P, Vadivukkarasi S, Saravanan G. Restorative potentiality of S-allylcysteine against diabetic nephropathy through attenuation of oxidative stress and inflammation in streptozotocin–nicotinamide-induced diabetic rats. Eur J Nutr 2019; 58(6): 2425-37.
[http://dx.doi.org/10.1007/s00394-018-1795-x] [PMID: 30062492]

[28] Uddandrao VVS, Parim B, Ramavat R, *et al.* Effect of S-allylcysteine against diabetic nephropathy *via* inhibition of MEK1/2-ERK1/2-RSK2 signalling pathway in streptozotocin-nicotinamide-induced

diabetic rats. Arch Physiol Biochem 2020; 1-9.
[http://dx.doi.org/10.1080/13813455.2020.1811731] [PMID: 32862702]

[29] Naidu PB, Sathibabu Uddandrao VV, Naik RR, *et al.* Effects of S-Allylcysteine on Biomarkers of the Polyol Pathway in Rats with Type 2 Diabetes. Can J Diabetes 2016; 40(5): 442-8.
[http://dx.doi.org/10.1016/j.jcjd.2016.03.006] [PMID: 27373435]

[30] Zucker LM, Zucker TF. Fatty, a new mutation in the rat. J Hered 1961; 52(6): 275-8.
[http://dx.doi.org/10.1093/oxfordjournals.jhered.a107093]

[31] Kava R, Greenwood MRC, Johnson PR. Zucker (fa/fa) Rat. ILAR J 1990; 32(3): 4-8.
[http://dx.doi.org/10.1093/ilar.32.3.4]

[32] Chua SC Jr, White DW, Wu-Peng XS, *et al.* Phenotype of fatty due to Gln269Pro mutation in the leptin receptor (Lepr). Diabetes 1996; 45(8): 1141-3.
[http://dx.doi.org/10.2337/diab.45.8.1141] [PMID: 8690163]

[33] Friedman JE, de Venté JE, Peterson RG, Dohm GL. Altered expression of muscle glucose transporter GLUT-4 in diabetic fatty Zucker rats (ZDF/Drt-fa). Am J Physiol 1991; 261(6 Pt 1): E782-8.
[PMID: 1767839]

[34] Wohlfart P, Lin J, Dietrich N, *et al.* Expression patterning reveals retinal inflammation as a minor factor in experimental retinopathy of ZDF rats. Acta Diabetol 2014; 51(4): 553-8.
[http://dx.doi.org/10.1007/s00592-013-0550-2] [PMID: 24477469]

[35] Yokoi N, Hoshino M, Hidaka S, *et al.* A novel rat model of type 2 diabetes: the Zucker fatty diabetes mellitus ZFDM rat. J Diabetes Res 2013; 2013: 1-9.
[http://dx.doi.org/10.1155/2013/103731] [PMID: 23671847]

[36] Goto Y, Kakizaki M. The spontaneous-diabetes rat: A model of noninsulin dependent diabetes mellitus. Proc Jpn Acad, Ser B, Phys Biol Sci 1981; 57(10): 381-4.
[http://dx.doi.org/10.2183/pjab.57.381]

[37] Portha B, Giroix MH, Tourrel-Cuzin C, Le-Stunff H, Movassat J. The GK rat: a prototype for the study of non-overweight type 2 diabetes. Ani Models in Diab Res 2012; 933: 125-59.
[http://dx.doi.org/10.1007/978-1-62703-068-7_9] [PMID: 22893405]

[38] Harishankar N, Vajreswari A, Giridharan NV. WNIN/GR-Ob - an insulin-resistant obese rat model from inbred WNIN strain. Indian J Med Res 2011; 134(3): 320-9.
[PMID: 21985815]

[39] Liao J, Huang W, Liu G. Animal models of coronary heart disease. Biomed Res J 2017; 31(1): 3.

[40] Giridharan NV. Glucose & energy homeostasis: Lessons from animal studies. Indian J Med Res 2018; 148(5): 659-69.
[http://dx.doi.org/10.4103/ijmr.IJMR_1737_18] [PMID: 30666991]

[41] Pleger ST, Most P, Boucher M, *et al.* Stable myocardial-specific AAV6-S100A1 gene therapy results in chronic functional heart failure rescue. Circulation 2007; 115(19): 2506-15.
[http://dx.doi.org/10.1161/CIRCULATIONAHA.106.671701] [PMID: 17470693]

[42] Patten RD, Hall-Porter MR. Small animal models of heart failure: development of novel therapies, past and present. Circ Heart Fail 2009; 2(2): 138-44.
[http://dx.doi.org/10.1161/CIRCHEARTFAILURE.108.839761] [PMID: 19808329]

[43] Miyamoto MI, del Monte F, Schmidt U, *et al.* Adenoviral gene transfer of SERCA2a improves left ventricular function in aortic-banded rats in transition to heart failure. Proc Natl Acad Sci USA 2000; 97(2): 793-8.
[http://dx.doi.org/10.1073/pnas.97.2.793] [PMID: 10639159]

[44] Breckenridge R. Heart failure and mouse models. Dis Model Mech 2010; 3(3-4): 138-43.
[http://dx.doi.org/10.1242/dmm.005017] [PMID: 20212081]

[45] https://www.criver.com/sites/default/files/resource-files/Left-Coronary-Artery-Ligation.pdf

[46] Weinberg EO, Schoen FJ, George D, *et al.* Angiotensin-converting enzyme inhibition prolongs survival and modifies the transition to heart failure in rats with pressure overload hypertrophy due to ascending aortic stenosis. Circulation 1994; 90(3): 1410-22.
[http://dx.doi.org/10.1161/01.CIR.90.3.1410] [PMID: 8087951]

[47] Nakahara T, Tanimoto T, Petrov AD, Ishikawa K, Strauss HW, Narula J. Rat model of cardiotoxic drug-induced cardiomyopathy. Experimental Models of Cardiovascular Diseases. New York, NY: Humana Press 2018; pp. 221-32.
[http://dx.doi.org/10.1007/978-1-4939-8597-5_17]

[48] Hearse DJ, Sutherland FJ. Experimental models for the study of cardiovascular function and disease. Pharmacol Res 2000; 41(6): 597-603.
[http://dx.doi.org/10.1006/phrs.1999.0651] [PMID: 10816328]

[49] Ganderup NC, Harvey W, Mortensen JT, Harrouk W. The minipig as nonrodent species in toxicology--where are we now? Int J Toxicol 2012; 31(6): 507-28.
[http://dx.doi.org/10.1177/1091581812462039] [PMID: 23134714]

[50] Milani-Nejad N, Janssen PML. Small and large animal models in cardiac contraction research: Advantages and disadvantages. Pharmacol Ther 2014; 141(3): 235-49.
[http://dx.doi.org/10.1016/j.pharmthera.2013.10.007] [PMID: 24140081]

[51] Swindle MM, Makin A, Herron AJ, Clubb FJ Jr, Frazier KS. Swine as models in biomedical research and toxicology testing. Vet Pathol 2012; 49(2): 344-56.
[http://dx.doi.org/10.1177/0300985811402846] [PMID: 21441112]

[52] Mersman H. The pig: a concise source of information.Swine in Cardiovascular Research, A Comparative Anatomic and Physiologic Overview of the Porcine Heart. Boca Raton, FL: CRC Press 1986; Vol. 1: pp. 1-9.

[53] Crick SJ, Sheppard MN, Ho SY, Gebstein L, Anderson RH. Anatomy of the pig heart: comparisons with normal human cardiac structure. J Anat 1998; 193(1): 105-19.
[http://dx.doi.org/10.1046/j.1469-7580.1998.19310105.x] [PMID: 9758141]

[54] Xanthos T, Bassiakou E, Koudouna E, *et al.* Baseline hemodynamics in anesthetized landrace-large white swine: reference values for research in cardiac arrest and cardiopulmonary resuscitation models. J Am Assoc Lab Anim Sci 2007; 46(5): 21-5.
[PMID: 17877323]

[55] Lelovas PP, Kostomitsopoulos NG, Xanthos TT. A comparative anatomic and physiologic overview of the porcine heart. J Am Assoc Lab Anim Sci 2014; 53(5): 432-8.
[PMID: 25255064]

[56] Hamamdzic D, Wilensky RL. Porcine models of accelerated coronary atherosclerosis: role of diabetes mellitus and hypercholesterolemia. J Diabetes Res 2013; 2013: 1-7.
[http://dx.doi.org/10.1155/2013/761415] [PMID: 23844374]

[57] Granada J, Kaluza G, Wilensky R, Biedermann B, Schwartz R, Falk E. Porcine models of coronary atherosclerosis and vulnerable plaque for imaging and interventional research. EuroIntervention 2009; 5(1): 140-8.
[http://dx.doi.org/10.4244/EIJV5I1A22] [PMID: 19577996]

[58] Crisóstomo V, Sun F, Maynar M, *et al.* Common swine models of cardiovascular disease for research and training. Lab Anim (NY) 2016; 45(2): 67-74.
[http://dx.doi.org/10.1038/laban.935] [PMID: 26814353]

[59] Gerrity RG, Natarajan R, Nadler JL, Kimsey T. Diabetes-induced accelerated atherosclerosis in swine. Diabetes 2001; 50(7): 1654-65.
[http://dx.doi.org/10.2337/diabetes.50.7.1654] [PMID: 11423488]

[60] Hasler-Rapacz JO, Nichols TC, Griggs TR, Bellinger DA, Rapacz J. Familial and diet-induced hypercholesterolemia in swine. Lipid, ApoB, and ApoA-I concentrations and distributions in plasma

and lipoprotein subfractions. Arterioscler Thromb 1994; 14(6): 923-30.
[http://dx.doi.org/10.1161/01.ATV.14.6.923] [PMID: 8199183]

[61]   Davis BT, Wang XJ, Rohret JA, *et al.* Targeted disruption of LDLR causes hypercholesterolemia and atherosclerosis in Yucatan miniature pigs. PLoS One 2014; 9(4): e93457.
[http://dx.doi.org/10.1371/journal.pone.0093457] [PMID: 24691380]

[62]   Li Y, Fuchimoto D, Sudo M, Haruta H, Lin QF, Takayama T, *et al.* Development of human-like advanced coronary plaques in low-density lipoprotein receptor knockout pigs and justification for statin treatment before formation of atherosclerotic plaques. J Am Heart Assoc 2016; 5(4): 002779.

[63]   Tahara S, Chamié D, Baibars M, Alraies C, Costa M. Optical coherence tomography endpoints in stent clinical investigations: strut coverage. Int J Cardiovasc Imaging 2011; 27(2): 271-87.
[http://dx.doi.org/10.1007/s10554-011-9796-3] [PMID: 21394615]

[64]   Won H, Kim JS, Shin DH, *et al.* Serial changes of neointimal tissue after everolimus-eluting stent implantation in porcine coronary artery: an optical coherence tomography analysis. BioMed Res Int 2014; 2014: 1-8.
[http://dx.doi.org/10.1155/2014/851676] [PMID: 25309929]

[65]   Schwartz RS, Edelman E, Virmani R, *et al.* Drug-eluting stents in preclinical studies: updated consensus recommendations for preclinical evaluation. Circ Cardiovasc Interv 2008; 1(2): 143-53.
[http://dx.doi.org/10.1161/CIRCINTERVENTIONS.108.789974] [PMID: 20031669]

[66]   Bikou O, Watanabe S, Hajjar RJ, Ishikawa K. A pig model of myocardial infarction: catheter-based approaches. Experimental Models of Cardiovascular Diseases. New York, NY: Humana Press 2018; pp. 281-94.
[http://dx.doi.org/10.1007/978-1-4939-8597-5_22]

[67]   Weaver ME, Pantely GA, Bristow JD, Ladley HD. A quantitative study of the anatomy and distribution of coronary arteries in swine in comparison with other animals and man. Cardiovasc Res 1986; 20(12): 907-17.
[http://dx.doi.org/10.1093/cvr/20.12.907] [PMID: 3802126]

[68]   Wilson JR, Douglas P, Hickey WF, *et al.* Experimental congestive heart failure produced by rapid ventricular pacing in the dog: cardiac effects. Circulation 1987; 75(4): 857-67.
[http://dx.doi.org/10.1161/01.CIR.75.4.857] [PMID: 3829344]

[69]   Sabbah HN, Stein PD, Kono T, *et al.* A canine model of chronic heart failure produced by multiple sequential coronary microembolizations. Am J Physiol 1991; 260(4 Pt 2): H1379-84.
[PMID: 1826414]

[70]   McDonald KM, Francis GS, Carlyle PF, *et al.* Hemodynamic, left ventricular structural and hormonal changes after discrete myocardial damage in the dog. J Am Coll Cardiol 1992; 19(2): 460-7.
[http://dx.doi.org/10.1016/0735-1097(92)90506-I] [PMID: 1732376]

[71]   Recchia FA, Lionetti V. Animal models of dilated cardiomyopathy for translational research. Vet Res Commun 2007; 31(S1) (Suppl. 1): 35-41.
[http://dx.doi.org/10.1007/s11259-007-0005-8] [PMID: 17682844]

[72]   Freeman LM, Rush JE. Nutrition and cardiomyopathy: Lessons from spontaneous animal models. Curr Heart Fail Rep 2007; 4(2): 84-90.
[http://dx.doi.org/10.1007/s11897-007-0005-6] [PMID: 17521500]

[73]   Basso C, Fox PR, Meurs KM, *et al.* Arrhythmogenic right ventricular cardiomyopathy causing sudden cardiac death in boxer dogs: a new animal model of human disease. Circulation 2004; 109(9): 1180-5.
[http://dx.doi.org/10.1161/01.CIR.0000118494.07530.65] [PMID: 14993138]

[74]   Cassano M, Berardi E, Crippa S, *et al.* Alteration of cardiac progenitor cell potency in GRMD dogs. Cell Transplant 2012; 21(9): 1945-67.
[http://dx.doi.org/10.3727/096368912X638919] [PMID: 22513051]

[75]   Leroux AA, Moonen ML, Pierard LA, Kolh P, Amory H. Animal models of mitral regurgitation

induced by mitral valve chordae tendineae rupture. J Heart Valve Dis 2012; 21(4): 416-23.
[PMID: 22953665]

[76]   Kelley ST, Malekan R, Gorman JH III, *et al.* Restraining infarct expansion preserves left ventricular geometry and function after acute anteroapical infarction. Circulation 1999; 99(1): 135-42.
[http://dx.doi.org/10.1161/01.CIR.99.1.135] [PMID: 9884390]

[77]   Devlin G, Matthews K, McCracken G, *et al.* An ovine model of chronic stable heart failure. J Card Fail 2000; 6(2): 140-3.
[http://dx.doi.org/10.1016/S1071-9164(00)90016-2] [PMID: 10908088]

[78]   Moorjani N, Catarino P, El-Sayed R, *et al.* A pressure overload model to track the molecular biology of heart failure. Eur J Cardiothorac Surg 2003; 24(6): 920-5.
[http://dx.doi.org/10.1016/S1010-7940(03)00514-1] [PMID: 14643809]

[79]   Byrne MJ, Raman JS, Alferness CA, Esler MD, Kaye DM, Power JM. An ovine model of tachycardia-induced degenerative dilated cardiomyopathy and heart failure with prolonged onset. J Card Fail 2002; 8(2): 108-15.
[http://dx.doi.org/10.1054/jcaf.2002.32323] [PMID: 12016635]

[80]   Emmert MY, Weber B, Wolint P, *et al.* Intramyocardial transplantation and tracking of human mesenchymal stem cells in a novel intra-uterine pre-immune fetal sheep myocardial infarction model: a proof of concept study. PLoS One 2013; 8(3): e57759.
[http://dx.doi.org/10.1371/journal.pone.0057759] [PMID: 23533575]

[81]   Killingsworth CR, Walcott GP, Gamblin TL, Girouard LTSD, Smith WM, Ideker R. Chronic myocardial infarction is a substrate for bradycardia-induced spontaneous tachyarrhythmias and sudden death in conscious animals. J Cardiovasc Electrophysiol 2006; 17(2): 189-97.
[http://dx.doi.org/10.1111/j.1540-8167.2005.00336.x] [PMID: 16533257]

Application of 21ˢᵗ Century Genetic Engineering Tools and CRISPR-Cas9 Technologies to Treat Most Advanced Cardiovascular Diseases of Humans

J. Venkateshwara Rao[1, *], R. Ravindar Naik[2], S. Venkanna[1] and **N. Ramesh Kumar[3]**

[1] *Department of Zoology, Osmania University, Hyderabad, Telangana, India*

[2] *ICMR-National Animal Resource Facility for Biomedical Research, Genome Valley, Shamir pet, Hyderabad, 500101, India*

[3] *Department of Genetics, Osmania University, Hyderabad, Telangana, India*

Abstract: 21ˢᵗ Century Genome-editing technologies have been rapidly emerging as the most powerful tool capable of creating genetically altered cells or organisms for explicit gene functions and mechanisms for causing several human ailments. While clinical gene therapy celebrates its first taste of success, with several products approved for clinical usage and several thousands of them awaiting stages in pipelines, unfortunately, there are no gene therapy treatment methods available for many cardiovascular diseases (CVD). Despite sustained medical advances over the last 50 years in CVD, the main cause of death is still uncertain in the developed world. The management of genetic expression by using small molecule RNA therapeutics and the development of accurate gene corrections may lead to several applications, such as cardiac revitalization after myocardial infarctions and gene corrections for the inherited cardiomyopathies but certainly with some limitations. CRISPR/Cas9 technology can be utilized to realign DNA modifications ranging from a single base pair to multiplepairs of mutations in both *in vitro* and *in vivo* models. This book chapter emphasizes various types of applications by CRISPR technologies in cardio-vascular research, and genome-editing novel therapies for future medicines.

Keywords: CRISPR/Cas9, Myocardial infarction, Gene Therapy, Myocardial infarction, Induced pluripotent stem cells (iPSCs).

---

* **Corresponding author J. Venkateshwara Rao:** Department of Zoology, Osmania University, Hyderabad, Telangana, India; E-mail: venbio@gmail.com

1. INTRODUCTION

Gene editing technologies are promising methods to investigate disease mechanisms at the gene level. By employing these technologies, scientists could introduce, modify or remove mutations at specific locations or points of the target gene and can make a successful model disease organism to prevent the incidence of many diseases. In 1996, the First and Second generations of Gene Technologies *i.e.*, transcription activator-like effector nucleases (TALEN's) and zinc-finger nucleases (ZFN's) evolved independently. However, the high costs and also low efficiencies involved in their procedure have restricted their accessibility and usage in various applications [1]. In 2013, CRISPR technology emerged as the 3rd generation of gene-correcting methods and has been quickly put to use by various scientists for its merits of high efficacy, speed, and cost reduction [2]. In recent times, this modern CRISPR technology has been applied to many fields such as agriculture, drug design, and discovery and medical research [3].

Exploring the genetic basis of several diseases will enable significant inputs into medical research. The successful finishing of the Human Genome Project (HGP) and the DNA sequencing knowledge extracted from several patients have allowed us to understand the relationships between genetic components and human diseases [4]. Alternations and genetic mutations in over 3000 genes that are linked to many diseases and disorders in humans have already been studied [5].

In contrast to cancer and diabetes, which are multifactorial illnesses brought on by a variety of genetic alterations and environmental factors, Huntington's disease, Thalassemia, Sickle Cell Anemia, and Cystic Fibrosis are monogenetic genetic disorders caused by the mutation of a single gene [6]. Unfortunately, there are many disorders without appropriate treatments. However, Genomic therapies can offer potential and effective therapeutic tools to fight many genetic diseases [4] and it is now the first and foremost choice of many medical practitioners and incorporates refinement of target genetic corrections by using precise gene editors. Genetic therapies sketchily include the deletion of a faulty gene or group of genetic alterations by incorporation of external DNA and correcting the changed gene at the inherent site [7]. Despite the benefits of this technology, there are several flaws and challenges associated with the applications that make the insertion of exogenous DNA risky. Some of the negative outcomes with unwanted implications include the insertion and activation of off-target gene modifications and erroneous findings generated by the induced genes. Additionally, only a few hereditary diseases are still the exclusive beneficiaries of direct applications nowadays [7].

However, gene correction creates a completely new field for modifying human genetics and gene therapy. It is a novel approach that modifies certain target sequences with alterations that are target-oriented and exact. Future research on genetically based medications may provide new therapeutic approaches for treating a variety of human ailments [7]. The primary method of gene correction involves DNA double-strand breaks (DSB) induction and endogenous cellular repair processes [8]. These cut breaks are classically repaired by either of two major pathways: Non-Homologous End Joining (NHEJ) or Homology-based repair (HDR). To target gene-editing technologies, the most critical component is the identification of precise DSB. Currently, four major methods are employed to initiate target-specific DSB's which include Zinc finger nucleases (ZFNs), engineered mega nucleases, Transcription Activator-Like Effector Nuclease (TALENs), and most recently CRISPR/Cas9 systems [7, 8]. The precise targeting of genetic changes in cultured cells, plants, and animals has been made possible by these new methods. CRISPR technologies are superior to other genome-editing techniques because they are less complicated and do not require expensive designed enzymes for each each DNA target locus [8]. In CRISPR technology, the exact results could be achieved by target-oriented RNA and a restriction enzyme mixture represented briefly as Cas9, which is one of the best and most remarkable gene-editing platforms [1]. For the past few decades, the CRISPR system is being applied to many biomedical problems, aimed at developing new curing technologies for monogenic and as well as for multi-factorial diseases [7].

Thus, CRISPR/Cas9 technology can be used in the development of various animal disease models for research purposes to represent diseases or to understand disease progress pathways, by mutating or silencing the relevant genes [2]. However, recently, the horizons of the CRISPR tool were expanded for correcting genes of human embryos as well. The path-breaking discovery of the ability to repair a mutation in the (OCT4 gene)4 octamer-binding transcription factors, a gene involved in the development of the human placenta in ahuman embryo using CRISPR/Cas9 technology, implies immense clinical potential in the future for treating human genetic diseases [3].

Although CRISPR technologies have been identified as the most successful gene therapy tools currently, some problems have surfaced like its reproducible capabilities and human ethical issues, chiefly concerning editing human germ lines [3]. Several impacts of off-side target cleavages are the primary setbacks of the target system and may restrict its usage for some of the therapeutic applications. In light of this, this review emphasizes the current state and future prospects of CRISPR uses in individualized medicine. The review also focuses on the use of CRISPR technologies as the primary therapeutic tool for a number of human diseases and disorders and summarizes its applications in gene therapies, with a focus on monogenic diseases like haemophilia, thalassemia, cystic fibrosis, *etc.*, and multifactorial diseases like diabetes, cancers, and cardiovascular diseases.

2. THE CRISPR/CAS9 PROTEIN TECHNOLOGY

The CRISPR/Cas9 complex was first observed in Escherichia coli in 1987 [9]. In 2007, the immunological mechanism of microbes was found, specifically in prokaryotic microorganisms [10]. In archaea and bacteria, the CRISPR/Cas 9 protein mechanism is a highly accurate machinery that permits the acquired immunity [11]. Doudna and her colleague Charpentier have done extensive work in developing the technique for genome editing which has brought about the creation of CRISPR technologyand were awarded a Nobel prize in 2020 [1]. Especially in several microbes, CRISPR technology is represented by gene location, where it provides information about acquired immunity, which is invaded by manymicroorganisms, viruses, and bacterial plasmids by directing nucleic acids in specific locations. Similar activities draw attention to the creation of highly precise and strong immunological barriers against a similar type of infections inside the cell. It is extremely surprising to know that a cell has some memory before every infection [12]. In the period when a microbe infected by an external DNA- bearing entity, incorporated with exogenous DNA, forms non-contagious repeats or tandems separated by variable special sequences known as spacers [13]. When such microbes are repeatedly targeted by viruses or bacteria-bearing entities of the CRISPR sequences will help in the creation of complementary (cRNA) genes by using the already inserted sequences. The complementary RNA which is created for adaptive immunity has two components, *viz.*, the CrRNA (CRISPR RNA) and the trans-activating RNA (tracrRNA) [9]. These two make highly specific splicing mechanisms. The tracer element of CRISPER helps to mature crRNA and helps the CRISPR/Cas9related (Cas) proteins to spot the target with a complementary strand of DNA. The entire RNA complex acts as a guide to the Cas9 protein complex to reach the target site and helps in the splicing of DNA at the precise site locations,thereby eliminating the incorporation of the external DNA molecule into the main genomic content of microorganisms.

The creation of blunt-edged DSB at onsite locations in external genes helps in achieving its target. Once the DSB is created, the cell will guide the DNA to overhaul itself by choosing one of the two pathways to prevent further damage prevalent to DNA moleculesinthe outside environment [9]. At this moment, the molecular mechanisms will command the cell to proceed with the NHEJ (Non-homologous end-joining of fragments) or with HDR (Homology- directed repairing mechanisms). While the former is a fast and modest process that essentially permits the separated components of the DNA molecule to bind to each other, it is far less efficient and can make more errors due to the frame-shift mutations [14].

By trendyin a recordnumber of the cases, the cell chooses to follow the homology-directed repair mechanism which works well with high accuracy and indulges in the use of homologue DNA or gene template molecule. By using double chromosomes or depending on the diploidcharacter of the cells, this procedurecan be implemented effortlessly and can also be artificially stimulated in living cells, to activate the CRISPR technologies [15].

Another mechanism employed for repairing DSB is the micro homology-mediated base paring method [16]. Such a repairing mechanism is present in association with alternate with NHEJ mechanisms which may not depend on Ku protein functions or recombination factors [17]. In addition to what was said above, CRISPER's micro homology-based base-pairing technique has created effective marking and identification mechanisms that will aid in the routine evaluation of the native proteins found in cells [18].

3. APPLICATION OF CRISPR/CAS9 TECHNOLOGY AS A THERAPEUTIC TOOL FOR HUMAN DISEASES

Two key factors have been taken into consideration while introducing CRISPR technology to the biomedical sector. One is the diagnosis of diseases, and the other is the treatment of illnesses with hereditary linkages [19]. CRISPR technologies are used in a variety of sectors and have been studied utilising this technology within the animal models, and as a result, its potential is now acknowledged on a global scale [20]. In addition, the use of genome editing tools severely competes with natural genome editing itself. Chen and his colleagues [21] have represented that this system may be used for the determination of the visualization of genes and associated key elements. Their efforts on telomers and sub-nuclear location of membrane mucin gene (MUC4) clearly reveal the dynamic behavior of MUC4 loci on sister chromatids. This will give a clear picture of the recombinations during chromatid exchange.

3.1. Cystic Fibrosis (CF)

The genetic anomaly or condition is characterised by abnormally high levels of sticky liquid discharges in the liver and pancreas' blood vessels as well as in the lungs' air passages [21 - 24]. Multiple organ dysfunctions brought on by CF occur together with significant airway blockage in the lungs when a person passes away

[24]. CF is mainly caused by changes in the cystic-fibrosis transmembrane (CFTR) genes [25, 26] and the electrolytic homeostasis of epithelial cells is disrupted by mutations in CFTR proteins which function as the main channel of anions, which in turn can be controlled by kinase-A-dependent phosphorylation in the cell membrane. The stability of the CFTR gene is impaired by the deletion of homozygous F508 loci, which leads to deletion at position 508 of phenylalanine in the nucleotide attachment domain that thereafter affects the protein refolding mechanisms, functions, expressions, and stabilities of the CFTR gene [27]. The mutation in F508 is successfully corrected by CRISPR/Ca9-mediated homologous recombination in intestinal stem cells extracted from CF patients and displays the capacity of a changed allele in the organoid system. The CFTR exon 11/intron 11 were targeted by single-guide RNAs (sgRNAs) with a contributor plasmid encoding wild or raw type CFTR sequences in patient organoids *i.e.*, small, and large intestines. This study was used as proof to study the safety of clinical studies [28, 29].

3.2. Sickle Cell Anemia

(SCA) is a serious monogenic type of disorder that results in irregular sickle cell-shaped erythrocytes. The sickle cells are severely affected due to diminished oxygen-carrying capacity, resulting in the total impairment of the functionality of red blood cells [30]. A single point mutation of the β-haemoglobin gene (HBB) responsible for causing SCA is characterized by a sickle form of hemoglobin (HbS) protein. A Single Nucleotide mutation (SNP) from A to T in the codon of the 6th amino acid replaces Glutamic acid (Glu) withValine (Val), and this modification is responsible for HbS [31]. Thus, in this case, genome editing is to be recommended to repair the HbS protein by the new therapy. The CRISPR is a well-proved gene-editing technology and has resulted in over 18% of gene modifications in blood marrow-derived CD34[+] cells procured from the SCA patients *in vitro*. Similarly, CRISPR technology has also set adjusted bone marrow-derived CD34[+] hemopoietic stem and progenitor cells from sickle cell patients in making a native type of hemoglobin. Initially, CRISPR has an advanced impact on β-globin gene damage compared with TALENs, which was analyzed by genome modifying tools [32]. An Optimized CRISPR/Cas9 system was developed by Park *et al* [31] to attain nearly 30% HDF in CD34[+] cells. Additionally, the efficiency of correction has been further increased by the optimization of the CRISPR technique to produce wild-type β-globin. The CRISPR technologies can be used to correct Glu to Val mutation which causes sickle cell disease, by using patient-derived stem and progenitor cells. This new type of homologous recombination method on HBB predicts successful therapies for β-hemoglobinopathies [33].

3.3. Thalassemia

The most common genetic disorder categorized by the reduction or absence of production of subunit β (HB β -chain) of hemoglobin (HB) is β-thalassemia, which has a worldwide distribution [34]. More than 200 different point mutations are responsible for causing thalassemia diseases but it is rare to see deletions in the HBB gene [34]. In Southeast Asians, the (C>T) IVS2-654 mutation is quite common. A site-specific correction can be attained by the patient-derived iPSc using the CRISPR method [35 - 37]. Similarly, CD41/42 mutations can be corrected by CRISPR/Cas9 in β-al iPSCs. The total exome sequencing has revealed that the mutation burden is minimum after treatment with CRISPR/CAS9, reserved full pluripotency, and exhibited a normal karyotype. The human native iPSCs extracted from the urinary cells of β thalassemia patients are treated with CRISPR/Cas9 technology. The native iPSCs demonstrated more gene correction capabilities than primed iPSCs. The native iPSCs were highly qualified for hematopoietic cell differentiation capabilities, thereby providing an outstanding source for additional clinical applications [38]. The HBB mutations were successfully fixed in iPSCs isolated from thalassemia patients using CRISPR/Cas9 and Piggy/Bac transposon systems. This method of correction is a surprising accomplishment; there were no off-target effects, and the cells demonstrated regular karyotypes with complete pluripotency [39]. The CRISPR technique is the most promising technology being utilised to correct iPSC cells' β-cells and enhance patients' hematopoietic capacities [40]. The updated β-al cells showed normal karyotypes, complete pluripotency as hESCs, and predominantly did not show any non-targets with a full reestablishment for HBB expression in comparison to controls [40].

3.4. Huntington's Disease

(HD) is a dominant autosomal, advanced neurogenerative disease exhibiting specific phenotypic expressions including dystonia, non-coordination, chorea, deterioration of cognitive functions, and interactive disorders [41]. HD is primarily triggered by repeated expressions of CAG present in the hunting gene (HTT), which results in an elongated polyglutamine chain tract in Huntington's protein [42]. The latest advancements in research show the use of genetic tool kits to counteract or deactivate the HTT mutant gene which is responsible for triggering the disease. Tailored personalized development of CRISPR/Cas9 technology should be used to selectively study the mutated gene responsible for HD, effectively implementing it in a person with an allele-dominant gene associated with HD disease. This personalized system relies heavily on the usage of double gRNA/PAM (protospacer adjacent motifs)-modifying SNP-platform linked allele-specific CRISPR system, to carry out knockout of gene mutations. Transcription of mutant HTT mRNA can be selectively prevented by using PAM-altered mutant varieties. The strong need for personalized treatment is revealed by haplotypes associated with HD [43]. Research efforts were made to separate and overexpress the HD gene with positive outcomes [44]. The existence of SNPs has made scientists opt to utilize CRISPR/Cas9 technologies in the HTT locus to lower the expression levels of mutant HTT in genetic alleles in HD fibroblast [45]. After allele-specific HTT expression of exon-1 is eliminated by SNP encouraged in the removal of N-terminal & C-terminal protein portions, the promoter of HTT is associated with a common set of guides in the region of intron-1. The sgRNA and Cas9 complexes are quite effective in treating *in vivo* HD animal models, nevertheless [46]. It has been observed that inactivating the HTT gene causes embryonic fatalities in mice, although CRISPR-based therapeutic approaches eliminated HTT expressions and decreased early neuropathology.

3.5. Duchenne Muscular Dystrophy

(DMD) is another fatal recessive X-linked degenerative disease [47], for which a mutation in the dystrophin gene is responsible [43]. The dystrophin gene was knocked-out effectively by employing CRISPR technologies through iPSC's from sick persons [48]. By using multiplex gene-editing capabilities, the capability of CRISPR technologies enables a single, enormous piece of deletion that can cure up to 62% of the flaws in DMD-related mutations. The exon region may be targeted using CRISPR technology to create shifts within exons or reduce deletions in one or more exons, allowing for the simultaneous emergence of a shared phenotype in human myoblasts [48]. By employing CRISPR to remove the exon region from a patient's generated iPSCs, the dystrophin protein can be restored. Skeletal muscle cells from developed iPSCs using CRISPR showed full-length expression of the dystrophin protein [24].

3.6. Hemophilia

is an X-linked genetic illness that has two kinds, Hemophilia A and Hemophilia B. These disorders are identified by a deficiency in the blood clotting proteins VIII & IX, respectively [49]. The F8 gene's intron 1 and intron 22 inversions (140 kbp and 600 kbp, respectively) are thought to cause the most severe haemophilia cases. CRISPR techniques have effectively repaired the mutations detected in the F8 area, returning chromosomal to WT conditions in iPSCs produced from patients [50]. Hemophilia B's severe form is caused by the Y371S mutation, which has been rectified by a mutation at the Y371D location in the human F9 locus of the gene. This mutation is revised by CRISPR in mice disease models and is widely acknowledged as being highly potent in therapeutic innovations [51].

3.7. Chronic Granulomatous Disorders (CGD)

are immunological deficiencies that are often observed and characterized by defective phagocytes that are incapable of producing reactive oxygen species (ROS) and NADPH-based oxidase [52]. As a result, phagocytic cells may lose their ability to eliminate infectious microorganisms including bacteria, viruses, and fungi that lead to infections and chronic inflammations and may endanger the lives of patients [53]. The majority of cases of CGD fall into one of two categories, with the first being X-linked granulomatous disease, which accounts for 65–70% of deaths in the United States and is caused by an X-linked chromosomal mutation connected to the gp91 phox gene [54]. A collection of changes associated to the p40phox, p22phox, p67phox, and p47phox genes cause the second condition, a chronic granulomatous autosomal disease, to appear [55].

Keller [56] conducted extensive studies to treat CGD in association with gene therapy methods for years. By using CRISPR/Cas9 technologies to correct endogenous genes through homologous mending processes, Flynn *et al.* [57] sought to cure CGD in 2015. In iPS-derived phagocytes extracted from a CGD individual who was suffocating due to an intron-based alteration in the gene CYBB using CRISPR/Cas9 technology, successful repair of oxidative volumes was found. A recent academic study [58] by De Ravin *et al.* used CRISPR/Cas9 technology to address changes in the blood stem cells of CGD patients.

4. MULTIFACTORIAL DISEASES

Monogenic illnesses are already complex, but multifactorial disorders are considerably more so. A significant portion of deaths globally are caused by multifactorial illnesses including cancer, diabetes, and mostly cardiovascular diseases, which we shall cover in this chapter. According to Todd's definition [59], the incidence of the disease is a plausible interplay of environment alleles at several loci interspersed across the length of the genome. Therefore, due to the very complicated nature of these illnesses, the intense study should be concentrated on treating this condition in order to find the best preventative measures. With new capabilities that provide new promise for effectively resolving many questions in this area, CRISPR/Cas9 has come along as a blessing in this circumstance.

4.1. Cancer

Contrary to monogenetic illnesses, cancer is characterised by a large number of genetic alterations and a series of serial genome changes that result in uncontrolled cell proliferation, a reduction in apoptosis, and changes in the epigenetic controls of gene expression [60, 61]. In their ground-breaking study, Hu *et al.* [62] examined the high-risk papillomavirus (HP-HPV), a serious hazard and the primary cause of human cervical cancer. Modifications connected to the E6 or E7 genes, which are primarily responsible for controlling cancer's malignant tendencies, are brought on by HPV infection [63, 64]. The apoptotic process and regulation of HPV-positive Caski and SiHa cells, but not HPV-negative HEK293 and C33A cells, were clearly promoted by the use of CRISPR technologies (HPV16-E7 combined with guided RNA-CRISPR), which destroyed the DNA of HPV16 loci E7 at specific sites.

4.2. Cardiovascular Diseases (CVD)

The leading cause of disease and mortality worldwide continues to be cardiovascular diseases. The most recent statistical analyses show that 31% of global causalities are attributable to CVD alone. In the USA, there were 900,000 recorded fatalities in 2017 from CVD alone. To put it bluntly, 1 in 3 fatalities are caused by CVD [65]. In this aspect, the diseases were ratified and remodeled using genomic and therapeutic tools, with the construction of animal models playing a major role. By designing research mice models to understand illness prediction and pathogenesis information related to CVD, the use of the CRISPR/Cas9 processes has increased optimism. ApoE (Apolipoprotein E) and LDLR (low-density lipoprotein receptor) genes were concurrently targeted by the use of the CRISPR system, and the knockout organisms are produced in one leap, thus creating a role model to study CVD [66 - 69]. Studies have received a lot of assistance to clarify and modify mutations linked to a high prevalence of CVD.

Proprotein convertase subtilisin/kexin type 9 (PCSK9) gene was discovered to be the cause of elevated blood levels of PCSK9 proteins, which in turn causes a high production of low-density lipoprotein cholesterol (LDL-C) by acting provocatively on LDL-located receptors, which was observed to be a positively changed form with loss of functionalities. By adopting these two points, they make highly specific splicing mechanisms. LDL levels have been found reduced due to the functional loss in the PCSK9 gene and the therapy using this method is more than 50% successful. It reduced glucose levels in plasma by 30-40%. Further, there are virtually no threats of off-target mutations in 10 selected sites [70]. The revised version of CRISRR/Cas9, known as Base Editor 3 (BE3), was introduced in February 2018 and offers a variety of features. The bases of genomes may be changed with great ease using base editors, which can switch cytosine to thymine and vice versa at specific sites. Using a gene-editing technique, the function of the Angiopoietin-like 3 gene (ANFPTL3) is eliminated with little blood TGA and LDL levels and a low-level congenital heart diseases (CHD) threat [71].

5. APPLICATIONS OF CRISPR/CAS9 IN CARDIAC RESEARCH

Genetic variations are mainly responsible for cardiac diseases. In adult patients, it is very difficult to assess the role of specific mutations relating to the environment and responsible for the pathogenesis of cardiac diseases. Currently, with the CRISPR/Cas9 genome-editing technologies, we can identify the disease-involving genes responsible for congenital heart diseases such as Fallor's teratology and acquired coronary heart diseases. CRISPR/Cas9 is the only system that runs at a low cost and has highly efficient platforms to investigate the genetic regulatory mechanisms in CVD, offering deep insights into genes in CHD. The most common birth defects include Atrioventricular canal defects and pulmonary atresia, which involve a series of location-based heart defects, especially in Cyanotic congenital heart disease. Heart development is clearly studied in the animal models like Zebrafish. It is a see-through fetus that allows pinpoint reflection in the larval heart and provides an easy understanding of several cardiac inputs. Knock-out of the mmp21 gene was observed in Zebra Fish in 2015 by CRISPR gene technology. Mainly heart-twisting defects were found in these models, suggesting that mmp21 is the most useful for the proper growth of cardiac structures [72, 73]. The developmental process of the heart in mutant zebrafish was observed on a real-time basis by researchers and heart lopping demerits were observed between 1- 2 hours post-fertilisation. Similarly, in the same year, the Dab2 locus in Zebrafish was targeted to elucidate the functional role of Dab2 in the proliferation of cardiomyocytes, besides differentiation [74].

Researchers are successfully applying CRISPR/Cas9 to more than one target simultaneously using s1-pr2 and s-pns2, which encode for the transporter and receptors of sphingosine-1 phosphate (S1-P) respectively. In genetically modified embryos, both genes are crucial for proper cardiac development with combined cardiac phenotypes as expected [19, 75, 76]. Valvular heart disease (VHD) is one of the common cardiac diseases apart from cyanotic congenital heart diseases connected to dysplasia of cardiac structures [20]. In 2017, induced pluripotent stem cells (iPSCs), a derivation of myocardial cells, destroyed the production of GATA4 by severely impairing the function of endothelial cells converting into typical mesenchymal cells, which is the key process throughout the embryonic stage of the heart [22]. Long QT-syndrome (LQTS) is a well-known inherited arrhythmia that can be diagnosed in iPSCs by using CRISPR/Cas9 technology. Prolongation of action potential in myocardial cells caused the destruction of activity of normal channels in patients and those whose electrocardiograms are characterized by extended QT interphase have shown similarities. Genetic testing is the most acceptable methodology for the diagnosis and prediction of LQTS and more than 15 subsets of this disease have already been diagnosed by these methods, as traditional examinations cannot properly diagnose LQTS.

The hERG-based channel gene KCNH2 that codes for myocardial cells, which are separated from iPSCs from diagnosis of variations with questionable diagnosis, has mutations at the T9831 location. Editing extended densities of hERG K+ and shortening the action potential length allowed researchers to explore the mechanics of LQTS. Utilizing these verified mutations, the study generated probable LQTS [29]. A large number of loci in genes [77] related to coronary heart disease were identified by using Genome-wide association studies (GWAS). The beginning of coronary disease has a large inclination to familial combinations. CRISPR/Cas9 technology mainly aids in the recognition of the target gene in those particular locations. In 2019, researchers used CRISPR-based technologies to delete a gene associated with the TNF-sensitive regulatory factor and analyse how AIDA influences atherosclerosis in patients [31].

5.1. Gene Therapy for CVD

The fast development of CRISPR/Cas9 platforms offers abundant opportunities for genetic therapy, including correction of mutant genes or interfering functions of disease-causing genes. The target gene therapy-based treatments are not only limited to cardiomyocytes but extended to the fetus, endothelial-based cells, and smooth muscle fibers which are the main agents involved in the formation of the heart system. One of the most common and sudden causes of death in humans is hypertrophic cardiomyopathy. Mutations in the MYBPC3 gene are responsible for these diseases [78]. The correction of mutations in MYBPC3 was attempted by a group of scientists in 2017 by CRISPR/Cas9- based technology in human embryos [36]. The amalgamations of sperms from males transferring a mutated MYBPC3 gene and similarly ova donated by healthy women have resulted in healthy embryos without any in-born defects of the disease. Homology-directed repair, along with CRISPR/Cas9 technologies, has resulted in the formation of DSBs which are helpful in recombination. This kind of practice is mainly at the laboratory stage of development at present, but mutation-based genes were completely rectified and off-target side effects are rare, even though uncertainties are still there in editing embryos.

Many researchers have experimented with gene corrections in matured cardiomyocytes to observe the evolution of cardiac diseases. Gene mutations were found to be the major source of arrhythmia. Sudden occurrence of arrhythmia can be to some extent prevented through outdated therapies like anti-arrhythmia drugs or electrophysiological therapies. Now, CRISPR/Cas9 technologies have been developed to cure arrhythmia in experimental animals *in vivo* on an accurate basis. The cardiac syndrome is a dominant autosomal disease, caused by the mutations in the loci of H530Rpresent in the PRKAG-2 gene loci by the non-catalytic of sub-unit Gamma-2 of (PRKAG-2), which is activated by protein-kinase AMP. The gene PRKAG-2 is responsible for a cardiac disorder, which progresses toward ventricular fibrillation, a highly fatal form of arrhythmia [37].

Researchers have successfully corrected this mutation by using an injection of CRISPR-based adeno-associated virus (AAV)-based transfer system by a knockout mutation in H530R / PRKAG2 regions in mice in 2016 and restored the function of the heart. This is a commendable achievement in replacing traditional therapies because classical heart transplantations are extremely costly and fraught with substantial risk during surgeries [38]. These experiments were conducted in post-natal mice easier than in the earlier stage of embryos, which was less challenging and closer to real-time situations. AVV is the most capable vector for gene delivery in cardiac-based research works. It has the capability of continuous expression in cardiac muscle cells and at the same time, has a very little inflammatory reaction, compared to adenovirus vectors. In modern times, scientists have found several ways to use the variants of the AVV, of which AAV9 is one of the most suitable transferring vehicles to infect cardiomyocytes. Apart from using cardiomyocytes for gene editing by the CRISPR/Cas9 system, some extra cells related to cardiac diseases such as smooth muscle cells or endothelial cells are suitable target candidates for gene therapy Necrotic cardiomyocytes cannot be regenerated by scientists in laboratories but the beginning of coronary heart disease may be reversed by using gene correction technology by bringing them into a low lipoprotein range. Low-density lipoprotein cholesterol levels can be inhibited by using pro-protein convertase (PCSK9) subtilisin/kexin type 9, which plays a key role in the metabolic regulation of the liver [39].

A reduction in the blood cholesterol level approximately by 30% without off-target effects was observed in 2014 by scientists by introducing loss of function-based mutation in the PCSK9 gene into the liver cells of mice through adenoviral-based CRISPR technologies. The target of making PCSK9 disruption can be achieved by NHEJ, which was demonstrated by an effective procedure in monkeys and mice [43]. It was found that the capability of gene editing by CRISPR/Cas9 is more than 50%, making it ready for future applications. Lipid-like nanoparticles are another approach used by other scientists to introduce mutated genes through CRISPR technologies into the liver cells [44]. This latest tool raises the immunogenicity of the AVV, but the range of Pcsk9 gene expression changes considerably in gene-corrected mice, which confirms that the trustworthiness of this new carrier vehicle should be improved in the near future. The suppression of the agnoprotein-like 3 (ANGPLT3) gene can lead to a lowering of cholesterol, indicating that the lipoprotein lipase inhibitors may be responsible for the rise of cholesterol levels in the blood. Chadwick and co-workers presented the mutated function loss of the Ang-ptl3 gene by using an ADV-based vector platform using CRISPR in 5-week-old mice, which showed much lesser levels of cholesterol production than Pcsk9-based mice [79].

5.2. The Future of CRISPR/Cas9 Genome Editing in Cardiac Research

Cardiac research was accelerated by using CRISPR/Cas9 technology [48]. The technology is causing a boom in the field of cardiac tissue engineering to facilitate further applications. Most of the organs used for transplantation nowadays come from terminally ill patients or accidental deaths. PERV, an endogenous retrovirus, has hindered clinical applications in pigs for porcine-based organs because of the potential risks of immune rejections after transplantations. Inactivation of whole-genome PERV was achieved by Luhan Yang in 2017 using CIRSPR technology, which prohibited viral infection and condensed safety issues concerned with pig organs for Xeno transplantations [50]. It was assumed that the dangers involved in eno transplantations with pig organs are greatly lowered because of the CRISPR technology-based editing technologies and a large number of clinical trials have been performed in monkeys for further studies.

In general, in modern times, there is much controversy and prophecies relating to genome-editing technologies. Off-target effects are one of the challenging issues in genome-editing technologies. The design of sgRNA may bind with the off-target DNA sequences, thereby familiarizing unpredictable gene mutations [57, 80]. Thus, off-targeting may promote high instabilities in genes and disrupt the functionalities of the normal genome [59]. Scientists are trying several ways to address a similar set of problems. Banasik and co-workers worked on the precise identification of off- target destruction by employing (LDLVs) integrase defective lentiviral vectors, which are more practical and active than *in silico* predictions or *in vitro* selections [23, 80, 81]. Skanner and Huang further improvised the CRISPR technology by employing a double strategy, in which paired sgRNAs were modelled and PAM applied *in toto* from tail-to-tail orientations [25]. A new Cas9- based protein was discovered in Staphylococcus aureus instead of Pyogenic coccus by the team led by Feng Zhang, which has more enhanced specificity toward the target locus [82]. A novel method known as " Prime Editing" was developed by Dravid Liu and his team recently, to deal with such problems. This method is a combination of the prime editing base guide of RNA comprising sgRNA and RNA-based template and engineered by Cas9 with reverse transcriptase enzyme as a fusion protein, used for target site on reverse transcription [30]. The Cas9 and sgRNA-enabled technologies enable the precise cleavage of single-strand and reverse transcriptase-introduced mutations according to the sequence aligned in the RNA template. DNA cleavage followed by repair will help us modify the sequence of the complementary strands.

Theoretically, this method can correct 90% of the diseases promoting mutations in human beings by its accuracy, efficiency, and fewer non-target effects, compared to classical homology-directed repair (HDR) mechanisms. The improvements in these methods will help us develop novel and much safer genome editing tools which will directly employ Cas9-grounded technologies for clinical usage in the near future. The origins of CCR5-edited babies in 2018 sounded an alarm in the contemporary scientific world concerning modifications of human embryos and raised ethical concerns. Germ cell gene-editing is different from somatic cell gene-editing because any mutations in reproductive cells could be transmitted to the next generations, which can be unquestionably dangerous to them. There is still huge scope for clinical application by using gene-correcting technologies in humans. Updated rules and regulations should be implemented for the right use of these technologies to avoid unethical exploitation of these advanced technologies [83].

6. CHALLENGES OF APPLICATION OF CRISPR/CAS9

Gaps and inefficient delivery methods, off-target effects, and human ethical considerations have been recognized as the major barriers to spreading CRISPR/Cas9 technologies in medical applications [84].

6.1. Delivery Systems of CRISPR/Cas9

The transport of CRISPR technologies to the target cells is the biggest challenge for the system. The major advantages of the CRISPR/Cas9 tool are effective delivery of mutated genes, and ensuring that the desired tissue or cell is reached by this method [83]. Many viral or physical methods were explored for the effective delivery of CRISPR-engineered genes to target sites. The Physical System of delivery comprises the usage of subsequent techniques: mechanical cell deformations, cell-penetrating peptides, electroporation methods, hydrodynamic delivery methods, DNA nano clews, micro-injection, and transduction methods induced by osmocytosis and propane betaine [84]. The advantage of physical methods is that they are highly safe to use, compared to viral-based vectors, where there is no issue of size limitations in DNA. Their convenience and cost-effectiveness is evidenced in their robust usage in various applications [84]. Physical delivery of CRISPR/Cas9 is already proved to be very effective in the production of knockout animal models and cell lines. However, relatively poor delivery issues have been reported in *in vivo* experiments [84]. But viral vector systems are being recognised as the most effective systems to deliver DNA/RNA *in vivo* or *in vitro* to mammalian cells. Hence, plasmid-based delivery systems are made possible using CRISPR-Cas9 to reach the mammalian cell lines effectively [84]. There are basically two types of viral systems used in genetic transduction studies, the AAV and the Lenti Virus [85]. To overcome the delivery-based problems, efforts were made with the usage of dual impact AAVs that have the capacities to deliver separately sgRNA and Cas-9 encoding DNA [86]. Moreover, the simultaneous injection of two AAVs into one target cell is a highly exciting task. Lentivirus-mediated CRISPR technologies have proved highly successful in both *in vitro* and *in vivo* systems [87]. The highest benefit of lentivirus is the high infection efficiencies even in non-dividing cells, which is vital for gene corrections even in cells like the brain and liver [84].

6.2. Off-target Effects

The low competence of HDR is one of the drawbacks, compared to that of CRISPR/Cas-9-based technologies [83]. NHEJ is highly efficient compared to the HDR and is highly fit for the generation of indels with knockout and knock-in mutations. The efficiency of HDR has been optimized in recent times. Recent developments include the production of the CRISPR nickase enzyme using mutant Cas9. The application of this improvised system is far more accurate and effective in lowering the number of non-target effects substantially [88]. Moreover, it is one of the major complex issues in reducing the off-target when using CRISPR/Cas9 tools. The intensity of HDR over NHEJ is four to five folds higher in comparison, which was evaluated by Chu *et al.* [89] by the silencing of KU70, KU80, and DNA ligase IV genes using adopting ligase IV inhibitors and expression of adenovirus 4 EB1B55 K and E4 or F6 proteins. Disruption of genes occur in AGAP011377, AGAP005958 and AGAP007280 genes through the CRISPR technologies to bring female sterility to reduce malaria carrier mosquitos in the phenomenal drive to control vector populations [90, 91].

6.3. Ethical Issues

For the treatment of many diseases, CRISPR/Cas9 is becoming an effective therapeutic tool. However, there are major ethical limitations that should be addressed while using CRISPR in clinical or pre-clinical trials [90]. The principal ethical limitations of the CRISPR/Cas9 tool are its potential and technical limitations in various human applications. The occurrence of off-target evaluations in competitive editing procedures and guidelines and limited execution of its efficacy inhibited have inhibited the application of CRISPR in the various experiment-based methods [90]. It is very indeterminate to define whether the mutated organism has changed forever or been corrected temporarily [90]. The search for further applications is needed because the truth of the genetic makeup and biological phenotypes and genotypes is not fully yet understood [90]. Since the implementation of the CRISPR/Cas9 tool in 2012, its level of improvement has reached to its fullest level within a relatively short time. One of the prime aspects of this technology is that we do not understand the full scale of its long-term effects in negotiating mutations in living organisms. We do not fully understand the complication of these gene alterations and how to correct them, especially the adverse effects caused by the implementation of these tools. Despite all the positive precautions, we may end up producing new-fangled epidemics by creating new species that are more companionable to contagious pathogens.

Sometimes, the integration of new genes into living organisms may change non-invasive forms to more invasive forms for pathogens, which may lead to the eradication of local species within a few years. Therefore, it is very essential to understand the advantages of the use of the CRISPR/Cas9 tool kit but at the same time, we have to look at some of the demerits during its implementation, so that we can reap maximum benefits from the tool. The modification of the human germ line is a big concern with ethical implications in the implementation of CRISPR/Cas9 technology. Many scientists still opine that we are not yet ready to deal with human embryos and it involves a big concern about ethical issues at all levels.

6.4. Emerging CRISPR Technologies

As the popularity of CRISPR/Cas9 usage is increasing constantly, so does the quest for improving the efficiency of the tool. With time, increasingly new approaches have been added to the existing ones to improve the caliber of CRISPR-based technologies. A novel approach in CRISPR technologies is based on base editing, which can very precisely change one nucleotide to another in RNA or DNA without introducing any double-strand DNA breaks [92]. These new improvements of base correctors are carried out through various combinations of unique nucleobasede aminases with Cpf1 or Cas9 proteins and using them in various applications with robust practice in recent times [93]. Scientists have been working further to improvise the CRISPR/Cas9 system by checking non-specific interactions between the target DNA and Cas9 protein. Nakade *et al.* [94] identified the usage of alternately changed forms of CRISPR/Cas9 such as SpCas9-HF and eSpCas9. The introduction of CRISPR-Cpf1 in the CRISPR/Cas9 tool has several advantages such as extremely low cost, high efficacy, and several factors which may not be achieved by the normal system. The modified CRISPR technology will allow DNA cleavage with a single nick of crRNA and produce cohesive regions of ends with 4 or 5 nucleotide projections permitting multiplex genome corrections and many other advantages not attained with CRISPR technologies [95].

CONCLUSION

The CRISPR technology is a highly flexible and unique gene manipulating tool compromising guide RNA sequence (sg RNA) and also DNA-splicing protein complex. The sgRNA development allowed scientists to develop very specific DSB at the desired location by the direction of guide RNA, as desired. Genomic medicine is future medicine because of the immense potential of this new technology as defective genes can be corrected by the tool effectively.

With the help of CRISPR/Cas9 technology, scientists are trying to rectify both monogenic and multi-factorial genes. These efforts are helpful not only to rectify the mutations but also to construct human or animal models that help in understating the pathology of diseases and their development. The huge amount of data collected in various genomic databases helps us understand deep insights into disease etiology and pathogenesis-related issues. Despite the utilization of many gene-editing tools such as TALENs, ZNFs, and RGENs, CRISPR technologies have made it possible to reach the goal faster primarily because of their easy usage and high flexibility options. However, one must be fully conscious of its limits while planning research with CRISPR/Cas9. Without undermining the potential uses of this genetic tool in the future, scientists should strive to use this technology in a variety of ways while overcoming any potential restrictions.

CONSENT FOR PUBLICATION

Not applicable.

CONFLICT OF INTEREST

The author declares no conflict of interest, financial or otherwise.

ACKNOWLEDGEMENTS

Declared none.

REFERENCES

[1]   Doudna JA, Charpentier E. The new frontier of genome engineering with CRISPR-Cas9. Science 2014; 346(6213): 1258096.
[http://dx.doi.org/10.1126/science.1258096] [PMID: 25430774]

[2]   Rodriguez E. Ethical issues in genome editing using the CRISPR/Cas9 system. J Clin Res Bioeth 2016; 7(266): 10-4172.

[3]   Fogarty NME, McCarthy A, Snijders KE, *et al.* Genome editing reveals a role for OCT4 in human embryogenesis. Nature 2017; 550(7674): 67-73.
[http://dx.doi.org/10.1038/nature24033] [PMID: 28953884]

[4]   Risch N, Merikangas K. The future of genetic studies of complex human diseases. Science 1996; 273(5281): 1516-7.
[http://dx.doi.org/10.1126/science.273.5281.1516] [PMID: 8801636]

[5]   Cox DBT, Platt RJ, Zhang F. Therapeutic genome editing: prospects and challenges. Nat Med 2015; 21(2): 121-31.
[http://dx.doi.org/10.1038/nm.3793] [PMID: 25654603]

[6]   Janssens ACJW, van Duijn CM. Genome-based prediction of common diseases: advances and prospects. Hum Mol Genet 2008; 17(R2): R166-73.
[http://dx.doi.org/10.1093/hmg/ddn250] [PMID: 18852206]

[7]   Maeder ML, Gersbach CA. Genome-editing Technologies for Gene and Cell Therapy. Mol Ther 2016; 24(3): 430-46.
[http://dx.doi.org/10.1038/mt.2016.10] [PMID: 26755333]

[8]   Porteus MH. Towards a new era in medicine: therapeutic genome editing. Genome Biol 2015; 16(1): 286.
[http://dx.doi.org/10.1186/s13059-015-0859-y] [PMID: 26694713]

[9]   Ishino Y, Shinagawa H, Makino K, Amemura M, Nakata A. Nucleotide sequence of the iap gene, responsible for alkaline phosphatase isozyme conversion in *Escherichia coli*, and identification of the gene product. J Bacteriol 1987; 169(12): 5429-33.
[http://dx.doi.org/10.1128/jb.169.12.5429-5433.1987] [PMID: 3316184]

[10]   Barrangou R, Fremaux C, Deveau H, *et al.* CRISPR provides acquired resistance against viruses in prokaryotes. Science 2007; 315(5819): 1709-12.
[http://dx.doi.org/10.1126/science.1138140] [PMID: 17379808]

[11]   Horvath P, Barrangou R. CRISPR/Cas, the immune system of bacteria and archaea. Science 2010; 327(5962): 167-70.
[http://dx.doi.org/10.1126/science.1179555] [PMID: 20056882]

[12]   Chen Y, Zheng Y, Kang Y, *et al.* Functional disruption of the dystrophin gene in rhesus monkey using CRISPR/Cas9. Hum Mol Genet 2015; 24(13): 3764-74.
[http://dx.doi.org/10.1093/hmg/ddv120] [PMID: 25859012]

[13]   Gupta RM, Musunuru K. Expanding the genetic editing tool kit: ZFNs, TALENs, and CRISPR-Cas9. J Clin Invest 2014; 124(10): 4154-61.
[http://dx.doi.org/10.1172/JCI72992] [PMID: 25271723]

[14]   Irion U, Krauss J, Nüsslein-Volhard C. Precise and efficient genome editing in zebrafish using the CRISPR/Cas9 system. Development 2014; 141(24): 4827-30.
[http://dx.doi.org/10.1242/dev.115584] [PMID: 25411213]

[15]   Hai T, Teng F, Guo R, Li W, Zhou Q. One-step generation of knockout pigs by zygote injection of CRISPR/Cas system. Cell Res 2014; 24(3): 372-5.
[http://dx.doi.org/10.1038/cr.2014.11] [PMID: 24481528]

[16]   Seol JH, Shim EY, Lee SE. Microhomology-mediated end joining: Good, bad and ugly. Mutat Res 2018; 809: 81-7.
[http://dx.doi.org/10.1016/j.mrfmmm.2017.07.002] [PMID: 28754468]

[17]   Ata H, Ekstrom TL, Martínez-Gálvez G, *et al.* Robust activation of microhomology-mediated end joining for precision gene editing applications. PLoS Genet 2018; 14(9): e1007652.
[http://dx.doi.org/10.1371/journal.pgen.1007652] [PMID: 30208061]

[18]   Lin DW, Chung BP, Huang JW, Wang X, Huang L, Kaiser P. Microhomology-based CRISPR tagging tools for protein tracking, purification, and depletion. J Biol Chem 2019; 294(28): 10877-85.
[http://dx.doi.org/10.1074/jbc.RA119.008422] [PMID: 31138654]

[19]   Long C, Amoasii L, Mireault AA, *et al.* Postnatal genome editing partially restores dystrophin expression in a mouse model of muscular dystrophy. Science 2016; 351(6271): 400-3.
[http://dx.doi.org/10.1126/science.aad5725] [PMID: 26721683]

[20]   Yang W, Tu Z, Sun Q, Li XJ. CRISPR/Cas9: Implications for Modeling and Therapy of Neurodegenerative Diseases. Front Mol Neurosci 2016; 9: 30.
[http://dx.doi.org/10.3389/fnmol.2016.00030] [PMID: 27199655]

[21]   Chen B, Gilbert LA, Cimini BA, *et al.* Dynamic imaging of genomic loci in living human cells by an optimized CRISPR/Cas system. Cell 2013; 155(7): 1479-91.
[http://dx.doi.org/10.1016/j.cell.2013.12.001] [PMID: 24360272]

[22]   Rodwell C, Aym'e S. 2014 Report on the State of the Art of Rare Disease Activities in Europe, Part II: Key Developments in the Field of Rare Diseases in Europe in 2013. Brussels, Belgium: European Union 2014.

[23]   Cutting GR. Cystic fibrosis genetics: from molecular understanding to clinical application. Nat Rev Genet 2015; 16(1): 45-56.
[http://dx.doi.org/10.1038/nrg3849] [PMID: 25404111]

[24]   Li HL, Fujimoto N, Sasakawa N, *et al.* Precise correction of the dystrophin gene in duchenne muscular dystrophy patient induced pluripotent stem cells by TALEN and CRISPR-Cas9. Stem Cell Reports 2015; 4(1): 143-54.
[http://dx.doi.org/10.1016/j.stemcr.2014.10.013] [PMID: 25434822]

[25]   Kerem BS, Rommens JM, Buchanan JA, *et al.* Identification of the cystic fibrosis gene: genetic analysis. Science 1989; 245(4922): 1073-80.
[http://dx.doi.org/10.1126/science.2570460] [PMID: 2570460]

[26]   Rogan MP, Stoltz DA, Hornick DB. Cystic fibrosis transmembrane conductance regulator intracellular processing, trafficking, and opportunities for mutation-specific treatment. Chest 2011; 139(6): 1480-90.
[http://dx.doi.org/10.1378/chest.10-2077] [PMID: 21652558]

[27]   Mall MA, Hartl D. CFTR: cystic fibrosis and beyond. Eur Respir J 2014; 44(4): 1042-54.
[http://dx.doi.org/10.1183/09031936.00228013] [PMID: 24925916]

[28]   Schwank G, Koo BK, Sasselli V, *et al.* Functional repair of CFTR by CRISPR/Cas9 in intestinal stem cell organoids of cystic fibrosis patients. Cell Stem Cell 2013; 13(6): 653-8.
[http://dx.doi.org/10.1016/j.stem.2013.11.002] [PMID: 24315439]

[29]   Firth AL, Menon T, Parker GS, *et al.* Functional Gene Correction for Cystic Fibrosis in Lung Epithelial Cells Generated from Patient iPSCs. Cell Rep 2015; 12(9): 1385-90.
[http://dx.doi.org/10.1016/j.celrep.2015.07.062] [PMID: 26299960]

[30]   Ware RE, de Montalembert M, Tshilolo L, Abboud MR. Sickle cell disease. Lancet 2017; 390(10091):

311-23.
[http://dx.doi.org/10.1016/S0140-6736(17)30193-9] [PMID: 28159390]

[31]   Park SH, Lee CM, Deshmukh H, Bao G. Therapeutic CRISPR/Cas9 genome editing for treating sickle cell disease. Blood 2016; 128(22): 4703.
[http://dx.doi.org/10.1182/blood.V128.22.4703.4703]

[32]   Hoban MD, Lumaquin D, Kuo CY, *et al.* CRISPR/Cas9-Mediated Correction of the Sickle Mutation in Human CD34+ cells. Mol Ther 2016; 24(9): 1561-9.
[http://dx.doi.org/10.1038/mt.2016.148] [PMID: 27406980]

[33]   Dever DP, Bak RO, Reinisch A, *et al.* CRISPR/Cas9 β-globin gene targeting in human haematopoietic stem cells. Nature 2016; 539(7629): 384-9.
[http://dx.doi.org/10.1038/nature20134] [PMID: 27820943]

[34]   Cao A, Kan YW. The prevention of thalassemia. Cold Spring Harb Perspect Med 2013; 3(2): a011775.
[http://dx.doi.org/10.1101/cshperspect.a011775] [PMID: 23378598]

[35]   Saxena R, Jain PK, Thomas E, Verma IC. Prenatal diagnosis of β-thalassaemia: experience in a developing country. Prenat Diagn 1998; 18(1): 1-7.
[http://dx.doi.org/10.1002/(SICI)1097-0223(199801)18:1<1::AID-PD209>3.0.CO;2-Y]   [PMID: 9483634]

[36]   Xu P, Tong Y, Liu X, *et al.* Both TALENs and CRISPR/Cas9 directly target the HBB IVS2–654 (C > T) mutation in β-thalassemia-derived iPSCs. Sci Rep 2015; 5(1): 12065.
[http://dx.doi.org/10.1038/srep12065] [PMID: 26156589]

[37]   Niu X, He W, Song B, *et al.* Combining Single Strand Oligodeoxynucleotides and CRISPR/Cas9 to Correct Gene Mutations in β-Thalassemia-induced Pluripotent Stem Cells. J Biol Chem 2016; 291(32): 16576-85.
[http://dx.doi.org/10.1074/jbc.M116.719237] [PMID: 27288406]

[38]   Yang Y, Zhang X, Yi L, *et al.* Naïve Induced Pluripotent Stem Cells Generated From β-Thalassemia Fibroblasts Allow Efficient Gene Correction With CRISPR/Cas9. Stem Cells Transl Med 2016; 5(1): 8-19.
[http://dx.doi.org/10.5966/sctm.2015-0157] [PMID: 26676643]

[39]   Xie F, Ye L, Chang JC, *et al.* Seamless gene correction of β-thalassemia mutations in patient-specific iPSCs using CRISPR/Cas9 and *piggyBac.* Genome Res 2014; 24(9): 1526-33.
[http://dx.doi.org/10.1101/gr.173427.114] [PMID: 25096406]

[40]   Song B, Fan Y, He W, *et al.* Improved hematopoietic differentiation efficiency of gene-corrected beta-thalassemia induced pluripotent stem cells by CRISPR/Cas9 system. Stem Cells Dev 2015; 24(9): 1053-65.
[http://dx.doi.org/10.1089/scd.2014.0347] [PMID: 25517294]

[41]   Martin JB, Gusella JF. Huntington's disease. Pathogenesis and management. N Engl J Med 1986; 315(20): 1267-76.
[http://dx.doi.org/10.1056/NEJM198611133152006] [PMID: 2877396]

[42]   Warby SC, Montpetit A, Hayden AR, *et al.* CAG expansion in the Huntington disease gene is associated with a specific and targetable predisposing haplogroup. Am J Hum Genet 2009; 84(3): 351-66.
[http://dx.doi.org/10.1016/j.ajhg.2009.02.003] [PMID: 19249009]

[43]   Shin JW, Kim KH, Chao MJ, *et al.* Permanent inactivation of Huntington's disease mutation by personalized allele-specific CRISPR/Cas9. Hum Mol Genet 2016; 25(20): ddw286.
[http://dx.doi.org/10.1093/hmg/ddw286] [PMID: 28172889]

[44]   Monteys AM, Ebanks SA, Keiser MS, Davidson BL. CRISPR/Cas9 Editing of the Mutant Huntingtin Allele *In Vitro* and *In Vivo.* Mol Ther 2017; 25(1): 12-23.
[http://dx.doi.org/10.1016/j.ymthe.2016.11.010] [PMID: 28129107]

[45]   Yang S, Chang R, Yang H, *et al.* CRISPR/Cas9-mediated gene editing ameliorates neurotoxicity in mouse model of Huntington's disease. J Clin Invest 2017; 127(7): 2719-24.
[http://dx.doi.org/10.1172/JCI92087] [PMID: 28628038]

[46]   Kolli N, Lu M, Maiti P, Rossignol J, Dunbar G. CRISPR-Cas9 Mediated Gene-Silencing of the Mutant Huntingtin Gene in an *In Vitro* Model of Huntington's Disease. Int J Mol Sci 2017; 18(4): 754.
[http://dx.doi.org/10.3390/ijms18040754] [PMID: 28368337]

[47]   Cohn RD, Campbell KP. Molecular basis of muscular dystrophies. Muscle Nerve 2000; 23(10): 1456-71.
[http://dx.doi.org/10.1002/1097-4598(200010)23:10<1456::AID-MUS2>3.0.CO;2-T]   [PMID: 11003781]

[48]   Ousterout DG, Kabadi AM, Thakore PI, Majoros WH, Reddy TE, Gersbach CA. Multiplex CRISPR/Cas9-based genome editing for correction of dystrophin mutations that cause Duchenne muscular dystrophy. Nat Commun 2015; 6(1): 6244.
[http://dx.doi.org/10.1038/ncomms7244] [PMID: 25692716]

[49]   Bowen DJ. Haemophilia A and haemophilia B: molecular insights. Mol Pathol 2002; 55(2): 127-44.
[http://dx.doi.org/10.1136/mp.55.2.127] [PMID: 11950963]

[50]   Park CY, Kim DH, Son JS, *et al.* Functional Correction of Large Factor VIII Gene Chromosomal Inversions in Hemophilia A Patient-Derived iPSCs Using CRISPR-Cas9. Cell Stem Cell 2015; 17(2): 213-20.
[http://dx.doi.org/10.1016/j.stem.2015.07.001] [PMID: 26212079]

[51]   Guan Y, Ma Y, Li Q, *et al.* CRISPR /Cas9 mediated somatic correction of a novel coagulator factor IX gene mutation ameliorates hemophilia in mouse. EMBO Mol Med 2016; 8(5): 477-88.
[http://dx.doi.org/10.15252/emmm.201506039] [PMID: 26964564]

[52]   van den Berg JM, van Koppen E, Åhlin A, *et al.* Chronic granulomatous disease: the European experience. PLoS One 2009; 4(4): e5234.
[http://dx.doi.org/10.1371/journal.pone.0005234] [PMID: 19381301]

[53]   Rosenzweig SD. Inflammatory manifestations in chronic granulomatous disease (CGD). J Clin Immunol 2008; 28(S1) (Suppl. 1): 67-72.
[http://dx.doi.org/10.1007/s10875-007-9160-5] [PMID: 18193341]

[54]   Song E, Jaishankar GB, Saleh H, Jithpratuck W, Sahni R, Krishnaswamy G. Chronic granulomatous disease: a review of the infectious and inflammatory complications. Clin Mol Allergy 2011; 9(1): 10.
[http://dx.doi.org/10.1186/1476-7961-9-10] [PMID: 21624140]

[55]   Kuhns DB, Alvord WG, Heller T, *et al.* Residual NADPH oxidase and survival in chronic granulomatous disease. N Engl J Med 2010; 363(27): 2600-10.
[http://dx.doi.org/10.1056/NEJMoa1007097] [PMID: 21190454]

[56]   Keller MD, Notarangelo LD, Malech HL. Future of Care for Patients With Chronic Granulomatous Disease: Gene Therapy and Targeted Molecular Medicine. J Pediatric Infect Dis Soc 2018; 7 (Suppl. 1): S40-4.
[http://dx.doi.org/10.1093/jpids/piy011] [PMID: 29746676]

[57]   Flynn R, Grundmann A, Renz P, *et al.* CRISPR-mediated genotypic and phenotypic correction of a chronic granulomatous disease mutation in human iPS cells. Exp Hematol 2015; 43(10): 838-848.e3.
[http://dx.doi.org/10.1016/j.exphem.2015.06.002] [PMID: 26101162]

[58]   De Ravin SS, Li L, Wu X, *et al.* CRISPR-Cas9 gene repair of hematopoietic stem cells from patients with X-linked chronic granulomatous disease. Sci Transl Med 2017; 9(372): eaah3480.
[http://dx.doi.org/10.1126/scitranslmed.aah3480] [PMID: 28077679]

[59]   Todd JA. From genome to aetiology in a multifactorial disease, type 1 diabetes. BioEssays 1999; 21(2): 164-74.
[http://dx.doi.org/10.1002/(SICI)1521-1878(199902)21:2<164::AID-BIES10>3.0.CO;2-4]   [PMID:

10193189]

[60]   Olsen J, Overvad K. The concept of multifactorial etiology of cancer. Pharmacol Toxicol 1993; 72 (Suppl. 1): 33-8.
[http://dx.doi.org/10.1111/j.1600-0773.1993.tb01666.x] [PMID: 8474986]

[61]   Yi L, Li J. CRISPR-Cas9 therapeutics in cancer: promising strategies and present challenges. Biochim Biophys Acta 2016; 1866(2): 197-207.
[PMID: 27641687]

[62]   Hu Z, Yu L, Zhu D, *et al.* Disruption of HPV16-E7 by CRISPR/Cas system induces apoptosis and growth inhibition in HPV16 positive human cervical cancer cells. BioMed Res Int 2014; 2014: 1-9.
[http://dx.doi.org/10.1155/2014/612823] [PMID: 25136604]

[63]   Mathers CD, Loncar D. Projections of global mortality and burden of disease from 2002 to 2030. PLoS Med 2006; 3(11): e442.
[http://dx.doi.org/10.1371/journal.pmed.0030442] [PMID: 17132052]

[64]   Lian YF, Yuan J, Cui Q, *et al.* Upregulation of KLHDC4 Predicts a Poor Prognosis in Human Nasopharyngeal Carcinoma. PLoS One 2016; 11(3): e0152820.
[http://dx.doi.org/10.1371/journal.pone.0152820] [PMID: 27030985]

[65]   Benjamin EJ, Blaha MJ, Chiuve SE, *et al.* Heart Disease and Stroke Statistics—2017 Update: A Report From the American Heart Association. Circulation 2017; 135(10): e146-603.
[http://dx.doi.org/10.1161/CIR.0000000000000485] [PMID: 28122885]

[66]   Miano JM, Zhu QM, Lowenstein CJ. A CRISPR Path to Engineering New Genetic Mouse Models for Cardiovascular Research. Arterioscler Thromb Vasc Biol 2016; 36(6): 1058-75.
[http://dx.doi.org/10.1161/ATVBAHA.116.304790] [PMID: 27102963]

[67]   Li Y, Song YH, Liu B, Yu XY. The potential application and challenge of powerful CRISPR/Cas9 system in cardiovascular research. Int J Cardiol 2017; 227: 191-3.
[http://dx.doi.org/10.1016/j.ijcard.2016.11.177] [PMID: 27847153]

[68]   Kenshi H, Manu B, Eva B, Patrick S, Micah LB, An X, *et al.* CRISPR-mediated insertions or deletions of the human LMNA homolog in zebrafish as a model of early-onset cardiac conduction disease. Circulation 2017; 136: 17178.

[69]   Huang L, Hua Z, Xiao H, *et al.* CRISPR/Cas9-mediated *ApoE* -/- and *LDLR* -/- double gene knockout in pigs elevates serum LDL-C and TC levels. Oncotarget 2017; 8(23): 37751-60.
[http://dx.doi.org/10.18632/oncotarget.17154] [PMID: 28465483]

[70]   Ding Q, Strong A, Patel KM, *et al.* Permanent alteration of PCSK9 with *in vivo* CRISPR-Cas9 genome editing. Circ Res 2014; 115(5): 488-92.
[http://dx.doi.org/10.1161/CIRCRESAHA.115.304351] [PMID: 24916110]

[71]   Chadwick AC, Evitt NH, Lv W, Musunuru K. Reduced Blood Lipid Levels With *In vivo* CRISPR-Cas9 Base Editing of ANGPTL3. Circulation 2018; 137(9): 975-7.
[http://dx.doi.org/10.1161/CIRCULATIONAHA.117.031335] [PMID: 29483174]

[72]   Bogdanove AJ, Voytas DF. TAL effectors: customizable proteins for DNA targeting. Science 2011; 333(6051): 1843-6.
[http://dx.doi.org/10.1126/science.1204094] [PMID: 21960622]

[73]   Kim S, Kim D, Cho SW, Kim J, Kim JS. Highly efficient RNA-guided genome editing in human cells *via* delivery of purified Cas9 ribonucleoproteins. Genome Res 2014; 24(6): 1012-9.
[http://dx.doi.org/10.1101/gr.171322.113] [PMID: 24696461]

[74]   Urnov FD, Rebar EJ, Holmes MC, Zhang HS, Gregory PD. Genome editing with engineered zinc finger nucleases. Nat Rev Genet 2010; 11(9): 636-46.
[http://dx.doi.org/10.1038/nrg2842] [PMID: 20717154]

[75]   Lee JK, Jeong E, Lee J, *et al.* Directed evolution of CRISPR-Cas9 to increase its specificity. Nat

Commun 2018; 9(1): 3048.
[http://dx.doi.org/10.1038/s41467-018-05477-x] [PMID: 30082838]

[76] Kocak DD, Josephs EA, Bhandarkar V, Adkar SS, Kwon JB, Gersbach CA. Increasing the specificity of CRISPR systems with engineered RNA secondary structures. Nat Biotechnol 2019; 37(6): 657-66.
[http://dx.doi.org/10.1038/s41587-019-0095-1] [PMID: 30988504]

[77] Hoban MD, Lumaquin D, Kuo CY, *et al.* CRISPR/Cas9-Mediated Correction of the Sickle Mutation in Human CD34+ cells. Mol Ther 2016; 24(9): 1561-9.
[http://dx.doi.org/10.1038/mt.2016.148] [PMID: 27406980]

[78] Dever DP, Bak RO, Reinisch A, *et al.* CRISPR/Cas9 β-globin gene targeting in human haematopoietic stem cells. Nature 2016; 539(7629): 384-9.
[http://dx.doi.org/10.1038/nature20134] [PMID: 27820943]

[79] Yang S, Chang R, Yang H, *et al.* CRISPR/Cas9-mediated gene editing ameliorates neurotoxicity in mouse model of Huntington's disease. J Clin Invest 2017; 127(7): 2719-24.
[http://dx.doi.org/10.1172/JCI92087] [PMID: 28628038]

[80] Guan Y, Ma Y, Li Q, *et al.* CRISPR /Cas9□mediated somatic correction of a novel coagulator factor IX gene mutation ameliorates hemophilia in mouse. EMBO Mol Med 2016; 8(5): 477-88.
[http://dx.doi.org/10.15252/emmm.201506039] [PMID: 26964564]

[81] Mall MA, Hartl D. CFTR: cystic fibrosis and beyond. Eur Respir J 2014; 44(4): 1042-54.
[http://dx.doi.org/10.1183/09031936.00228013] [PMID: 24925916]

[82] Rogan MP, Stoltz DA, Hornick DB. Cystic fibrosis transmembrane conductance regulator intracellular processing, trafficking, and opportunities for mutation-specific treatment. Chest 2011; 139(6): 1480-90.
[http://dx.doi.org/10.1378/chest.10-2077] [PMID: 21652558]

[83] Roy B, Zhao J, Yang C, *et al.* CRISPR/Cascade 9-Mediated Genome Editing-Challenges and Opportunities. Front Genet 2018; 9: 240.
[http://dx.doi.org/10.3389/fgene.2018.00240] [PMID: 30026755]

[84] Liu C, Zhang L, Liu H, Cheng K. Delivery strategies of the CRISPR-Cas9 gene-editing system for therapeutic applications. J Control Release 2017; 266: 17-26.
[http://dx.doi.org/10.1016/j.jconrel.2017.09.012] [PMID: 28911805]

[85] Grimm D, Lee JS, Wang L, *et al. In vitro* and *in vivo* gene therapy vector evolution *via* multispecies interbreeding and retargeting of adeno-associated viruses. J Virol 2008; 82(12): 5887-911.
[http://dx.doi.org/10.1128/JVI.00254-08] [PMID: 18400866]

[86] Zetsche B, Volz SE, Zhang F. A split-Cas9 architecture for inducible genome editing and transcription modulation. Nat Biotechnol 2015; 33(2): 139-42.
[http://dx.doi.org/10.1038/nbt.3149] [PMID: 25643054]

[87] Zufferey R, Dull T, Mandel RJ, *et al.* Self-inactivating lentivirus vector for safe and efficient *in vivo* gene delivery. J Virol 1998; 72(12): 9873-80.
[http://dx.doi.org/10.1128/JVI.72.12.9873-9880.1998] [PMID: 9811723]

[88] Ran FA, Hsu PD, Wright J, Agarwala V, Scott DA, Zhang F. Genome engineering using the CRISPR-Cas9 system. Nat Protoc 2013; 8(11): 2281-308.
[http://dx.doi.org/10.1038/nprot.2013.143] [PMID: 24157548]

[89] Chu VT, Weber T, Wefers B, *et al.* Increasing the efficiency of homology-directed repair for CRISPR-Cas9-induced precise gene editing in mammalian cells. Nat Biotechnol 2015; 33(5): 543-8.
[http://dx.doi.org/10.1038/nbt.3198] [PMID: 25803306]

[90] Brokowski C, Adli M. CRISPR Ethics: Moral Considerations for Applications of a Powerful Tool. J Mol Biol 2019; 431(1): 88-101.
[http://dx.doi.org/10.1016/j.jmb.2018.05.044] [PMID: 29885329]

[91]   Hammond A, Galizi R, Kyrou K, *et al.* A CRISPR-Cas9 gene drive system targeting female reproduction in the malaria mosquito vector Anopheles gambiae. Nat Biotechnol 2016; 34(1): 78-83.
        [http://dx.doi.org/10.1038/nbt.3439] [PMID: 26641531]

[92]   Molla KA, Yang Y. CRISPR/Cas-Mediated Base Editing: Technical Considerations and Practical Applications. Trends Biotechnol 2019; 37(10): 1121-42.
        [http://dx.doi.org/10.1016/j.tibtech.2019.03.008] [PMID: 30995964]

[93]   Yang B, Yang L, Chen J. Development and Application of Base Editors. CRISPR J 2019; 2(2): 91-104.
        [http://dx.doi.org/10.1089/crispr.2019.0001] [PMID: 30998092]

[94]   Nakade S, Yamamoto T, Sakuma T. Cas9, Cpf1 and C2c1/2/3—What's next? Bioengineered 2017; 8(3): 265-73.
        [http://dx.doi.org/10.1080/21655979.2017.1282018] [PMID: 28140746]

[95]   Mbugua MM, Hill SA, Morris DP, McMurry JL. Simultaneous delivery of CRISPR/cas and donor DNA using cell-penetrating peptide-adaptors. FASEB J 2019; 33(S1): 620-5.
        [http://dx.doi.org/10.1096/fasebj.2019.33.1_supplement.620.5]

Role of Vyana Vayu in CardioVascular System, Etiopathogenesis and Therapeutic Strategies: An Ayurveda Perspective

Savitri Vasudev Baikampady[1,*], **C. S. Hiremath**[1], **Reeta Varyani**[1] and **Venketesh**[2]

[1] *Department of Cardiology, Sri Sathya Sai Institute of Higher Medical Sciences, EPIP Area, Whitefield, Bangalore, India*

[2] *Department of Biosciences, Sri Sathya Sai Institute of Higher Learning, Prashanthi Nilayam, Puttaparthy, Andhra Pradesh, India*

Abstract: A systems approach to health is the hallmark of Ayurveda. It believes in preventing disease and maintaining and restoring health. The entire concept stands on three fundamental functional units-*Vata, Pitta and Kapha,* where *Vata,* mobilizes the other two units. Depending on their locations, *Vata (Vayu) is* classified into five subtypes, where each has its distinct role to perform. *Vyana Vayu* (VV), an important subtype of Vata, is synthesized in myocytes and responsible for the genesis of the action potential. A key regulator in contractile functions, VV propels out nutrients from the heart. It not only mediates intracrine and paracrine activities but modulates the vascular tone too. Wherever there is scope to flow, VV has its unique role to contribute. Ancient scholars of *Ayurveda* have identified its ubiquitous role in the endogenous system, where all the activities depend on VV. Hence, preventing VV from any stimulus is of paramount importance since they consequently lead to various cardio vascular diseases (CVD). Classical texts have addressed the prognosis in six discrete phases where each phase can be avoided strategically. Highlighting the precipitants that attenuate VV, we focus on addressing those phases along with curative measures so that the functions of *Vyana Vayu* can be restored.

Keywords: Contractile functions, Phases of prognosis, Preventive cardiology, Vascular tone, *Vyana Vayu.*

1. INTRODUCTION

A systems approach to health is the hallmark of *Ayurveda*. It carries the rich tradition of knowledge with epistemological values based on life principles more

* **Corresponding author Savitri Vasudev Baikampady:** Department of Cardiology, Sri Sathya Sai Institute of Higher Medical Sciences, EPIP Area, Whitefield, Bangalore, India; E-mail: ayurvedsavitur@yahoo.co.in

Dr. V. V. Sathibabu Uddandrao & Dr. Parim Brahma Naidu (Eds.)

than 3500 years from date [1]. Theories and concepts postulated by *Ayurveda* scholars are valid even today despite the absence of diagnostic tools and gadgets during their times. It has a comprehensive outlook towards every individual that embraces physical, physiological, and spiritual components. Expressed in Sanskrit, there is a need to comprehend the knowledge and translate it scientifically in the present state-of-art as its affluent intellectual property cannot be possessed only by Sanskrit scholars. Its proficiency lies in the appropriate use for mankind.

The entire concept of *Ayurveda* stands on three fundamental pathophysiological units-*Vata, Pitta and Kapha,* where *Vata,* mobilizes the other two. *Vata* is expounded to hold the living system [2], comprising gaseous components, moving through a specific cavity [3]. The gamut of its action is always associated with locomotion (*Gati*). Based on the extent of operations, *Vata* is classified into five subtypes, where each constitutes an independent system with a distinct role to perform [4]. Even though each subtype is confined to perform in a given territory, the *Vyana Vayu* (VV), a unique subtype of *Vata* has a wider role to perform throughout the body. VV is an indigenous component of the heart (*Hrdaya*), responsible for contractile functions. It is due to VV that the heart relentlessly (*Ajasram*) pumps out required nutrients to fulfill the metabolic demands. Diffuse (*Krutsna dehachari*) in nature, VV plays a central role in maintaining homeostasis in the circulatory system (*Rasasamvahana*). It protects the cardiovascular system (CVS) and metabolic system (MS) through anti-inflammatory and anti-oxidant properties [5 - 8]. The slightest imbalance in the bioavailability of VV can give rise to serious pathological conditions. Several intrinsic and extrinsic factors (IEF) can exasperate the balanced state, invoking the pre-determinants of cardiovascular and metabolic disorders (CMD) [9]. Deleterious effects on CMD can be negated if VV's intrinsic properties are preserved. Hence, knowledge of the realm of VV on CVS and MS could provide an alternative approach to detect the prognosis of CMD with complications. Since every cardiac patient has the potential to develop heart failure, there is a need to explore new areas on predisposing factors that leads to CMD prognosis.

If the etiological elements are not curtailed in time, CVD will remain to be the leading cause of death for the next ten years of more than 100 million populations [10, 11]. There is a general agreement that these factors are modifiably associated with environment and lifestyle. WHO has initiated several awareness programs to abridge CVD and its risks, but despite this awareness, there has not been any decline in the number of CVD cases. Technological advancements have considerably improved survival rates from acute cardiovascular events, but surviving inhabitants with compromised functions of the heart have simultaneously increased.

Hence, intending to prevent CMD prognosis and improving the quality of life of survived victims, we explore the knowledge of Ayurveda to extend the horizon of etiology and provide a broader scope for prevention. This can be understood in six discrete phases of pathogenesis where each phase can be strategically avoided. This chapter highlights the analysis of *Vyana Vayu* from physiological and etiopathological aspects, followed by concomitant contemporary concepts and therapeutic strategies.

2. A PREAMBLE TO VATA

The very existence of *Vata* in the endogenous system denotes life. Whether voluntary or involuntary, all actions are governed by *Vata*, right from attending to gross functions such as breathing, swallowing food, belching, sneezing, coughing or excretion of wastes, and many more [12]. It contributes to the manifestation of shape, cell division, cell signaling, and cognition [13]. Processes involving conduction of impulse, metabolite transport, scavenging of free radicals, apoptosis, and necrosis are all governed by it [14]. Due to its gaseous property, it acquires a natural tendency to arid (*Ruksha*). This prevents the cellular components from over-lubrication, at the same time facilitates apoptosis appropriately. Highly unstable (*Chala*), subtle (*Sukhma*), and dynamic nature of Vata varies with time and places of action [15, 16]. Even though it maintains the body's thermal equilibrium by cooling *(Sheeta),* it is highly sensitive to extreme temperatures [17]. Its proficiency is best demonstrated with optimum bioavailability (*Sama*) but becomes pathologic and devastating otherwise *(Vruddhi. Kshaya)* [18]. Whether intracellular or extracellular, the quantum of its kinetic nature is demonstrated through diverse actions.

2.1. Vyana Vayu

The human system is uniquely designed, where all actions are performed through well-defined, well-coordinated, intact, and enclosed channels (*Srotas*) [19]. VV is believed to be activated and spread indefinitely across these intact channels, where ever there is scope to flow. VV facilitates cell trafficking, membrane trafficking, and the exchange of blood to and from the heart (*Gamanaagaman kriya*) and establishes communication between the substrate and circulating metabolite. Whether an organ designed for a specific task or a circulating channel carrying metabolites to the target tissue, VV has its extensive role to perform in it. This is possible only if VV is expressed on the surface of any flowing channel. Classical authors have unanimously expounded on the diffuse nature of VV that originates and regulates several functions from the heart (*Hrdaya*). Whether the intracrine or paracrine, Vata must be functional in space. Furthermore, whether within the chambers of the heart or luminal vascular surface, VV is expressed on the substrate that communicates with bodily fluid through the endocardium and endothelium. It maintains homeostasis by establishing communication with the underlying tissue and the flowing metabolite [20]. It is believed that VV is very agile (*Yugapat*) and rapid (*Mahajava*), participating in several physiological processes other than the heart [21]. Due to its subtle and rapid nature, it is highly reactive and oxidant. VV has a unique cleansing property that enables the heart and circulating channels to be protected from antagonistic elements by promoting free radical scavenging activity (*Vishodhana*) [7].

VV is expressed in three states; declined, optimum and proliferative states [22]. Appropriate expression of VV is of paramount importance since its depletion or over expression can be daunting to the system, where its impairment not only leads to morbidity in CVS but has the potential to debilitate metabolic strength too.

2.1.1. Role of Vyana Vayu in the Heart

Vyana Vayu is situated in the heart, responsible for the majority of cardiac functions [23]. Its gaseous origin is articulated in the endocardium. Its swift and relentless (*Ajasram*) movement enables the heart to meet the metabolic demands of the body. VV initiates the triggering mechanism that marks the onset of the action potential through excitation and contraction coupling.

Its controlled release in the cardiac muscle facilitates the actions of contraction and expansion of the heart muscles (*Akunchana & Prasarana bhava*) [5]. The ventricular squeeze enables the blood to move upwards (*Utkshepana*) and its relaxation allows the same to move downwards (*Apakshepana*), facilitated by VV. This happens as a well-coordinated response through systolic and diastolic movements where the nourishing metabolite is ejected out from the heart, only at the mercy of VV (*Vikshepana*) [23]. The metabolic demands of the body solely depend upon the cardiac output (*Vikshipta Rasa*) [8]. Uniquely designed in the heart, it performs a cyclic maneuver (*Parivruttistu chakravat*), where every cardiac cycle achieves completion due to an efficient VV. This indicates that VV can sense charges in extracellular compartments mediating the intracrine and paracrine activities enabling cell trafficking (*Gamana Aagaman kriya*) [23]. VV coordinates with its counterpart (*Pran Vayu*) and influences neighboring cells to modify physiologically by conducting impulses and generating energy [24]. This constant endeavor is symbiotic throughout one's lifespan (*Kalatah Sada*).

The slightest impairment in the normal expression of VV can alter the homeostasis through its actions turning pathological. Disturbances in any of the above functions of VV can potentially impair cardiac performance compromising with cardiac contractility. Disorders of arrhythmia and contractile dysfunctions are caused due to deranged VV.

2.1.2. Role of Vyana Vayu in Vasculature (Dhamani and Sira)

The diffuse nature of VV is demonstrated in places other than the myocardium. After propelling out nutrients from the heart to meet the demands of metabolizing tissue, VV is expedited out by ejecting nourishing metabolite through hitting (*Akshepana*) due to its constant pulsating nature (*Praspandanam*). Facilitated through the arteries (*Dhamanies*), branching out from the heart, VV is responsible to circulate (*Vahan*) and nourish (*Tarpan*) not only the metabolizing tissue but exercising muscle too. It gratifies them by ensuring a normal flow [5]. Moreover, VV ensures the prompt flow of blood without coagulation (*Rakta Sraavan*), thereby preventing unnecessary clogging. Whether through a circulating blood vessel or any organ, VV can be influenced by both the environments, extracellular (flowing metabolites) as well as intracellular. Being interphase also contributes to maintaining homeostasis by balancing between the extracellular environment, hemodynamic forces, and permeability. Speed, volume, and flow of bodily fluid across a channel are directly proportional to the production of VV to meet the demand. Hence, the appropriate vascular tone is obtained by maintaining pressure and volume not only within the chambers of the heart but along the circulating vessels too. Vasodilation and vasoconstriction (*Akunchana and prasarana*) are important workings of VV in the vasculature. Its abnormal expression in the vessels causes vasoconstriction (*Sirakunchana*). This compromises the demands of the metabolizing tissue leading to several metabolic disorders [7].

Lipid metabolism is facilitated by VV. Apart from augmenting the tissues and bodily fluids (*Tarpan*), it maintains appropriate lubrication across the cell membrane by its controlled release since over expression dries up the underlying tissues by shrinking. It protects the environment by preventing it from any stimuli that compromise its functions. Moreover, it does so to protect from localized deposition of toxins (*dosha*) that result in edema (*Shoth*) [25]. The appropriate interplay of VV with lipids (*Meda dhatu*), prevents blood vessels from narrowing (*sirakunchana)* due to atherosclerotic deposits. Impairment in this communication can block the expression of VV by lipids (*Avruta VV by Meda*) [26].

2.1.3. Role of Vyana Vayu in Skeletal Muscles and other Organs

The complexity of VV on skeletal muscles needs to be better understood since all actions inside the body are performed by it. Proper expression of VV on muscles facilitates its appropriate contraction and expansion (*Akunchana and Prasarana*). Pain, trembling and rigidity of muscles are due to attenuated VV.

Opening and closure of eyelids (*Umnmesh Nimesh*), activation of the taste buds on the tongue (*Annaaswadana*), appropriate expression of sweat (*Sweda Sraavana*), and plotting of sperm to the site of fertilization (*Shukra Pratipadana*) are some of the functions regulated by VV [7] apart from the normal functions (Fig. **1**).

Testimonials in Table **1** mention attributes of *Vyana Vayu* when normal; they are quoted in verses from different chapters of various sections.

Table 1. Physiologic attributes of *Vyana Vayu*.

Sr. No.	Attributes of Vyana Vayu	Charaka Samhita	Susruta Samhita	Ashtanga Hridyam	Ashtang Sangraha
1	Gati	Chi: 28-9	Ni 1-17	Sut: 12- 7	Sha: 20-2
2	Utkshepana	-	-	Sut: 12-7	Sha: 20-2
3	Apakshepana	Chi: 28-9	-	Sut: 12/7	
4	Akunchana	-	Sha:7-3	Sha: 3-68	Sut: 20-2
5	Prasarana	Chi 28-9	Sha:7-3	-	-
6	Vikshepana	Chi: 15-36	Sut: 46-528 Utt: 39-85	Sha:3-68	Sha: 6-28
8	Krutsna Dehachara	Chi: 28-9	Ni: 1-17	Sut:12-7	-
9	Mahajava	-	-	Sut:12-7	-
10	Tarpan	-	Sha: 6-18 Sut: 14-3	-	-
11	Vahana	Vim: 5-3 Sut: 12-8	Sha:9-13 Sut: 1-17	Sha: 3-18 to39	-
13	Sraavan	-	Ni: 1-18	-	Sha:20-2
14	Ajasram	Chi: 15-36	-	Sha: 3-68 to 70	-
15	Praspandan	-	Sut: 15-1	-	-
16	Yugapat	Chi:15-36	-	Sha:3-68	-

References from popular texts of Ayurveda extracted from different sections; *Sut: Sutrasthan, Sha: Sharirasthan, Ni: Nidansthan, Chi: Chikitshasthan, Vi: Vimanasthan and Utt: Uttaratantra* with the chapter number followed by verses.

3. ETIOLOGY

Pathologic *Vyana Vayu* is one of the *Vata dosha*, where *dosha* is defined as a potential to incapacitate the surrounding and impair it. *Doshas* are physiologic when unperturbed but turn pathologic instantly when provoked. The rapid and volatile nature of VV gets provoked in the same way [27].

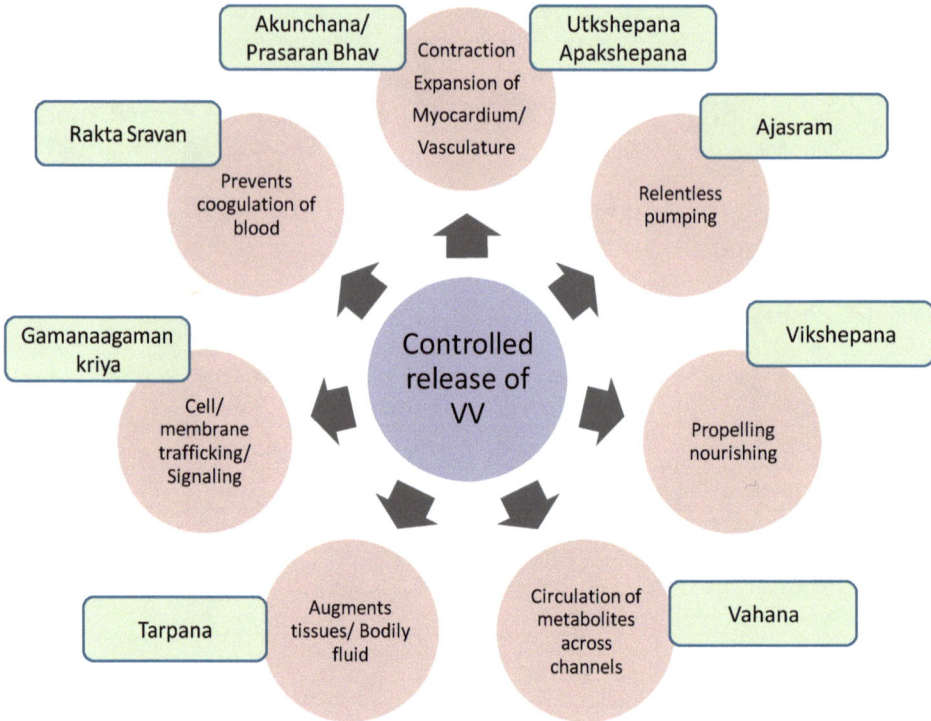

Fig. (1). Normal functions of Vyana Vayu.

Classical texts explicitly mention that functions of VV get altered due to many factors either by depletion (*kshaya*) or overexpression (*Vruddhi*) [18]. The bioavailability of VV depends upon the quality of bodily fluid (*Rasa and Rakta*) or bodily tissues (*Mansa and Meda*) along with the substrate that it is associated with. Since Charaka considers all intact channels synonymous with an organ system (*Srotas*), VV augments the flow across these intact channels (*Srothovahana*), where its disruption may lead to hypo or hyperactivity of the organ system with morbidities such as remodeling or fibrosis (*Atipravrutti*), obstruction (*Sanga*), twisting and enlargement (*granthi*) and flow reversal of bodily fluid or displacement of any anatomical structure (*Vimarga gamana*) (Fig. 2) [28].

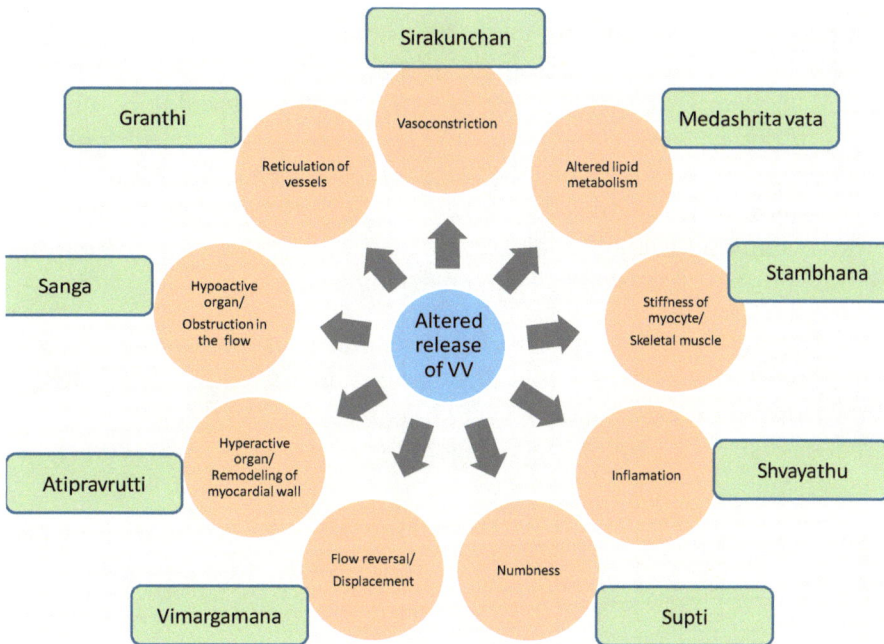

Fig. (2). Functions of vitiated Vyana Vayu.

Receptivity to any stimulus is based on intrinsic and extrinsic factors. Any factor that alters the thermoregulation associated with arid, rapid, and subtle (*sukshma*) qualities in the system disrupts the VV mechanism [17].

Intrinsic factors are genetically predetermined and include phenotypic constitution; one possesses it from the time of birth. This determines their physiological and psychological status [29]. Environment, diet, lifestyle, and stress are some of the VV's extrinsic components that can potentially incapacitate the weaker host [30].

With the help of its intrinsic properties to adapt to the state of equilibrium, it responds differently to extreme temperatures by accumulating and aggravating to protect the system either by inhibition leading to depletion or over-expressed due to proliferation.

It is necessary to maintain appropriate lubrication within and around the cell. Proper nutrition helps in bringing the same and prevents the organ system from disruption. Hence, food plays an important role in conserving the bioavailability of VV. As over expression can lead to inflammation of any interstitial tissue leading to cytokine storm (*khe varshamiva toyadah*) or promoting pathological dryness (*Ruksha),* causing necrosis of the cells around [25].

Overindulgence in food with pungent and astringent tastes (*Katu, Kashaya Ras*) disrupts VV by promoting pathological dryness and stiffness in the metabolizing tissues and skeletal organs, leading to stiffness of vasculature and hypo or dyskinesis of the muscles (*Stambhana*) [31]. Even though salt mitigates dryness and is advocated in various Vata disorders [32], excessive consumption inhibits VV through its secretory nature (*Syandana*), thereby disrupting the vascular tone. Addiction to smoking is another classic cause that augments the disruption of VV. They reduce intrinsic lubrication by intensifying dryness and stiffness.

VV gets disrupted by suppression of some natural urges leading to conduction abnormalities. Urges such as belching, excretion of flatus, feces, and semen, inhibit the normal expression of VV [12]. Yawning is facilitated by *Vyana Vayu* where repeated suppression of this maneuver can give rise to vasoconstriction and frequent twitches of the skeletal muscles [33].

Redundant walking (*Atigamana*), distorted activities (*Vishama Cheshta*), excessive mental stress (*Vishaada)* are few other causes of disruption of VV [34] (Fig. **2**).

4. PATHOGENESES

Frequent indulgence of the above etiological factors, individually or cumulatively, can turn VV pathologic and disturb the equilibrium of the body. The disease prognosis from pathological VV to various complications can be best explained in six distinct phases *(Kriya Kal)* [35, 36].

4.1. Stage of Accumulation (*Sanchaya*)

The body's state of equilibrium is always maintained by keeping the core internal lubrication and temperature optimum. At the same time temperature and moisture of cellular surroundings also needs to be maintained for sustained homeostasis. An increase in thermoregulation with reduced lubrication triggers VV to abnormally accumulate in the host (*Ushnena yukta rukshadyah*). This usually is a transient phase that progresses undetected.

4.2. Stage of Aggravation (*Prakopa*)

Constant stimulus allows the accumulated VV to proliferate and drift. In this phase, there is a decline in the thermoregulatory mechanism along with reduced lubrication within or around the cells. This phase can be identified strategically by critical introspection. By detecting a sudden change in the body demand during the stage of accumulation, there is an increased liking for opposite elements like demanding a cool environment with proper hydration. Pathologic thirst (Polydipsia) is one such example of this stage which often gets ignored [37]. Pain and cramps in the muscular region (*Udveshtana*), bloated abdomen (*Adhman*), and regurgitation (*Hrdayotkledana*) are due to proliferation of VV [38]. It is recommended to mildly increase the thermoregulation along with adequate water and fat-soluble lubrication to enable lipophilic permeability [39].

4.3. Stage of Dissemination (*Prasar*)

Stage of proliferation when left unattended leads to dissemination. This stage is associated with blood influenced in two ways; either a deluge in abnormally produced VV (*Vruddhi*) due to extrinsic factors or inhibition of VV (*kshaya*) due to increased lipid concentration.

The former disturbs the hemostasis whereas the latter alters homeostasis by hyperperfusion (*Pratarpan*) of fats on the tissues. Vascular tone is altered in both conditions [40].

It reacts to its other species quickly due to IEF and alters its subtle (*Sukshma*) nature. An increase in pathological dryness leads to stiffness (*Sthambhana*) of the vasculature that resists blood to flow swiftly and an increase in lipid concentration increases vasoconstriction or stenosis (*Sirakunchana*). This marks the onset of vascular and insulin resistance [41].

Detection of this state is challenging due to its transient nature. Circulation of raised lipid concentration in blood, altered mean arterial pressure [42], and glucose tolerance test (GTT) can predetermine this stage [43]. Apart from maintaining the core body temperature, this state can be reverted through appropriate diet and exercise.

4.4. Stage of Localization (*Sthanasamshraya*)

Influenced by intrinsic and extrinsic factors, the plotting of lipid-rich components occurs at weaker sites. Initially, the site responds to stimuli through inflammation either by deposition of lipids in the lumen of coronary or peripheral arteries or deposition of fats in the buttocks, chest, and abdomen. The scavenging property of VV is disrupted in this stage causing inflammation (*Shvayathu*), hypertrophy, ischemia, remodeling or fibrosis, cysts, or tumor in various domains [44].

This is an important phase of pathogeneses. All prodromal symptoms are expressed in this phase. Since the function of VV is widespread and regulates the majority of actions, its pre-symptoms too are widespread. Pathologic yawning before fever (*Jwara*) and progressive wasting disease (*Rajayakshma*), pathological belching before tumor [7], palpitation or missed beats before arrhythmia, pseudo hunger before obesity [45] are some of the pre-symptoms to established conditions of disrupted VV.

It has become easier to determine this stage due to advancements in technology. Electro and echocardiogram are important non-invasive tools to predict future or ongoing cardiac events at the same time raised levels in cardiac enzymes with inflammatory markers such as tumor necrosis factors, interleukins are popularly used for a prospective coronary event. Phyto-pharmacological interventions of antioxidants (*Vata Doshaghna*) are recommended in this state.

4.5. Stage of Manifestation (*Vyakta*)

This phase is an established morbid condition caused due to varied expression of VV. Clinical presentation and evaluations are distinct for each manifested disease and impossible to explicitly justify in this domain.

Obesity (*Atisthoulya*), diabetes mellitus (*Prameha*), myocardial infarction (*Hrd Marmaghat*), Arrhythmia (*Hrdrav*), PVD (*Sirakunchana*) are some of the established diseases from disrupted VV of this stage.

Imaging techniques such as Cardiac MRI, echocardiogram, and electrocardiogram to detect cardiac incompetency, glycosylated hemoglobin for diabetes, peripheral doppler test for PVD, and cardiac enzymes such as Troponins, Creatine-Phospho-Kinase-MB (CPKMB), Myoglobins are frequently used test to detect and confirm the eventual myocardial injury.

4.6. Stage of Complication (*Bheda*)

Emphasis on CVD complications (*Upadrava*) from VV deserves an independent section. The impact of deranged VV can be fatal. Details on signs and symptoms that predict death are elaborated in eight distinct chapters, by Charaka (*Indriya Sthana*) [46].

This stage is expressed as a syndrome with a cluster of diseases under the frame of deranged VV in multiple planes. It is a decompensated stage where the CVS and MS run at the cost of constant VV depletion and failing VV mechanism.

Dilated Cardiomyopathy (*Hrdvyas*), Atrial fibrillation (*Hrdrava*), Adam stroke syndrome (*Apatantraka*) [47], myoclonic twitches (*Akshepa*) [48] are some of the complications caused due to deranged VV.

5. CONCOMITANT CONCEPT

A similar concept in conventional science was explored using keywords – Gaseous component associated with contraction, expansion, ejection, heart, vasodilation, vasoconstriction, muscular stiffness, and metabolite transport to bodily tissues. It was found that endothelium-derived relaxing factor, identified as Nitric Oxide (NO) has a similar role to perform. It is believed to be a highly diffusible molecule with intrinsic oxidant properties and vital to the majority of cardiac functions. There is extensive evidence that confirms the contribution of NO in initiating the action potential. Due to its rapid movement, it is very difficult to determine NO concentration. NO is produced by many cells in the body but its expression in the myocardium and vascular endothelium is extremely important. Its slightest abnormal genesis can be detrimental to the circulatory system including the heart. The concentration of 0.05 micromole of NO brings a positive inotropic effect whereas NO concentration higher than 10 micromoles brings negative inotropic effects. NO at higher concentrations becomes cytotoxic [49]. It is reported that constant endothelial laminar or oscillatory flow at 12 dyn/cm^2 preserves endothelial functions [50]. There is a strong link between NO abundance, apoptosis, and fibrosis of cardiomyocytes. At the mitochondrial level, excessive NO concentration inhibits apoptosis and promotes necrosis through energy depletion [51] eventually leading to cell death and major organ failure.

NO is synthesized in almost all cardiac cell types that govern myocardial contraction and a key factor in excitation and contraction coupling [52]. Documented reports confirm that the concentration of NO in myocytes is inversely proportional to myocardial contractility [53]. On the contrary, its altered concentration is responsible for causing myocardial fibrosis and contractile dysfunctions [54]. The heart produces NO on a beat-to-beat basis in response to changes in coronary flow and myocardial loading [55].

NO arbitrates flow-mediated vasodilation and opposes vasoconstrictor effects. It counteracts vascular stiffness and lowers blood pressure. NO is a critical modulator of blood flow, vascular tone, and blood pressure. Physiologic NO reduces oxidative stress. It enhances endogenous antioxidant potential by producing Super Oxide Dismutase (SOD) in the endothelium, vascular smooth muscle cells, and myocytes.

NO has been the most researched molecule for the past few decades with more than 115,000 scientific articles published on it [56]. Even though it has diverse physiologic effects and operates in various organs other than the myocardium, it has a unifying effect of maintaining homeostasis. There are extensive reviews on NO's potent antioxidant, anti-inflammatory, antithrombotic and anti-atherogenic actions. NO plays a key role in cell metabolism and is instrumental in coordinating tissue energy demand with supply [57]. There are several vascular components involved in regulating these processes but not as critical as NO.

NO in Skeletal muscle plays a vital role in total body glucose and lipid homeostasis. Neurotransmission, cell growth, muscle metabolism, and excitation-contraction couplings [58].

6. CLINICAL IMPLICATIONS

There is no clinical radar screen available that can assess the working of VV or capture its bioavailability from any given site. Just as deregulation of NO signaling pathways is associated with the pathogenesis of many cardiovascular and metabolic disorders [59], disrupted VV too has daunting effects on the same CVS and MS. A deterred VV can be understood only through an impacted target site. Echocardiography is an important tool that gives comprehensive information on various attributes of *vyana vayu* where its impairment can be determined through velocity, turbulence, open and closure of valves, contraction, expansion, ejection, relentless pumping, and many more. Diseases related to disruption of VV are listed in Table **2**.

Table 2. Disorders of pathologic vyana vayu.

Domains	Disorders from Pathologic *Vyana Vayu*
Myocardium	Angina (*Hrtshool/ Hrdvyatha*) Ventricular ectopic beats (*Hrdayoparodh*) Myocardial injury (*Hrd marmaghat*) Dilated cardiomyopathy (*Hrd Vyas*) Arrhythmia (*Hrdrav*) Myocardial stiffness (*Hrtstambha*) Regurgitations (*Vimarga gamana*)
Metabolic	Ischemic Heart Disease (*Kutila sira*) Peripheral vascular disease (*Sirakunchan*) Hypertension (*Vyana bala vaishamya*) Varicose veins (*Siraja granthi*) Reticulated vessels (*Sirapratan*) Diabetes (*Prameha*) Obesity (*Atishoulya)*

(Table 2) cont.....

Domains	Disorders from Pathologic *Vyana Vayu*
Musculoskeletal	Adam stroke's syndrome (*Apatanaka/Apatantraka*) Paralysis (*Khanja*) Brachial neuralgia (*Khalli*) Myoclonal twitches (*Akshepaka*) Thigh muscle stiffness (*Urusthambha*)
Other disorders [34]	Loss of energy (*Utsah Bhransh*) Erectile dysfunctions (*Punstvopaghat*) Edema (*Shvayathu*) Pyrexia (*Jwara*) Trembling (*Kampa*) Numbness *(Angasupta)* Skin diseases (*Kushta*) Herpes Zoster (*Visarpa*)

Morbidities caused due to altered expressions of VV.

7. TREATMENT STRATEGIES

Conventionally, every treatment module has a targeted therapeutic approach. On the contrary, Ayurveda recommends viewing the same target comprehensively. Hence, considering the array of VV's role, the use of a legitimate regimen would certainly prevent a forthcoming disaster.

Refraining from etiological factors always remains a primary line of action to prevent disease prognosis [60]. Ayurveda advocates restoration of disrupted VV by mildly increasing the core body temperature associated with therapies that mitigates dryness, stiffness through nutrition and medication that promotes lipophilic permeability.

7.1. Diet

Planning a proper diet can benefit the appropriate expression of VV. A considerably hot drink (fortified or medicated) after morning meals is a targeted therapeutic approach to correct disrupted VV (*Vyanente pratarashasya*) [61]. This simple intervention promotes nourishment and saturation (*Preenayati*) [62]. Gruels and drinks of roasted grains (*Vilepi and Saktu*) promote life and strength. Charaka has indicated many Cardio-protective fruits, such as Mangifera indica, pomegranates, Garcinia cambogia, which concurrently are validated to be rich in flavonoids and promote free radical scavenging activity [63 - 65].

7.2. Exercise

Apart from curative measures through food and medication, appropriate exercise also has a positive impact on VV. Controlled and limited exercise can prevent further impairment of VV.

7.3. Pharmacological Approach

There are several formulations (single and polyherbal) cited in classical texts that are conducive to VV. Concurrently some of the formulations have been studied concerning NO concentration and reported to possess antioxidant properties conducive to the heart.

7.3.1. Terminalia Arjuna (TA)

An extensive in-depth study of TA, confirms its cardiogenic, vasodilating, anti-atherogenic, antidiabetic, antioxidant activities. The bark of TA is believed to possess at least fifteen types of tannins with related compounds, where tannins are regarded to enhance the synthesis of Nitric Oxide [66].

7.3.2. Innula Recemosa

(*Pushkarmool*) is a popular herb found in high altitudes. Charaka advocates its roots in acute coronary syndrome [67]. Usually, myocardial injury is caused as a consequence of multiple responses such as inflammatory cytokines, compromised circulatory and energy metabolism. It is reported to inhibit overexpression of NO because of alantolactone, which involves in various inhibitory signaling pathways such as interleukins and tumor necrosis factors [68].

7.3.3. Fagonia Arabica

Dissolving a thrombus in a blood vessel has always been a challenging task. Steptokinase and Urokinase have been popular drug of choice for lysis but have their limitations with fatal consequences. Fagonia Arabica (*Dhamasa*) is reported to possess thrombolytic properties *in vitro*, but its efficacy needs to be validated *in vivo* [69].

8. OMICS STUDY AND AYURVEDIC THERAPEUTIC STRATEGIES

There is a need to understand Ayurvedic therapeutic strategies using biomarkers and evaluate prognosis with the help of modern techniques. Genomics, transcriptomics, proteomics, and metabolomics (multi-omics), have been used to understand the genetic variations, changes in gene expression, protein expression, or changes in metabolic profile in CVD cases. Of these techniques, metabolomics offers the advantage of biomarker discovery. Since metabolites represent the sum of the interaction of genomics, transcriptomics, and proteomics; it is very close to the phenotype. Hence, metabolomic offers the scope for measuring metabolic profile in CMD and during treatment to understand the mechanistic aspects of Ayurveda formulations. Many of the current treatments in Ayurveda have not been analyzed using multi-omic techniques. Such multi-omic studies in the future will help gain insight into the holistic approach used in Ayurvedic treatment and understand it from a systems biology perspective.

CONCLUSION

Every minute action of Nitric Oxide corresponds to the functions of *Vyana Vayu* where they play a ubiquitous role in maintaining homeostasis in the endogenous system. Performing dynamically from the heart, they are responsible for regulating vascular tone, metabolite transfer, and tissue permeability. The slightest attenuation of VV can potentially damage the contractile stature of the myocardium along with the vasculature. Its deleterious effects on the musculoskeletal system can blunt its activities, halting quality of life. Hence, refraining from IEF can reverse the CMD prognosis to some extent by timely identifying transient stages and strategically intervening during each. Preserving the intrinsic properties of VV can help in restoring the equilibrium, reducing adverse events and enhancing the quality of life of the survived individual. With the help of metabolomic studies, evidence-based Ayurvedic formulations that correct the impaired Vyana Vayu can be validated.

10. HIGHLIGHTS

• *Vyana Vayu* regulates contractile functions of the heart and maintains appropriate vascular tone.

• It is responsible for the circulation and perfusion of bodily fluid across the channels, metabolizing tissue, and exercising muscle.

• Its abnormal and subnormal expression can damage the myocardium and circulatory elements.

• Concomitantly it resembles the functions of Nitric oxide in the endogenous system.

CONSENT FOR PUBLICATION

Not applicable.

CONFLICT OF INTEREST

The author declares no conflict of interest, financial or otherwise.

ACKNOWLEDGEMENTS

I owe special thanks to my mentor Dr. Shekhar Rao, Director, Chairman, and Professor of Cardiothoracic Vascular Surgery from Sri Sathya Sai Institute of Higher Medical Sciences, Whitefield, and Bangalore. I am also thankful to my guru, Vaidya Dilip P Gadgil, and Late Vaidyaraj Chandrashekhar Ganesh Joshi for guiding me to understand Ayurveda as it is.

This work was funded by the Ministry of Science and Technology, Government of India, Department of Science and Technology (Ref. No: SR/WOS-A/L--151/2018).

REFERENCES

[1]   Pandey MM, Rastogi S, Rawat AKS. Indian traditional ayurvedic system of medicine and nutritional supplementation. Evid Based Complement Alternat Med 2013; 2013: 1-12.
        [http://dx.doi.org/10.1155/2013/376327] [PMID: 23864888]

[2]   Shilpa S, Venkatesha Murthy CG. Development and standardization of Mysore Tridosha scale. Ayu 2011; 32(3): 308-14.
        [http://dx.doi.org/10.4103/0974-8520.93905] [PMID: 22529642]

[3]   Priyavat S. Caraka Samhita. Choukhambha Orientalia: Varanasi 1981.

[4]   Shrestha S, Suvedi KS, Adhikary R. Basic Principles in Shareera Kriya Vigyana (Physiology): An Appraisal. Journal of Ayurveda Campus 2020; 1(1): 45-53.
        [http://dx.doi.org/10.51648/jac.18]

[5]   Trikamji VY. Acharya Sushrutasamhita of Sri Dalhanacharya. 8th edition. Varanasi: Choukhambha Orientalia 1981; p. 261.

[6]   Vaidya ADA. Ashtanga Sangraha of Srimadvruddha Vagbhat with Indu critical notes. 1980.

[7]   Vaidya ADA. Ashtanga Sangraha of Srimadvruddha Vagbhat with Indu critical notes. Ayurvidya Mudrananalya. 1980.

[8]   Trikamji VY. Acharya Sushrutasamhita of Sri Dalhanacharya. Varanasi: Choukhambha Orientalia 1981; p. 253.

[9]   Sharma H, Chandola HM. Ayurvedic concept of obesity, metabolic syndrome, and diabetes mellitus. J Altern Complement Med 2011; 17(6): 549-52.
        [http://dx.doi.org/10.1089/acm.2010.0690] [PMID: 21649521]

[10]   Barquera S, Pedroza-Tobías A, Medina C, *et al.* Global Overview of the Epidemiology of Atherosclerotic Cardiovascular Disease. Arch Med Res 2015; 46(5): 328-38.
        [http://dx.doi.org/10.1016/j.arcmed.2015.06.006] [PMID: 26135634]

[11]   Kaptoge S, Pennells L, De Bacquer D, *et al.* World Health Organization cardiovascular disease risk

charts: revised models to estimate risk in 21 global regions. Lancet Glob Health 2019; 7(10): e1332-45.
[http://dx.doi.org/10.1016/S2214-109X(19)30318-3] [PMID: 31488387]

[12] Baikampady SV. Vata dynamics with special reference to cardiac disorders – A cross-disciplinary approach. J Ayurveda Integr Med 2020; 11(4): 432-9.
[http://dx.doi.org/10.1016/j.jaim.2020.10.005] [PMID: 33218848]

[13] Travis F, Wallace R. Dosha brain-types: A neural model of individual differences. J Ayurveda Integr Med 2015; 6(4): 280-5.
[http://dx.doi.org/10.4103/0975-9476.172385] [PMID: 26834428]

[14] Prasher B, Gibson G, Mukerji M. Genomic insights into ayurvedic and western approaches to personalized medicine. J Genet 2016; 95(1): 209-28.
[http://dx.doi.org/10.1007/s12041-015-0607-9] [PMID: 27019453]

[15] Vaidya YT. Acharya Charaksamhita of chakrapanidatta. Varanasi: Choukhambha Orientalia 2004; p. 16.

[16] Srikantha Murthy Prof. Vagbhat's Ashtanga Hrdayam. 7th edition., Varanasi: Choukhambha Orientalia 2010.

[17] Pt. Bhishagacharya harishastri paradkar vaidya. Astangahrdayam composed by Vagbhata and commentaries by arunadatta and hemadri. 2000.

[18] Vaidya YT. Acharya Charaksamhita of Chakrapanidatta. Varanasi: Choukhambha Orientalia 2004; p. 105.

[19] Byadgi P. Critical appraisal of Doshavaha Srotas. Ayu 2012; 33(3): 337-42.
[http://dx.doi.org/10.4103/0974-8520.108819] [PMID: 23723638]

[20] Vaidya YT. Acharya Charaksamhita of Chakrapanidatta. Varanasi: Choukhambha Orientalia 2004.

[21] Bhawsar P, Nampalliwar AR. Vyana vata-physiological understanding: a review. Int Ayurvedic Med J 2017; 5(11): 4258-63.

[22] Vaidya YT. Acharya Charaksamhita of Chakrapanidatta. Varanasi: Choukhambha Orientalia 2004; p. 105.

[23] Srikantha M. Vagbhat's Ashtanga Hrdayam. Varanasi: Choukhambha Orientalia 2010; p. 82.

[24] Menon M, Shukla A. Understanding hypertension in the light of Ayurveda. J Ayurveda Integr Med 2018; 9(4): 302-7.
[http://dx.doi.org/10.1016/j.jaim.2017.10.004] [PMID: 29153383]

[25] Pt. Bhishagacharya harishastri paradkar vaidya. Astangahrdayam composed by vagbhata and commentaries by arunadatta and hemadri. 2000; 400.

[26] Kundu S. A review On Concept Of Atisthoulya Vis-A-Vis Metabolic Syndrome: An Approach To Explore The Convectional Entity. Int J Res Ayurveda Pharm 2018, 9(5): 35-40.
[http://dx.doi.org/10.7897/2277-4343.095151]

[27] Balkrishna A, Pathak S, Kumar A, Mishra P, Balkrishna A. Ayurvedic doshas as predictors of sleep quality. Med Sci Monit 2015; 21: 1421-7.
[http://dx.doi.org/10.12659/MSM.893302] [PMID: 25982247]

[28] Khendkar V, Chandrakant J, Janardanrao PJ, Scholar PG. Physiological and Clinical Significance of Srotas. Int J Health Sci (Qassim) 2016; 6: 451.

[29] Rotti H, Raval R, Anchan S, *et al.* Determinants of prakriti, the human constitution types of Indian traditional medicine and its correlation with contemporary science. J Ayurveda Integr Med 2014; 5(3): 167-75.
[PMID: 25336848]

[30] Nath R, Mandal SK, Kumar MS. An analytical study of different clinical presentation of Diabetes

mellitus: Ayurveda perspective. Journal of Scientific and Innovative Research 2017; 6(2): 44-9.
[http://dx.doi.org/10.31254/jsir.2017.6201]

[31]   Vaidya YT. Acharya Charaksamhita of Chakrapanidatta. Varanasi: Choukhambha Orientalia 2004; p. 120.

[32]   Shenoy U S, Kumar B N A, Manjunatheshwara D, Kumar A. Rational usage of Lavana in the management of Vatavyadhi with respect to Sneha and its formulations. J Pharmacol 2020; 9(2): 146-8.
[http://dx.doi.org/10.31254/phyto.2020.920112]

[33]   Vaidya ADA. Ashtanga Sangraha of Srimadvruddha Vagbhat with Indu critical notes. Ayurvidya Mudrananalya. 1980; p. 396.

[34]   Vaidya ADA. Ashtanga Sangraha of Srimadvruddha Vagbhat with Indu critical notes. Ayurvidya Mudrananalya. 1980; p. 400.

[35]   Chauhan A, Semwal DK, Mishra SP, Semwal RB. Ayurvedic concept of Shatkriyakala : a traditional knowledge of cancer pathogenesis and therapy. J Integr Med 2017; 15(2): 88-94.
[http://dx.doi.org/10.1016/S2095-4964(17)60311-X] [PMID: 28285613]

[36]   Vaidya YT. Acharya Sushrutasamhita of Sri Dalhanacharya. 8th edition. Varanasi: Choukhambha Orientalia 1981; pp. 103-6.

[37]   Gupta M, Pujar R, Gopikrishna S, Vijnana V, Dharmasthala S, Hassan H, *et al.* Understanding of thirst mechanism in ayurveda. Int J Pharm Pharm Sci 2020; 9(2): 1238-47.

[38]   Vaidya YT. Acharya Sushrutasamhita of Sri Dalhanacharya. Varanasi: Choukhambha Orientalia 1981; p. 70.

[39]   Pt. Bhishagacharya harishastri paradkar vaidya. Astangahrdayam composed by vagbhata and commentaries by arunadatta and hemadri. 2000; 211.

[40]   Vaidya Y. Acharya Sushrutasamhita of Sri Dalhanacharya. Varanasi: Choukhambha Orientalia 1981; p. 253.

[41]   Vaidya YT. Acharya Sushrutasamhita of Sri Dalhanacharya. Varanasi: Choukhambha Orientalia 1981; p. 261.

[42]   Šuláková T, Feber J. Should mean arterial pressure be included in the definition of ambulatory hypertension in children? Pediatr Nephrol 2013; 28(7): 1105-12.
[http://dx.doi.org/10.1007/s00467-012-2382-7] [PMID: 23340855]

[43]   Jagannathan R, Neves JS, Dorcely B, *et al.* The oral glucose tolerance test: 100 years later. Diabetes Metab Syndr Obes 2020; 13: 3787-805.
[http://dx.doi.org/10.2147/DMSO.S246062] [PMID: 33116727]

[44]   Asthana AK, Asthana M, Sharma G. Critical Review of Shatkriyakala and Its Significance. Int Ayurvedic Med J 2018; 6(10): 2300-4.

[45]   Shukla A, Baghel AS, Vyas M. Lifestyle related factors associated with *Sthaulya* (obesity) - A cross-sectional survey study. Ayu 2016; 37(3): 174-83.
[http://dx.doi.org/10.4103/ayu.AYU_87_16] [PMID: 29491669]

[46]   Vaidya YT. Acharya Charaksamhita of chakrapanidatta. Varanasi: Choukhambha Orientalia 2004; pp. 343-75.

[47]   Sharma MR. Critical study on apatantraka. Ann Ayurvedic Med 2012; 1(3): 109-12.

[48]   Vaidya YT. Acharya Sushrutsamhita of Sri Dalhanacharya. Varanasi: Choukhambha Orientalia 1981; p. 262.

[49]   Levine AB, Punihaole D, Levine TB. Characterization of the role of nitric oxide and its clinical applications. Cardiology 2012; 122(1): 55-68.
[http://dx.doi.org/10.1159/000338150] [PMID: 22722323]

[50]   Dhawan SS, Avati Nanjundappa RP, Branch JR, *et al.* Shear stress and plaque development. Expert Rev Cardiovasc Ther 2010; 8(4): 545-56.
[http://dx.doi.org/10.1586/erc.10.28] [PMID: 20397828]

[51]   Crouser ED. Mitochondrial dysfunction in septic shock and multiple organ dysfunction syndrome. Mitochondrion 2004; 4(5-6): 729-41.
[http://dx.doi.org/10.1016/j.mito.2004.07.023] [PMID: 16120428]

[52]   Ziolo MT, Kohr MJ, Wang H. Nitric oxide signaling and the regulation of myocardial function. J Mol Cell Cardiol 2008; 45(5): 625-32.
[http://dx.doi.org/10.1016/j.yjmcc.2008.07.015] [PMID: 18722380]

[53]   Mohan P, Brutsaert DL, Paulus WJ, Sys SU. Myocardial contractile response to nitric oxide and cGMP. Circulation 1996; 93(6): 1223-9.
[http://dx.doi.org/10.1161/01.CIR.93.6.1223] [PMID: 8653845]

[54]   Kleinbongard P, Dejam A, Lauer T, *et al.* Plasma nitrite reflects constitutive nitric oxide synthase activity in mammals. Free Radic Biol Med 2003; 35(7): 790-6.
[http://dx.doi.org/10.1016/S0891-5849(03)00406-4] [PMID: 14583343]

[55]   Drexler H. Nitric oxide synthases in the failing human heart: a doubled-edged sword? Circulation 1999; 99(23): 2972-5.
[http://dx.doi.org/10.1161/01.CIR.99.23.2972] [PMID: 10368111]

[56]   Ignarro LJ. Preface to this special journal issue on nitric oxide chemistry and biology. Arch Pharm Res 2009; 32(8): 1099-101.
[http://dx.doi.org/10.1007/s12272-009-1800-2] [PMID: 19727601]

[57]   Spier SA, Delp MD, Stallone JN, Dominguez JM II, Muller-Delp JM. Exercise training enhances flow-induced vasodilation in skeletal muscle resistance arteries of aged rats: role of PGI $_2$ and nitric oxide. Am J Physiol Heart Circ Physiol 2007; 292(6): H3119-27.
[http://dx.doi.org/10.1152/ajpheart.00588.2006] [PMID: 17337602]

[58]   Kingwell BA. Nitric oxide□mediated metabolic regulation during exercise: effects of training in health and cardiovascular disease. FASEB J 2000; 14(12): 1685-96.
[http://dx.doi.org/10.1096/fj.99-0896rev] [PMID: 10973917]

[59]   Clementi E, Nisoli E. Nitric oxide and mitochondrial biogenesis: A key to long-term regulation of cellular metabolism. Comp Biochem Physiol A Mol Integr Physiol 2005; 142(2): 102-10.
[http://dx.doi.org/10.1016/j.cbpb.2005.04.022] [PMID: 16091305]

[60]   Raut A. Integrative endeavor for renaissance in Ayurveda. J Ayurveda Integr Med 2011; 2(1): 5-8.
[http://dx.doi.org/10.4103/0975-9476.78179] [PMID: 21731380]

[61]   Junjarwad A, Savalgi P, Vyas M. Critical review on Bhaishajya Kaala (time of drug administration) in Ayurveda. Ayu 2013; 34(1): 6-10.
[http://dx.doi.org/10.4103/0974-8520.115436] [PMID: 24049398]

[62]   Vaidya YT. Acharya Charaksamhita of chakrapanidatta. Varanasi: Choukhambha Orientalia 2004; p. 172.

[63]   Kim H, Moon JY, Kim H, *et al.* Antioxidant and antiproliferative activities of mango (*Mangifera indica* L.) flesh and peel. Food Chem 2010; 121(2): 429-36.
[http://dx.doi.org/10.1016/j.foodchem.2009.12.060]

[64]   Noda Y, Kaneyuki T, Mori A, Packer L. Antioxidant activities of pomegranate fruit extract and its anthocyanidins: delphinidin, cyanidin, and pelargonidin. J Agric Food Chem 2002; 50(1): 166-71.
[http://dx.doi.org/10.1021/jf0108765] [PMID: 11754562]

[65]   Sripradha R, Sridhar MG, Maithilikarpagaselvi N. Antihyperlipidemic and antioxidant activities of the ethanolic extract of Garcinia cambogia on high fat diet-fed rats. J Complement Integr Med 2016; 13(1): 9-16.

[http://dx.doi.org/10.1515/jcim-2015-0020] [PMID: 26595408]

[66] Amalraj A, Gopi S. Medicinal properties of *Terminalia arjuna (Roxb.) Wight & Arn.*: A review. J Tradit Complement Med 2017; 7(1): 65-78.
[http://dx.doi.org/10.1016/j.jtcme.2016.02.003] [PMID: 28053890]

[67] Vaidya YT. Acharya Charaksamhita of Chakrapanidatta. Varanasi: Choukhambha Orientalia 2004; pp. 602-3.

[68] Tavares WR, Seca AML. Inula L. secondary metabolites against oxidative stress-related human diseases. Antioxidants 2019; 8(5): 122.
[http://dx.doi.org/10.3390/antiox8050122] [PMID: 31064136]

[69] Prasad S, Kashyap RS, Deopujari JY, Purohit HJ, Taori GM, Daginawala HF. Effect of Fagonia Arabica (Dhamasa) on *in vitro* thrombolysis. BMC Complement Altern Med 2007; 7(1): 36.
[http://dx.doi.org/10.1186/1472-6882-7-36] [PMID: 17986325]

CHAPTER 7

Nutraceuticals: The Potential Agents to Rescue Human Race from Cardiovascular Diseases (CVDs)

Sreedevi Gandham[1], **Ghali. EN.Hanuma Kumar**[2] and **Balaji Meriga**[2,*]

[1] *Department of ECE, Siddhartha Educational Academy Group of Institutions, Tirupati, Andhrapradesh, India*

[2] *Department of Biochemistry, Sri Venkateswara University, Tirupati, Andhrapradesh, India*

Abstract: Cardiovascular disease(CVD) is the foremost global health problem that accounts for the highest rate of morbidity, mortality and huge healthcare costs. Food habits and lifestyles predominantly affect the functioning of the cardiovascular system either directly or indirectly through risk factors like hypertension, obesity, dyslipidemia, diabetes, *etc*. Decreased physical activity, increased sedentariness, and growing fast food culture are some of the apparent reasons that make the disease impact more on the younger generation. Several plant species have been reported in ethnomedicine for their therapeutic efficacies against CVDs and other diseases. Even though some preclinical and clinical studies have demonstrated the beneficial effects of dietary plant components in the prevention and treatment of CVDs, they are limited to selected study groups. Therefore, their scope and utility need to be broadened and applied to larger populations to reduce the public health burden of CVDs. Since nutraceutical approach is more preferable than other therapeutic methods, there is a growing interest in functional foods and diet based remedies. In the present chapter, we have presented the current scenario of CVDs, their pathophysiology, the therapeutic drugs available, the role of nutraceuticals in treating CVDs and their mode of action with a special emphasis on commonly used kitchen spices.

Keywords: CVDs, Dyslipidemia, Hypertension, Nutraceuticals, Phytocons-tituents, Spices.

1. INTRODUCTION

In recent decades, with advancements in science and technology, human lifestyle has changed dramatically in both developed and developing countries. The consumption of fast foods/energy dense foods, snacking frequency and late night

---

* **Corresponding author Balaji Meriga:** Department of Biochemistry, Sri Venkateswara University, Tirupati, Andhrapradesh, India; E-mail: balaji.meriga@gmail.com

Dr. V. V. Sathibabu Uddandrao & Dr. Parim Brahma Naidu (Eds.)

meals and snacks have increased. Simultaneously, physical excercise has considerably reduced due to increased conveyance facilities, availability of high end machinery, tools and electronic devices used in every sphere of human activity [1]. As a result, the environment sensed by the brain has become arrhythmic. Taken together, the incidence of CVDs and other metabolic syndrome disorders has been alarmingly rising across the globe [2].

Cardiovascular diseases (CVDs) are a cluster of disorders of blood vessels and heart, including peripheral heart disease, coronary heart disease, cerebrovascular disease (stroke), heart failure, heart attack, cardiomyopathies, congenital heart disease and dyslipidemias. CVDs majorly occur due to impairment in blood supply to organs like the heart or/and the brain because of atherosclerosis, thrombosis and high blood pressure. Fig. (**1**) shows some principle reasons for the occurrence of cardiovascular diseases. As per the WHO report in 2017, CVDs caused 31% annual deaths worldwide. According to the European cardiovascular disease statistics, more than 45% of deaths occur due to CVDs in Europe [3]. In the USA, about 50% of population suffers from one or other form of CVDs as per the American Heart Association report [4]. In India, with more than one billion population and with a high incidence of abdominal obesity, diabetes and hypertension, the CVD morbidity is on the brink of turning into an epidemic [5]. The annual number of deaths from CVDs in India is projected to rise from 2.26 million (1990) to 4.77 million or more by 2020 [4]. Worldwide distribution of various cardiovascular diseases is represented in Fig. (**2**).

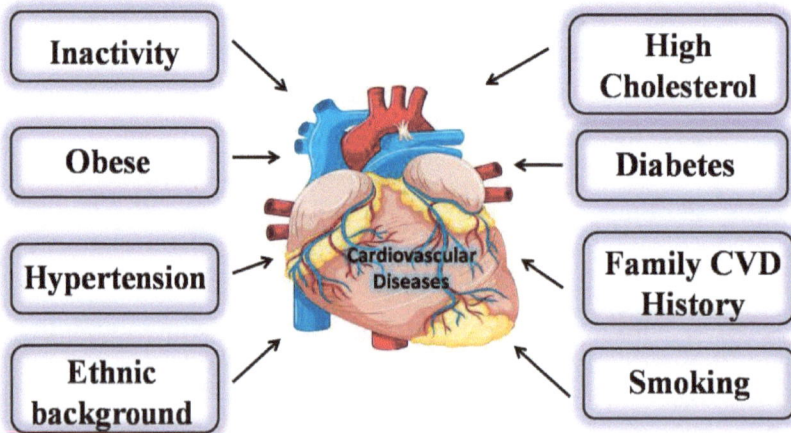

Fig. (1). Principle reasons of CVD.

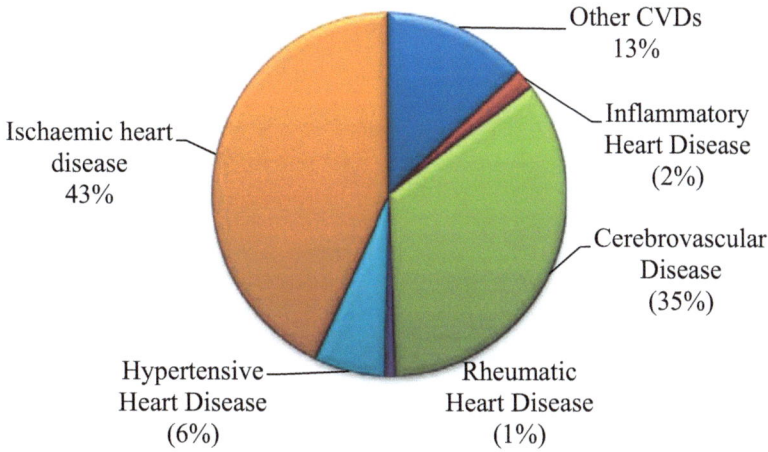

Fig. (2). Worldwide distribution of various CVD.

The common risk factors for CVDs include physical inactivity, obesity, hypertension, ethnic background, family CVD history, smoking, hyperlipidemia, elevated levels of low-density lipoprotein (LDL) cholesterol, reduced levels of high-density lipoprotein cholesterol (HDL) and diabetes [6]. Recent studies confirmed inflammation as a prominent risk factor which is indicated by high levels of highly sensitive C-reactive protein (hs-CRP) and interleukin-6 (IL-6) [7]. Basic symptoms include pain or discomfort in the centre of the chest, arms, left shoulder, jaw and elbows, difficulty in breathing, vomiting or feeling sick, faintness, dizziness and unconsciousness.

2. CVDS: PATHOPHYSIOLOGY

The main pathogenic process identified in CVD patients is atherosclerosis caused by the decreased or lessened blood flow in the blood vessels in the aorta and the arteries. Fig. (3) represents the narrowing of arteries due to plaque deposition. Atherosclerosis involves inflammation, endothelial dysfunction, immunologic phenomena and dyslipidemia [8]. A dysfunctional endothelial system causes the deposition of LDL particles and their conversion into oxidized LDL in the intima of blood vessel walls. They trigger the development of fatty plaques due to the accumulation of extracellular matrix and lipid-laden macrophages. It leads to further macrophage recruitment that becomes calcified and transition to atherosclerotic plaques. Over the years, gradual thickening of intima causes reduced blood flow or its complete occlusion to the heart or the brain, leading to myocardial infarction or stroke, respectively. Further, hypertension, if left unmanaged, leads to arteriosclerosis and damage to target organs. Therefore, it is known as a silent killer as it is a prominent risk factor for atherosclerosis, heart failure, stroke and other diseases like retinopathy, and nephropathy [9].

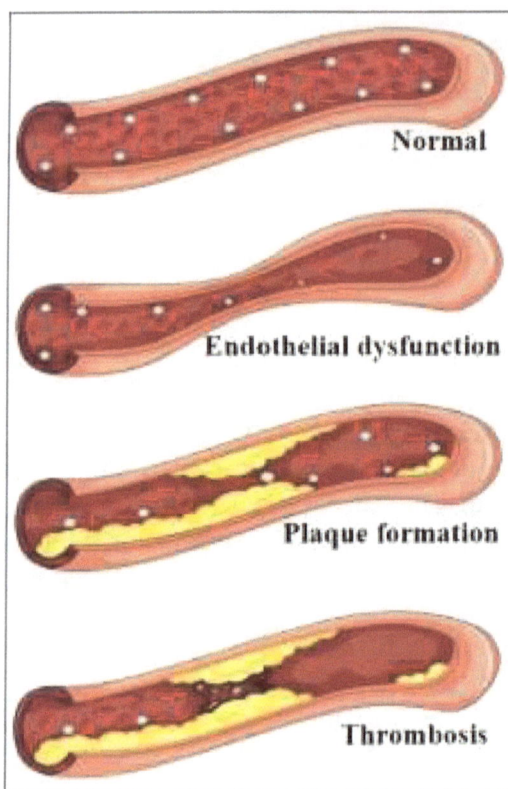

Fig. (3). Narrowing of arteries due to the deposition of plaque.

Apart from diet/lifestyle induced CVDs, genetics of atherosclerosis indicates that a positive family history is the main risk factor for predicting future atherosclerosis and related events for an individual [10]. ABO blood groups are the earliest genetic variants that are associated with an elevated risk of atherosclerosis. ABO blood group locus also influences the interactions of leukocyte and endothelial cells in the early stage of inflammation [10, 11]. Low-density lipoprotein receptor (LDLR), expressed by many cell types, is a cell surface protein that binds to apolipoprotein B (ApoB) and contributes to the uptake of low density lipoproteins (LDL) and intermediate density lipoproteins (IDL) from the blood. Apolipoprotein E (ApoE) is able to uptake chylomicron and

VLDL from the blood *via* the LDLR and LDL receptor related protein. Similarly increased apolipoprotein A (LPA) levels increase the risk of atherosclerosis and other associated diseases. In addition, other lipoprotein genes which are directly linked to LDL are also associated with the altered atherosclerotic risk.

Despite great scientific advancements in medical and health domains, CVDs still account for the highest mortality rate in the world. Therefore intense research efforts continue to develop new therapeutic options to effectively prevent/treat all types of CVDs. All member countries (194), under the leadership of WHO, introduced the "Global action plan for the prevention and control of non communicable diseases (NCDs) 2013-2020" including CVDs to reduce premature deaths from NCDs by 25% by 2025 [12]. Incidence of hypertension can be reduced by implementing some of the policies like population-wide policies to lessen the behavioural risk factors. The UN General Assembly convened a third high-level meeting on NCDs in 2018, and by 2025, took stock of national progress in attaining the voluntary global targets.

3. CVDS: TREATMENT OPTIONS

Apart from surgery, several synthetic drugs like antihypertensives, antiarrhythmics, lipid-lowering drugs, anti-platelet drugs, vitamin K antagonists *etc.*, have been developed to tackle CVDs [13]. Anticoagulants (blood thinners) including dabigatran (pradaxa), apixaban (eliquis), rivaroxaban (xarelto), heparin (various), edoxaban (savaysa), warfarin (coumadin), *etc*, decrease the clotting (coagulating) ability of the blood. Table **1** depicts the generic name, dosage and side effects of drugs used to treat CVDs.

Table 1. Drugs used to treat CVDs: Generic name, indications dosage and side effects.

Type of Drug	Generic Name	Indications	Dosage	Side Effects
ANTIHYPERTENSIVES				
ACE Inhibitors	Captopril, Monopril	Heart Failure	Captopril: 12.5 mg 3 times daily	Hypotension, upper Respiratory tract symptoms, altered liver function tests, blood disorders, dizziness, photosensitivity, headache, renal impairment.
		Hypertension	Captopril: 12.5 mg twice daily	
		Diabetic nephropathy	Captopril: 75-100 mg once daily	
		Prophylaxis Following MI	Captopril: 6.25 mg once daily	

(Table 1) cont.....

Type of Drug	Generic Name	Indications	Dosage	Side Effects
Diuretics	Furosemide	Resistant Hypertension	Furosemide: 40-80 mg once daily	Hepatic encephalopathy, rise in serum cholesterol, acute urinary retention, metabolic alkalosis, blood disorders, hypersensitivity reactions like pruritus, hypotension
		Oedema	Furosemide: 20-40 mg once daily	
Angiotensin Receptor Blockers	Losartan, Candesartan	Diabetic nephropathy	Losartan: 50 mg daily	Dizziness, headache, pruritus, malaise, palpitation, rash, gastro intestinal disturbances
		Left ventricular hypertrophy	Losartan: 12.5-150 mg daily	
		Hypertension	Losartan: 50 mg once daily	
Beta Blockers	Atenolol, Propranolol	Migraine	Atenolol: 50-200 mg daily	Sleep disturbances, dizziness, gastro intestinal disturbances, heart failure, hypotension, headache, purpurea, visual disturbances, dry eyes
		Arrhythmias	Atenolol: 50-100 mg daily	
		Angina	Atenolol: 100 mg once/twice daily	
		Hypertension	Atenolol: 25-50 mg daily	
Alpha Blockers	Prazosin, Doxazosin	Congestive Heart Failure	Prazosin: 4-20 mg daily	Postural Hypotension, asthenia, headache, palpitations, gastro intestinal symptoms, oedema
		Raynaud's Syndrome	Prazosin: 1-2 mg daily	
		Hypertension	Prazosin: 1-10 mg 2-3 times daily	
Calcium Channel Blockers	Nifedipine, Verapamil, Diltiazem	Raynaud's Syndrome	Nifedipine: 5-20 mg 3 times daily	Oedema, dizziness, asthenia, tremor, gastro intestinal disturbances, headache, lethargy, vertigo, visual disturbance, sweating, hypotension
		Angina (prophylaxis)	Nifedipine: 5-20 mg 3 times daily	
		Hypertension	Nifedipine: 20-30 mg once daily	

(Table 1) cont.....

ANTI-ARRHYTHMICS				
Class I (sodium channel blockers) & Class II (Beta blockers)	Flecainide, Lidocaine, Procainamide	Ventricular Arrhythmias	Flecainide: 50-100 mg twice daily	Peripheral neuropathy, hepatic dysfunction, leucopenia, increased sweating, rarely pneumonitis, asthenia, visual disturbances, dysponea, gastro intestinal disturbances, raise in antinuclear antibodies, photosensitivity, fever
Class III (Potassium channel blockers) & Class IV (Calcium channel blockers)	Amiodarone, Sotalol	Ventricular, Arrhythmias	Amiodarone: 200 mg 2-3 times daily	Taste and hepatic disturbances, tremor, hyperthyroidism, reversible comeal microdeposits, skin discoloration, peripheral neuropathy, ataxia, headache, aplastic anaemia, rash, respiratory distress syndrome, sweating
	Digoxin	Heart Failure	62.5-125 µg daily	Anorexia, vomiting, abdominal pain, nervous system disturbances, thrombocytopenia, anorexia, necrosis, psychosis.
		Supra-ventricular arrhythmias	125-150µg daily	
ANTI-PLATELET DRUGS				
Anti-thrombotics/ Antiplatelet agents	Aspirin	Pain / pyrexia	300-600 mg every 4-6 h as necessary	Gastro intestinal irritation, chest pain, hypertension, oedema, bronchospasm, gastro intestinal haemorrhage, hypertension, chest pain
		Prevention of cardiovascular disease	75 mg per day	
	Clopidogrel	Acute myocardial infarction	300 mg daily initially then 75 mg once/day	Headache, dizziness, dyspepsia, thrombocytopenic purpurea,

(Table 1) cont.....

-		Prevention of thrombotic events (esp. when warfarin not tolerated)	75 mg once/day	fatigue, blood disorders, nausea, oedema, rash, Stevens Johnson syndrome, hypersensitivity reactions
		Acute coronary syndrome	300 mg daily initially then 75 mg once/day	
	Ticragelor	Prevention of thrombotic events.	180 mg bolus then 90 mg twice daily	Dyspnoea, nausea, hypertension, dizziness, headache, cough, arrhythmias, hypotension, raise in serum creatinine, vertigo, haemorrhage, bruising
	Prasugrel	Prevention of thrombotic events.	60 mg bolus then 5-10 mg once daily	Hypertension, haemorrhage, headache, back pain, dizziness, arrhythmias, pyrexia, rash, oedema, hypercholesterolaema
VITAMIN K ANTAGONISTS				
	Warfarin	Prevention of thrombotic/ embolic events (esp. after prosthetic valve insertion)	5-10 mg initially then tailored to individual (usually 3-9 mg once daily at the same time)	Hepatic dysfunction, haemorrhage, pancreatitis, nausea, pyrexia, alopecia, vomiting, purpura, rash
	Acenocoumarol	Prevention of thrombotic/ embolic events (esp. after prosthetic valve insertion)	4 mg initially, followed by 1-8 mg daily	
LIPID-LOWERING DRUGS				
Statins	Simvastatin, Atorvastatin	Primary hyper-cholesterolaemia, combined hyperlipidaemia	Simvastatin: 10-20 mg once daily	Gastritis, headache, insomnia, eczema, oedema, diabetes mellitus, vertigo, bronchitis, urinary tract infection
		Prevention of cardiovascular events	20-40 mg once daily	
		Familial hyper-cholesterolaemia	Simvastatin: 40 mg once daily	

(Table 1) cont.....

Fibrates	Ezetimibe	Primary and familial hyper-cholesterolaemia	10 mg once daily	Abdominal pain, diarrhea, fatigue, headache, sinusitis, coughing hypersensitivity reactions like anaphylaxis, myopathy
	Gemfibrozil	Hyperlipidaemias of types IIa, IIb, III, IV and V	Gemfibrozil: 0.9-1.2 mg daily	Nausea, dyspepsia, abdominal pain, vomiting, headache, fatigue, pancreatitis, sexual dysfunction, myopathy, blurred vision, vertigo, alopecia, appendicitis

Antiplatelet agents and dual antiplatelet therapy (dapt), namely aspirin, ticagrelor (brilinta), clopidogrel (plavix), dipyridamole (persantine), prasugrel (effient) *etc*, prevent clots by preventing blood platelets from sticking together. Dapt involves a combinatorial treatment strategy which includes two types of antiplatelet agents (aspirin, p2y 12 inhibitor) at the same time to prevent the blood clot [14]. Angiotensin-converting enzyme (ACE) inhibitors include benazepril (lotensin), lisinopril (prinivil, zestril), enalapril (vasotec), captopril (capoten), fosinopril (monopril), trandolapril (mavik), moexipril (univasc), ramipril (altace), quinapril (accupril), perindopril (aceon), *etc*, which expand blood vessels and decrease resistance by lowering the levels of angiotensin II, allowing easy flow of blood and improving heart work efficiently [15].

Angiotensin II receptor blockers (or inhibitors) include eprosartan (teveten), azilsartan (edarbi), losartan (cozaar), candesartan (atacand), telmisartan (micardis), irbesartan (avapro), valsartan (diovan) and olmesartan (benicar). Rather than lowering angiotensin II levels, angiotensin II receptor blockers prevent this chemical from effecting heart and blood vessels. This maintains normal blood pressure [16]. Angiotensin receptor-neprilysin inhibitors (arnis) include entresto (sacubitril/valsartan) and neprilysin. Neprilysin is an enzyme that breaks down natural substances in the body and opens narrowed arteries [17]. By limiting the effect of neprilysin, entresto improves blood flow, artery opening, decreases strain on the heart, and reduces sodium (salt) retention.

Cholesterol-lowering medications like statins: atorvastatin (lipitor), pravastatin (pravachol), lovastatin (mevacor), pitavastatin (livalo), simvastatin (zocor), fluvastatin (lescol), rosuvastatin (crestor), nicotinic acids: niacin; combination statin and cholesterol absorption inhibitors: ezetimibe/simvastatin (vytorin); cholesterol absorption inhibitor: ezetimibe (zetia), *etc*, lower blood cholesterol levels [18]. Vasodilators include hydralazine (apresoline), isosorbide dinitrate (isordil), isosorbide mononitrate (imdur), minoxidil, *etc* that decrease blood pressure and relax blood vessels. A category of vasodilators called nitrates increases the supply of oxygen and blood to the heart and reduces workload on heart, thereby reducing chest pain (angina). Nitroglycerin can be absorbed or swallowed under the tongue as a pill (sublingual), in the form of spray and as a cream (topical application) [19]. Vascepa, farxiga and statins are some of the FDA approved drugs used to reduce cardiovascular risk among patients with elevated triglyceride levels, of which, farxiga improves glycemic control in adults with type 2 diabetes, and also reduces the risk of hospitalization for heart failure [USFDA, 2019].

4. PLANTS AND HERBS FOR TREATMENT OF CVDS

Over the past decades, pharmacological treatment of CVDs has increased greatly and several chemically synthesized drugs such as statins, beta-blockers, antiplatelets and ACE inhibitors have been prescribed and used in the treatment of CVDs. However, their effectiveness is limited owing to side effects upon long time usage and hence there is a relook into natural product based therapeutics to develop efficient alternative drugs or in adjunct therapy [20]. Plants are rich sources of several minerals, vitamins, micronutrients, oils and secondary metabolites. Different classes of phytochemicals like polyphenols, alkaloids, saponins, carotenoids, sterols, terpenoids, glycosides, *etc.* make plants and herbs as potential source of therapeutics. Plants and herbs in the form of extracts or as partially purified forms or pure compounds have been traditionally used from ancient times to treat human ailments including CVDs [21]. The main reason behind growing interests on plant based products is that they are viewed as natural, generally safe, inexpensive with no or minimal side effects and easy to consume. Furthermore, some of the plants and herbs are a part of dietary components as fruits, vegetables, spices and other edible items and work as functional foods/nutraceuticals/pharmaceuticals. However, more systematic research studies are required to evaluate their safety profile and add scientific validation to them. List of common nutraceuticals, their chemical constituents and mechanism of action are summarized and depicted in Table **2**.

Table 2. List of common nutraceuticals, used parts, chemical constituents and mechanism of action.

Plant Names	Parts Used	Chemical Constituents	Actions	References
Moringa oleifera (drumstick tree)	Leaves, pods	Saponins, alkaloids, Tannins, flavonoids, terpenes, carbohydrates, and cardiac glycosides	Antiinflammatory, cardioprotective, anticancer and antipyretic	[40]

(Table 2) cont.....

Plant Names	Parts Used	Chemical Constituents	Actions	References
Lagenaria siceraria (Bottle gourd)	Fruit	Sterols, saponins, flavonoids and terpenoids	Antioxidant, cardioprotective and antihyperlipidemic	[41]
Psidium guajava (gua)	Leaves, fruit	Phenolic, terpenoid, carotenoid, flavonoid and triterpene	Cardioprotective and antidiabetic	[42]
Aristotelia chilensis (Maqui berry)	Fruits	Phenolic compounds, flavonoids, delphinidin, anthocyanidins, gallate, quercetin, myricetin and rutin	Cardioprotective, anti-inflammatory, analgesic, and antioxidant	[43]
Olea europaea (olive)	Aerial parts	Flavonoids, flavanones, iridoids, secoiridoids, triterpenes and benzoic acid derivatives	Antidiabetic, anticancer and cardioprotective	[44]
Allium cepa (onion)	Leaves	Flavonoids, steroids and triterpenic acids	Cardioprotective, hypouricemic, antibacterial and antioxidant	[45]
Garcinia indica	Fruit	Garcinol, xanthochymol, isoxanthochymol, phenolic acids, hydroxycitric acid, flavonoids, anthocyanins, benzophenones, isogarcinol and tannins	Cardioprotective, hepatoprotective, antibacterial and antioxidant	[46]
Hairy fig (*Ficus hispida*)	Leaves	Alkaloids, mucilage, saponins, glycosides, flavonoids, gums, terpenes, phenols, sterols, triacontanol, b-amyrine acetate, lupeol acetate, b-sitosterol and b-amyrin	Cardioprotective, hepatoprotective, antipyretic and antiinflammatory	[47]
Crocus sativus (Saffron)	Flowers	Carotenoid compounds, crocetin, safranal, crocin, delphinidin, glucoside picrocrocin, petunidin and anthocyanins	Cardioprotective, anxiolytic, hypnotic and anticancer	[48]
Mucuna pruriens (Cowhage)	Seeds	Alkylamines, alkaloids, sterols, saponins, 6-methoxyharman, mucunadine, mucunain, and mucunine	Cardioprotective, neuroprotective and antidepressant	[49]
Cordia myxa	Fruit	Flavonoids, tannin and saponins	Cardioprotective, antiinflammatory and analgesic	[50]
Sesbania grandiflora (Agati)	Leaves	Alkaloids, tannin, flavonoids, steroid, glycosides, anthraquinone, terpenoids and pholobatannins	Antibacterial, cardioprotective and anxiolytic	[51]

4.1. Polyphenols

Polyphenols are among a wide variety of secondary metabolites and phytochemicals present in many plants, fruits and vegetables. Epidemiological studies indicate that the intake of diet rich in polyphenols decreases the risk of diabetes, CVDs, cancers and other chronic diseases. Around 8000 compounds under polyphenols have been identified in different plant species. They are classified in to four major groups like flavonoids, lignans, stilbenes and phenolic acids. Polyphenols are rich in grapes, berries, pears, apples, cherries, coffee, tea, red wine, legumes, chocolates and spices [22]. Polyphenols are involved in the defense mechanism against several pathogenic infections and diseases. They show antioxidant activity by donating an electron to the free radicals or ROS generated in the cells. Polyphenols manage blood pressure levels, improve HDL cholesterol levels, antioxidant status, exert anti-atherosclerotic effects and protect against platelet aggregation and myocardial ischemia [23].

4.2. Flavonoids

Many vegetables, fruits and beverages contain flavonoids. Flavonoids include other subclasses like flavanols, flavanones, flavonols, flavones, isoflavones, and anthocyanins. Dietary supplements play a crucial role in reducing the risk of cardiovascular diseases [24]. Flavonols represent bioactive compounds like quercetin, kaempferol, myricetin, isorhamnetin, *etc*, which are generally found in common dietary sources like onions, grapes, tea, bananas, apples, *etc*. Flavanones are rich in citrus fruits, grapes and pineapple and the examples are narigenin, and hesperidin. Catechins, epicatechins, and epicatechin gallate are the examples of flavonols and they are generally rich in teas and fruits. The importance of flavonoids' intake to treat cardiovascular diseases and a consequent decrease in mortality in US adults was demonstrated earlier [25]. Flavones include phytochemicals like apigenin, luteolin, *etc*, usually found in citrus fruits and apples [26]. Anthocynins are rich in berries and grapes and they include plant compounds like petunidin, malvidin, peonidin, *etc*. Isoflanones are rich in legumes and soybean and they include bioactive compounds like genistein, biochanin, daidzein, *etc*. Other polyphenols like resveratrol from red wine, curcumin in turmeric, lignans in flax seed, sesame seeds and whole grains have health promoting effects.

4.3. Carotenoids

Carotenoids are colored pigments that give yellow, orange, and red colors to plants, herbs and algae. They are rich in tomatoes, carrot, pumpkin, papaya, *etc*.

Examples include lycopene, lutein, zeaxanthine, *etc*. They have strong antioxidant, antilipidemic, antihypertensive, antiinflammatory activities and improve endothelial functions [27]. For instance, the consumption of lycopene reduces the incidence of myocardial infarction, angina pectoris and coronary insufficiency. It also reduces atherosclerosis, stroke, hypertension, *etc* [28].

4.4. Other Phytochemicals

Terpenoids like arjunolic acid from *Terminalia arjuna* [29] and gymnemic acid from *Gymnema sylvetris* [30] have been reported for their cardioprotective activities. Alkaloids like ajmaline and quinidine have antiarrhythmic and antihypertensive activities [31]. Saponins from ginseng and Allium species, *Terminalia arjuna*, *Glycyrrhiza glabra* and Astralagus species have been well studied for their cardioprotective potential [32]. Phytoestrogens, a group of plant constituents that elicit estrogen like biological response, possess antioxidant activity, influence the lipoprotein metabolism, increase vascular reactivity, decrease superoxide production and cardiovascular mortality, inhibit platelet aggregation and improve healthy lipid profile [33]. Mechanisms behind their protective role is due to the existence of their metal chelating property.

4.5. Vitamins

Intake of vitamin E and vitamin C offers cardiovascular protection and lowers blood pressure [34]. Vitamin C lowers the blood pressure by decreasing the binding affinity of the angiotensin (AT) receptors (AT1 and AT2). Vitamin D is another important vitamin synthesized in the skin after sunlight exposure. Vitamin D exerts immunoregulatory and antiinflammatory effects. Studies demonstrated that there is a strong relationship between cardiovascular diseases and vitamin D deficiency [35]. Vitamin D deficiency also increases recruitment of M1 macrophages, increases HDL cholesterol levels, decreases inflammatory processes and increases the protection against the development of atherosclerosis [36]. In addition to fruits and vegetables, some marine food provides vitamins and minerals to treat CVDs [37].

5. NUTRACEUTICALS TO TREAT CVDS

Life style interventions, in the form of regular physical exercise and supply of nutrients through diet, are a promising strategy for the prevention and management of cardiovascular diseases, hypertension and other metabolic disorders [38]. Dietary foods or their derivatives that provide health benefits are commonly known as nutraceuticals. The term "nutraceuticals" was introduced by Stephen DeFelice in 1989. They are largely herbal products, isolated nutrients or dietary supplements and/or processed foods like beverages, cereals and other food products that act directly as well as indirectly on the physiological and biochemical processes of the body and promotes health. Studies demonstrated that the intake of some of the low cost nutraceuticals improved control of blood pressure as a strategic management that aimed to prevent hypertension [39].

6. SPICES AS EFFECTIVE NUTRACEUTICALS TO TREAT CVDS

Spices are plant products that possess a variety of phytochemicals and are known for their disease preventing and health promoting properties. They have been in use since ancient times for their antiinflammatory, carminative, anti-flatulent and many other properties [52]. Spices contain a good amount of minerals like potassium, manganese, iron, magnesium, *etc*. Manganese and potassium are the essential components for metabolic activities, of which, manganese is used as a co-factor for the antioxidant enzyme and superoxide dismutase whereas potassium exists in body fluids and cells that help in controlling blood pressure and heart rate. Spices can be aromatic or pungent in flavors and peppery or slightly bitter in taste. The bioactive components present in the spices have numerous health benefits including smooth digestion, antiinflammatory, antihypertensive, antihyperlipidemic and anticlotting action (preventing clogging of platelets in the blood vessels), and thus help easing blood flow, preventing stroke and coronary artery disease [53].

6.1. Ginger (*Zingiber Officinale*)

Ginger is the dried rhizome of *Zingiber officinale* (Family Zingiberaceae), an herbaceous perennial species. The knotted and branched rhizome, commonly called the 'root' is the portion of ginger used as spice food and dietary supplement [54]. Ginger is reported to possess essential oils, phenolic compounds, flavonoids, carbohydrates, proteins, alkaloids, glycosides, saponins, steroids, terpenoids and tannin as the major phytochemical groups which play an important role in the medicinal property of this plant [55]. Two major groups like diarylheptanoids and gingerol-related compounds have been reported as bioactive components identified in this particular plant..

Zinger has been documented to be used as a carminative and an anti-flatulent in treating cold, headaches, stomach upset, diarrhoea, indigestion, arthritis, rheumatological conditions, and muscular discomfort. Ginger was reported to have antimicrobial, antifungal, antiviral, antioxidant, antiinflammatory and anticancer activities [56]. Therapeutic efficacy of *Z. officinale* is represented in Fig. (**4**). It was reported that the aqueous extract of fresh ginger exhibits hypotensive, endothelium-independent vasodilator and cardio-suppressant properties through its specific inhibitory action at the voltage-dependent calcium channels [57]. It could be possible that the cholinergic-mediated vascular effects of ginger are due to sesquiterpenes such as zingiberene, bisabolene, camphene, and phellandrene also known to be present in ginger. Cholinergic receptor mediated vasodilation is due to the release of NO from the endothelium and consequent increase of cGMP contents in the vascular smooth muscles in response to the activation of guanylyl cyclase. These results show that the aqueous extract of fresh ginger lowers blood pressure *via* endothelium-dependent (cholinergic) and endothelium-independent (Ca^{++}channel blocker) vasodilator pathways. In atria, an additional cardiotonic component emerged, sensitive to blockade of Ca^{++} release from cardiac SR evident only in the presence of cholinergic receptor blockade. Some of the gingerols showed an atropine resistant and endothelium-dependent vasodilator effects along with a Ca^{++} antagonist activity that was identified in the presence of 6-gingerol [58].

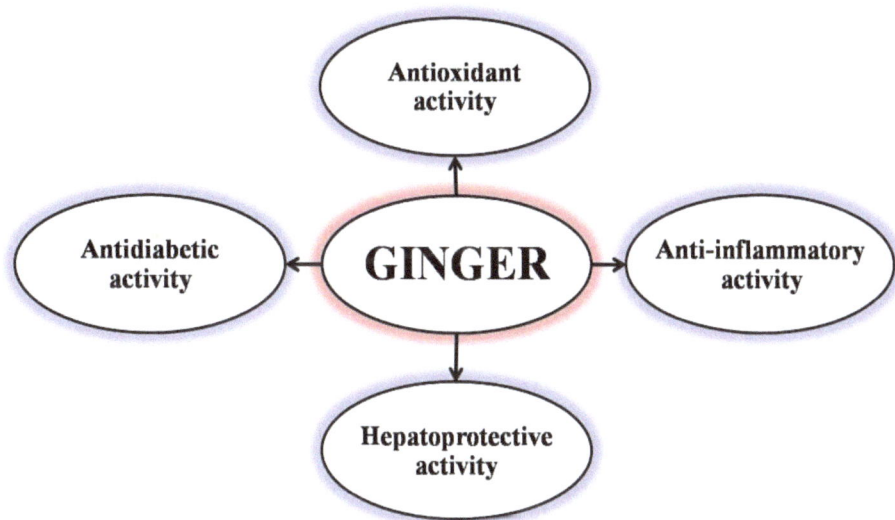

Fig. (4). Therapeutic activity of *Z. officinale*.

6.2. Turmeric *(Curcuma Longa)*

It is a rhizomatous perennial herb of Zingiberaceae family, commonly used in Indian, Chinese cuisine and traditional medicine. An array of phytochemicals are present in *Curcuma longa* such as saponins, steroids, tannins, anthocyanins, emodins, flavonoids, diterpenes, phytosterol, phenol, phlobatannin, leucoan- thocyanin, anthroquinone, chalcones, cardiac glycosides, and carbohydrates. Major phytochemical constituents are curcumin, demethoxycurcumin, bis- demethoxycurcumin, ar-tumerone, α-phellandrene, sabinene, geraniol, *etc* [59].

C. longa finds its place in both traditional and modern medicine. According to the Ayurvedic Pharmacopoeia of India, essential oil from rhizome of *C. longa* is used as a carminative, stomachic and tonic. Curcumin possesses antioxidant, antidiabetic, hypocholesterolemic activity and is reported to suppress tumor growth, inflammation and modulate cellular response of various immune cell types, such as T cells, B cells, macrophages, neutrophils, NK cells and dendritic cells [60] (Fig. **5**). Thus, turmeric has several beneficial effects and its bioactive components are known to play a key role in combating lifestyle based disorders.

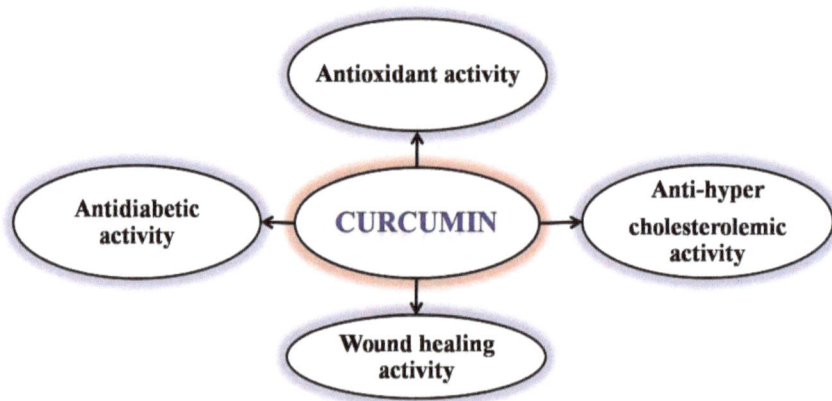

Fig. (5). Therapeutic activity of Curcumin.

6.3. Black pepper (*Piper Nigrum*)

It is famous as the spices king due to its pungent quality. Traditionally, black pepper is used as a spice in different kinds of food preparations. Peppers have been in use since centuries for its antiinflammatory, anti-obesity, anti-diabetic, anti carminativeand anti-flatulent properties [61]. Peppercorns comprise health benefiting essential oils like piperine and an amine alkaloid that gives strong spicy pungent property to the pepper.They are also an excellent source of many vital B- complex groups of vitamins such as pyridoxine, riboflavin, thiamin and niacin.

It contains several valuable compounds including phenolics, various derivatives of lignans, terpenes, chalcones, flavonoids, alkaloids and steroids. It also contains numerous monoterpenes hydrocarbons such as sabinene, pinene, terpenene, limonene, and mercene which altogether give aromatic property to the pepper

[62]. Some of the important compounds are piperine, piperolein, piperamide, piperamine, piperettine, piperenol, *etc.*

The active principles of pepper may uplift the gut motility and the digestion potential by enhancing the secretions of gastro-intestinal enzyme. Piperine also increases the absorption of selenium, B-complex vitamins, beta-carotene, and other nutrients from the food. Peppercorns are a good source of many anti-oxidant vitamins such as vitamin-C and vitamin-A. They are also rich in polyphenolic anti-oxidants like carotenes, cryptoxanthin, zeaxanthin, and lycopene. These compounds help the body in removing harmful free radicals and protect from cancers and diseases.These compounds have antiinflammatory, thermogenic, growth stimulatory, anti-thyroid and chemopreventive activities [63, 64] (Fig. **6**). Also, a study by Meriga *et al.* [65] depicted the antiobesity and antihyperlipidemic effects of piperonal of *Piper nigrum* in high-fat diet (HFD)-induced obese rats.

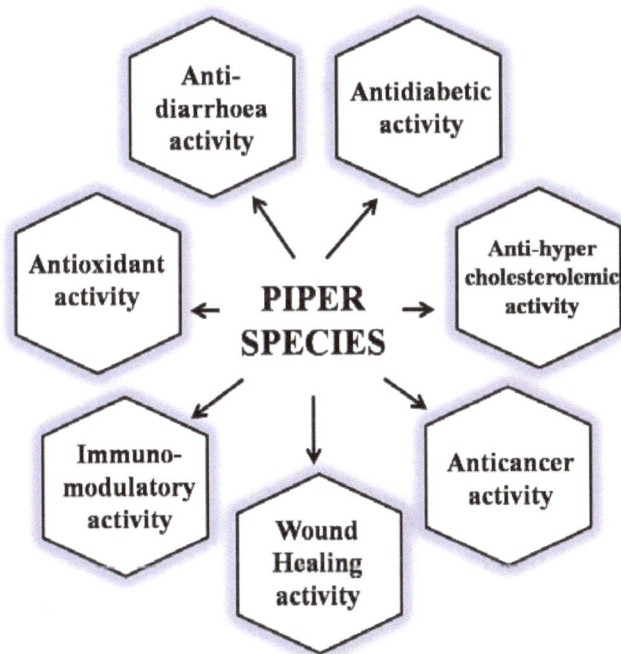

Fig. (6). Therapeutic activity of Piper species.

6.4. Coriander *(Coriandrum Sativum)*

Coriander belongs to carrot ancestors (Umbelliferae) and it is easily cultivated. Active constituents present in *Coriandrum sativum* are carbohydrates, reducing sugars, steroids, glycosides, triterpenes, and proteins. Coriander seeds contain petroselinic acid, linoleic acid, oleic acid, palmitic acid, monoterpenes, camphor, geraniol, coriandrin, dihydrocoriandrin, coriandronsA-E, flavonoids and essential oils. Various parts of this plant such as seeds, leaves, flowers and fruits, possess diuretic, antioxidant, ant-diabetic, anti-convulsant, sedative hypnotic, anti-microbial, anti-mutagenic and anthelmintic activity (Fig. **7**). It also possesses antihyperlipidemic activity and is used in the preparation of many house hold medicines to cure bed cold, seasonal fever, nausea, and stomach disorders [66].

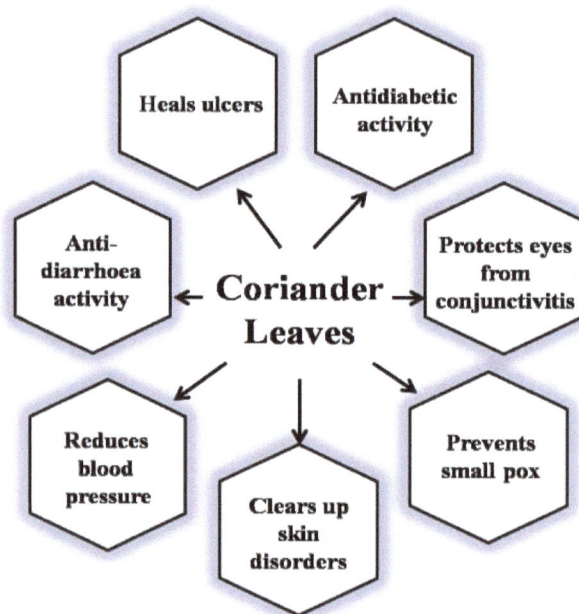

Fig. (7). Therapeutic activity of coriander leaves.

6.5. Cinnamon *(Cinnamomum Zeylanicum)*

Cinnamon is a spice obtained from the inner bark of several species of trees belonging to the genus cinnamomum. Although there are different species of cinnamon, *Cinnamomum zeylanicum* is categorised as true cinnamon when referred to as a spice. It is aromatic and used for cooking traditional Indian, Persian, and Turkish cuisines as a flavouring agent. Major components of cinnamon include cinnamaldehyde, cinnamic acid eugenol and coumarin [67]. Water-soluble polyphenolic compounds of cinnamon like epicatechin and catechin showed antioxidant, insulin potentiating and other related activities. Methyl chalcones of cinnamon increase the triacylglycerols lipase property, glycogen synthesis, phosphorylation of insulin receptor in adipocytes and skeletal muscles, and glucose uptake [68].

Literature suggests that cinnamon has potential pharmacological effects including antidiabetic, antioxidant, antiobese, and antihypercholesterolemic activities (Fig. **8**). Early studies suggested that cinnamon can be used effectively to lower blood glucose and cholesterol levels in type 2 diabetes mellitus [69]. It is demonstrated that consuming up to 6 grams of cinnamon per day reduces serum glucose, triglycerides, LDL cholesterol, and total cholesterol in people with type 2 diabetes, and the inclusion of cinnamon in the diet of people with type 2 diabetes will reduce risk factors associated with diabetes and cardiovascular diseases [70]. Cinnamon polyphenols enhance the uptake of glucose by showing insulin like properties in adipose tissue and skeletal muscles. These studies indicate that cinnamon is beneficial to treat lifestyle based disorders.

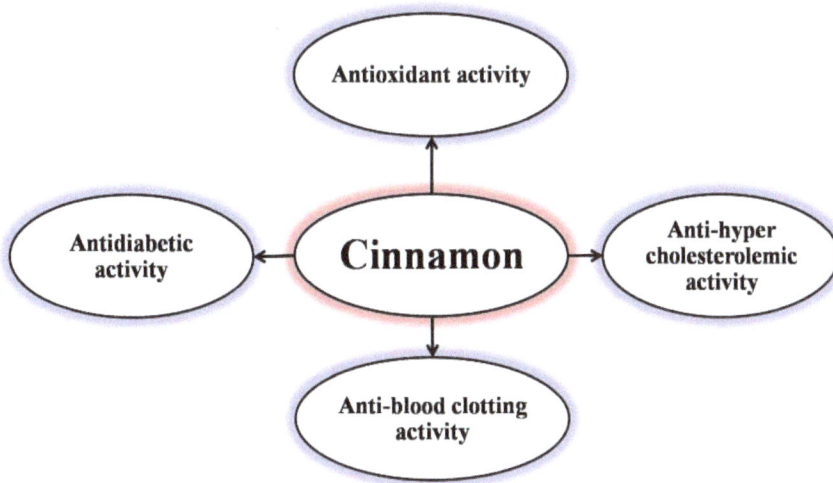

Fig. (8). Therapeutic activity of cinnamon.

6.6. Garlic *(Allium Sativum)*

Garlic is a strongly aromatic bulb crop, which belongs to the family Amaryllidaceae, and is renowned throughout the world for its distinctive flavour as well as its health-giving properties. Garlic, onions, leeks and chives are the members of the genus Allium, which comprises approximately 750 species. It is one of the most commonly used plants utilized both for medicinal purposes and culinary practices by providing flavor and taste to the final product. Garlic health promoting perspectives have been proven and it is recommended worldwide as a dietary supplement [71]. The nutritional composition of garlic bulb contains approximately 65% water, 28% carbohydrates, 2.3% organosulfur compounds, 2% protein, 1.2% free amino acids, and 1.5% fiber [72]. Dehydrated garlic and its oil are popular and are being sold as dietary supplements.

Both the aqueous and ethanol extracts of garlic were found to contain carbohydrates, reducing sugars, lipids, flavonoids, ketones, alkaloids, steroids and triterpenes. Important phytochemicals seen in *A. sativum* are quercetin, alliin, allicin, allyl alcohol, diallyl disulfide, ajoene, S-allyl cysteine, alliinase, allixin, allistatin-I, allistatin-II, β-phyllandrene, *etc* [73, 74].

Garlic and its sulfurous compounds are valuable for the treatment of many disorders related to the heart and blood vascular system like high blood pressure, high cholesterol, coronary heart disease, heart attack, and atherosclerosis. It also helps maintain healthy liver, combat stress, fatigue and treat some types of cancers [75]. Fig. **(9)** depicts therapeutic effects of garlic.

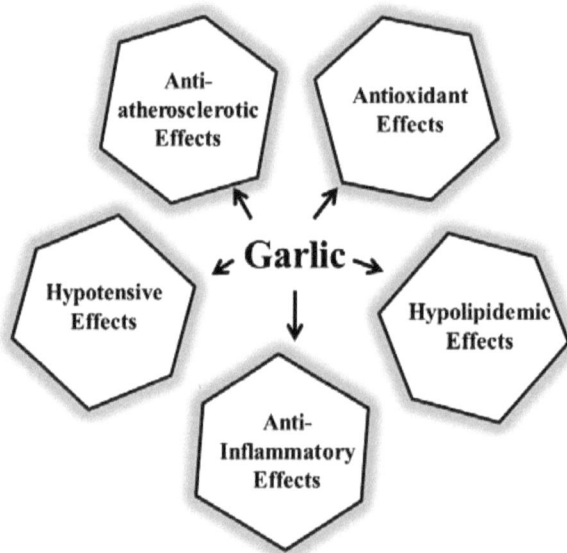

Fig. (9). Therapeutic effects of garlic.

6.7. Cloves *(Syzygium Aromaticum)*

Clove is a medium sized tree (8-12 m) belonging to the Mirtaceae family. Whole and ground cloves are used to enhance the flavor and nutritional value of many food. They are highly valued in medicine as a carminative and a stimulant, and are said to be a natural anthelmintic. The oil of clove is used extensively for flavoring many kinds of food products, such as meats, sausages, baked goods, confectionery, candies, table sauces, and pickles, and is also used extensively in perfumes, soaps and as a clearing agent in histological work [76]. Clove buds contain essential oil, which is dominated by eugenol, eugenyl acetate and β-caryophyllene; tannins like gallotannic acid; methyl salicylate (painkiller), flavonoids like eugenin, kaempferol, rhamnetin and eugenitin; triterpenoids like oleanolic acid, stigmasterol and campesterol.

The active principles in the clove are documented to have antidiabetic, hepatoprotective, antioxidant, anti-septic, local anesthetic, antiinflammatory, rubefacient (warming and soothing), carminative and anti-flatulent properties. It has also been successfully used for asthma and various allergic disorders [77]. Presence of sesquiterpenes in cloves confers potential anti-carcinogenic efficacies. In addition, the cloves are anti-mutagenic, antiviral, anti-thrombotic and anti-parasitic [78, 79] (Fig. **10**).

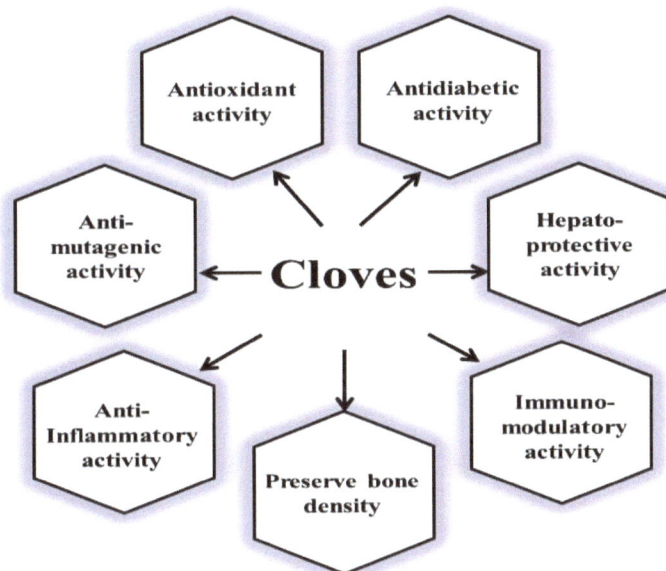

Fig. (10). Therapeutic activity of cloves.

6.8. Other Common Spices

The curry leaf tree (*Murraya koenigii*) is a member of the family **Rutaceae** and is native to **India** and **Sri Lanka**. The phytochemicals present in leaves include carbohydrates, tannins, alkaloids, steroids, triterpenoids and flavonoids. One of the most important phytochemicals Mahanimbine, when given orally, lowered the body weight gain as well as plasma TC and TG levels significantly. Thus, *M. koenigii* shows anti-diabetic, hypocholesterolemic and anti-lipid peroxidative activities [80]. The curry leaf powder is traditionally consumed by diabetics in southern part of India.

Brassica juncea is also known as mustard and belongs to the Cruciferae (Brassicaceae) family. Mustard seeds contain beta carotene, vitamin-A, C, K, B3, iron, selenium, fatty acids, calcium and magnesium and has several health benefits. It lowers cholesterol, helps to lose weight, slows down ageing, relieves rheumatoid, arthritic, and muscle pain. Mustard has potential pharmacological effects in treating cardiovascular diseases and diabetes [81].

Elettaria cardamomum, commonly known as green or true cardamom, is a herbaceous perennial plant in the ginger family "Zingiberaceae", native to southern India. Cardamom is a seed pod, known for its culinary and medicinal properties since centuries. Cardamom is rich in pinene, sabinene, myrcene, phellandrene, limonene, cymene, geraniol, *etc*. It decreases the level of total cholesterol, triglycerides, LDL-C, VLDL and has increased HDL-C levels. Cardamom is used to treat hyperglycemia, dyslipidemia, and hepatic steatosis [82].

Myristica fragrans, commonly known as Mace (Nutmeg) is a perennial edible plant belonging to the family Annanceae. Nutmeg contains terpene hydrocarbons (sabinene and pinenes, camphene, p-cymene, phellandrene, terpinene, limonene, myrcene), terpene derivatives (linalool, geraniol, terpineol) and phenylpropanoids (myristicin, elemicin, safrol, eugenol and eugenol derivatives). Of the latter group, myristicin (methoxy-safrole) is responsible for the hallucinogenic effect of nutmeg [83].

Moringa oleifera is reported to provide 7 times more vitamin C than oranges, 10 times more vitamin A than carrots, 17 times more calcium than milk, 9 times more protein than yoghurt, 15 times more potassium than bananas and 25 times more iron than spinach and it is also rich in phenolics and glucosinolates, hence it is called as miracle tree or super natural food. Almost each and every part of *Moringa* tree is useful for medicinal, functional food preparations and as nutraceuticals. Moringa leaves have multiple health benefits like antihyperlipidemic, antihypertensive, antihyperglycemic, cardioprotective, antiobesity, *etc* [84]. A study by Muni swamy *et al*. [85] demonstrated that on treatment of 3T3-L1 adipocytes with astragalin of *M. oleifera,* there was a significant suppression of adipogenesis and stimulation of lipolysis.

Capsicum annum commonly called as Red pepper is rich in bioactive compounds like capsinoids and capsaicin which are reported for antiobesity and cardioprotective activities. It was found that people who eat foods containing chilli powder at least 4 times a week are about 50% less likely to die of coronary heart disease or stroke [86].

7. NUTRACEUTICALS/SPICES: MODE OF ACTION

Atheroprotective properties like antioxidant, antiinflammatory, antidiabetic, antiatherogenic, anti-coagulant and antidyslipidemic are the major means through which spices offer protection against CVDs. However, the biochemical processes, signaling events and molecular mechanisms are not clearly understood; hence, need to be studied in-depth to establish the complete mode of action. Table **3** depicts a brief note on some known spices, their atheroprotective effects, and potential mechanism of actions.

Table 3. List of commonly used spices, atheroprotective effects and potential mechanisms.

Spices	Atheroprotective Effects	Potential Mechanism	References
Ginger	Antioxidation, Anti-inflammation.	(−) PI3K/AKT/mTOR signaling, (−) Lipid peroxidation, (+) Beclin1 expression to promote autophagy	[87]
Turmeric	Anti-oxidation, Anti-inflammation, Anti-diabetes, Anti-atherogenesis.	(−) M1 macrophage polarization and IL-6, TNF-α and IL-12 expression through inhibition of NF-kB activation and MAPKs (+) Free radical scavenging (+)LXRα and PPARγ transcription factors activity (+)cholesterol efflux and ABCA1 expression	[88, 89]
Black pepper	Anti-atherogenesis, Anti-oxidation.	(−) Lipid profile, LDL, including total cholesterol and triglycerides (−) ROS production and pp38 expression, (−) VSMCs proliferation *via* repressing pERK1/2, (+) ABCA1 expression	[90]
Coriander	Anti-inflammation, Anti-oxidation, Anti-dyslipidemia.	(−) Isoproterenol-induced ROS production, (−) LDL oxidation, (−) Total cholesterol, triglyceride and VLDL, plaque formation (−) LPS-stimulated PGE2 production and nitric oxide through NF-κB and MAPKs activation	[91, 92]
Cinnamon	Anti-coagulation, Anti-oxidation, Anti-inflammation, Anti-diabetes.	(−) CD36 and SRA expression, (−) Phagocytosis of LDL, (−) Platelet aggregation, (−) TNFα-activated VCAM-1 expression	[93]
Garlic	CVD protection, Anti-oxidation, Anti atherogenesis.	(−) Lipid profile, LDL, including total cholesterol and triglycerides (−) lipid accumulation in early stage of atherosclerosis and Inflammation, (+) cholesterol efflux through PPARγ/LXRα signalling and ABCA1 expression	[94, 95]

(Table 3) cont.....

Spices	Atheroprotective Effects	Potential Mechanism	References
Clove	Anti-oxidation, Anti-inflammation, Reduction of hyperlipidemia and hyperglycemia.	(−) LPS-induced IL-6 and IL-1β expression through NF-kB pathway	[96]

CONCLUSION

Balanced diet and regular physical activity certainly make people live a longer and healthy life. Plants and herbs, more particularly functional foods and nutraceuticals, have a promising role in the prevention and treatment of CVDs. Appropriate protective measures and treatment undeniably reduce the high risk and mortality caused by CVDs. Realizing the nutraceutical potential of plants, herbs and spices and making them part of dietary components along with lifestyle interventions have proven promising in this regard. Inclusion of functional foods in diet that have antihypertensive, antioxidant, antithrombotic, antihyperlipidemic, antihyperglycemic, antiadipogenic, immunoboosting, antiinflammatory and antiatherosclerotic properties, would certainly be beneficial in protecting people from CVDs and other ailments. This is mainly due to the abundance of a variety of phytochemicals, vitamins, minerals, polyunsaturated fatty acids and many more components in plants and herbs. In addition, spices play a leading role in maintaining healthy cardiovascualr system and protecting from other chronic ailments. Together, we conclude that nutraceuticals and their adequate supplementation in diet can rescue human race not only from cardiovascular diseases but also from other ailments.

CONSENT FOR PUBLICATION

Not applicable.

CONFLICT OF INTEREST

The author declares no conflict of interest, financial or otherwise.

ACKNOWLEDGEMENTS

Declared none.

REFERENCES

[1]   Duffey KJ, Rivera JA, Popkin BM. Snacking is prevalent in Mexico. J Nutr 2014; 144(11): 1843-9.
[http://dx.doi.org/10.3945/jn.114.198192] [PMID: 25332484]

[2]   Cornier MA, Dabelea D, Hernandez TL, *et al.* The metabolic syndrome. Endocr Rev 2008; 29(7): 777-822.
[http://dx.doi.org/10.1210/er.2008-0024] [PMID: 18971485]

[3]   Movsisyan NK, Vinciguerra M, Medina-Inojosa JR, Lopez-Jimenez F. Cardiovascular diseases in central and Eastern Europe: A call for more surveillance and evidence-based health promotion. Ann Glob Health 2020; 86(1): 21.
        [http://dx.doi.org/10.5334/aogh.2713] [PMID: 32166066]

[4]   Huffman MD, Prabhakaran D, Osmond C, *et al.* Incidence of cardiovascular risk factors in an Indian urban cohort results from the New Delhi birth cohort. J Am Coll Cardiol 2011; 57(17): 1765-74.
        [http://dx.doi.org/10.1016/j.jacc.2010.09.083] [PMID: 21511113]

[5]   Krishnan MN. Coronary heart disease and risk factors in India – On the brink of an epidemic? Indian Heart J 2012; 64(4): 364-7.
        [http://dx.doi.org/10.1016/j.ihj.2012.07.001] [PMID: 22929818]

[6]   Hajar R. Risk factors for coronary artery disease: Historical perspectives. Heart Views 2017; 18(3): 109-14.
        [http://dx.doi.org/10.4103/HEARTVIEWS.HEARTVIEWS_106_17] [PMID: 29184622]

[7]   Sproston NR, Ashworth JJ. Role of C-reactive protein at sites of inflammation and infection. Front Immunol 2018; 9: 754.
        [http://dx.doi.org/10.3389/fimmu.2018.00754] [PMID: 29706967]

[8]   Scott J. Pathophysiology and biochemistry of cardiovascular disease. Curr Opin Genet Dev 2004; 14(3): 271-9.
        [http://dx.doi.org/10.1016/j.gde.2004.04.012] [PMID: 15172670]

[9]   Seidman MA, Mitchell RN, Stone JR. Pathophysiology of atherosclerosis. Cellular and molecular pathobiology of cardiovascular disease. Cambridge: Academic Press 2014; 12: pp. 221-37.
        [http://dx.doi.org/10.1016/B978-0-12-405206-2.00012-0]

[10]   Biros E, Karan M, Golledge J. Genetic variation and atherosclerosis. Curr Genomics 2008; 9(1): 29-42.
        [http://dx.doi.org/10.2174/138920208783884856] [PMID: 19424482]

[11]   Liumbruno GM, Franchini M. Beyond immunohaematology: the role of the ABO blood group in human diseases. Blood Transfus 2013; 11(4): 491-9.
        [PMID: 24120598]

[12]   World Health Organization. Sixty-fifth World Health Assembly resolutions, decisions, annexes. 2012.

[13]   Frishman WH, Beravol P, Carosella C. Alternative and complementary medicine for preventing and treating cardiovascular disease. Dis Mon 2009; 55(3): 121-92.
        [http://dx.doi.org/10.1016/j.disamonth.2008.12.002] [PMID: 19215737]

[14]   Thachil J. Antiplatelet therapy – a summary for the general physicians. Clin Med (Lond) 2016; 16(2): 152-60.
        [http://dx.doi.org/10.7861/clinmedicine.16-2-152] [PMID: 27037385]

[15]   Kaufman MB. ACE inhibitor-related angioedema: Are your patients at risk? P&T 2013; 38(3): 170-2.
        [PMID: 23641138]

[16]   Warner KK, Visconti JA, Tschampel MM. Angiotensin II receptor blockers in patients with ACE inhibitor-induced angioedema. Ann Pharmacother 2000; 34(4): 526-8.
        [http://dx.doi.org/10.1345/aph.19294] [PMID: 10772441]

[17]   Ambrosy AP, Mentz RJ, Fiuzat M, *et al.* The role of angiotensin receptor–neprilysin inhibitors in cardiovascular disease—existing evidence, knowledge gaps, and future directions. Eur J Heart Fail 2018; 20(6): 963-72.
        [http://dx.doi.org/10.1002/ejhf.1159] [PMID: 29464817]

[18]   Feingold KR. Cholesterol lowering drugs. Retrieved from MDTextcom, Inc Retrieved from Endotext, South Dartmouth (MA). 2021.

[19]   Hariri L, Patel J. Vasodilators. StatPearls Treasure Island. FL: Stat Pearls Publishing 2021.

[20]   Dutta D, Mahabir S, Pathak YV. Background to nutraceuticals and human 1907 health. In: Mahabir S, Pathak VS, Eds. Nutraceuticals and health Review of 1908 human Evidence. Boca Raton, FL: CRC Press 2014; pp. 3-12.

[21]   Shaito A, Thuan DTB, Phu HT, *et al.* Herbal medicine for cardiovascular diseases: Efficacy, mechanisms, and safety. Front Pharmacol 2020; 11: 422.
[http://dx.doi.org/10.3389/fphar.2020.00422] [PMID: 32317975]

[22]   Scalbert A, Manach C, Morand C, Rémésy C, Jiménez L. Dietary polyphenols and the prevention of diseases. Crit Rev Food Sci Nutr 2005; 45(4): 287-306.
[http://dx.doi.org/10.1080/1040869059096] [PMID: 16047496]

[23]   Pandey KB, Rizvi SI. Plant polyphenols as dietary antioxidants in human health and disease. Oxid Med Cell Longev 2009; 2(5): 270-8.
[http://dx.doi.org/10.4161/oxim.2.5.9498] [PMID: 20716914]

[24]   Durante A, Bronzato S. Dietary supplements and cardiovascular diseases. Int J Prev Med 2018; 9(1): 80.
[http://dx.doi.org/10.4103/ijpvm.IJPVM_179_17] [PMID: 30283612]

[25]   McCullough ML, Peterson JJ, Patel R, Jacques PF, Shah R, Dwyer JT. Flavonoid intake and cardiovascular disease mortality in a prospective cohort of US adults. Am J Clin Nutr 2012; 95(2): 454-64.
[http://dx.doi.org/10.3945/ajcn.111.016634] [PMID: 22218162]

[26]   Hertog MGL, Hollman PCH, van de Putte B. Content of potentially anticarcinogenic flavonoids of tea infusions, wines, and fruit juices. J Agric Food Chem 1993; 41(8): 1242-6.
[http://dx.doi.org/10.1021/jf00032a015]

[27]   Maria AG, Graziano R, Nicolantonio DO. Carotenoids: potential allies of cardiovascular health? Food Nutr Res 2015; 59(1): 26762.
[http://dx.doi.org/10.3402/fnr.v59.26762] [PMID: 25660385]

[28]   Mozos I, Stoian D, Caraba A, Malainer C, Horbańczuk JO, Atanasov AG. Lycopene and vascular health. Front Pharmacol 2018; 9: 521.
[http://dx.doi.org/10.3389/fphar.2018.00521] [PMID: 29875663]

[29]   Amalraj A, Gopi S. Medicinal properties of *Terminalia arjuna (Roxb.) Wight & Arn.*: A review. J Tradit Complement Med 2017; 7(1): 65-78.
[http://dx.doi.org/10.1016/j.jtcme.2016.02.003] [PMID: 28053890]

[30]   Akbar S. Gymnema sylvestre R. Br. (Apocynaceae). Handbook of 200 medicinal plants 2020. 2020.

[31]   Jain A, Sisodia J. Quinidine. StatPearls. Treasure Island, FL: StatPearls Publishing 2021.

[32]   Singh D, Chaudhuri PK. Structural characteristics, bioavailability and cardioprotective potential of saponins. Integr Med Res 2018; 7(1): 33-43.
[http://dx.doi.org/10.1016/j.imr.2018.01.003] [PMID: 29629289]

[33]   Hwang J, Wang J, Morazzoni P, Hodis HN, Sevanian A. The phytoestrogen equol increases nitric oxide availability by inhibiting superoxide production: an antioxidant mechanism for cell-mediated LDL modification. Free Radic Biol Med 2003; 34(10): 1271-82.
[http://dx.doi.org/10.1016/S0891-5849(03)00104-7] [PMID: 12726915]

[34]   Moser M, Chun O. Vitamin C and heart health: A review based on findings from epidemiologic studies. Int J Mol Sci 2016; 17(8): 1328.
[http://dx.doi.org/10.3390/ijms17081328] [PMID: 27529239]

[35]   Judd SE, Tangpricha V. Vitamin D deficiency and risk for cardiovascular disease. Am J Med Sci 2009; 338(1): 40-4.
[http://dx.doi.org/10.1097/MAJ.0b013e3181aaee91] [PMID: 19593102]

[36]   Yin K, You Y, Swier V, *et al.* Vitamin D protects against atherosclerosis *via* regulation of cholesterol

efflux and macrophage polarization in hypercholesterolemic swine. Arterioscler Thromb Vasc Biol 2015; 35(11): 2432-42.
[http://dx.doi.org/10.1161/ATVBAHA.115.306132] [PMID: 26381871]

[37]   Hosomi R, Yoshida M, Fukunaga K. Seafood consumption and components for health. Glob J Health Sci 2012; 4(3): 72-86.
[http://dx.doi.org/10.5539/gjhs.v4n3p72] [PMID: 22980234]

[38]   Willett WC, Koplan JP, Nugent R. Prevention of chronic disease by means of diet and lifestyle changes. In: Jamison DT, Breman JG, Measham AR, Eds. Co-published, Disease control priorities in developing countries. 2nd ed., Washington, DC: International Bank for Reconstruction and Development / the World Bank by Oxford University Press, New York 2006.

[39]   Quiara Lovatti A, Samuel Barbosa C. Role of nutraceuticals in the prevention and treatment of hypertension and cardiovascular diseases. J Hypertens Manag 2019; 5(1): 037.

[40]   Nandave M, Ojha SK, Joshi S, Kumari S, Arya DS. *Moringa oleifera* leaf extract prevents isoproterenol-induced myocardial damage in rats: evidence for an antioxidant, antiperoxidative, and cardioprotective intervention. J Med Food 2009; 12(1): 47-55.
[http://dx.doi.org/10.1089/jmf.2007.0563] [PMID: 19298195]

[41]   Upaganlawar A, Balaraman R. Cardioprotective effects of *Lagenaria siceraria* fruit juice on isoproterenol-induced myocardial infarction in Wistar rats: A biochemical and histoarchitecture study. J Young Pharm 2011; 3(4): 297-303.
[http://dx.doi.org/10.4103/0975-1483.90241] [PMID: 22224036]

[42]   Yamashiro S, Noguchi K, Matsuzaki T, *et al.* Cardioprotective effects of extracts from Psidium guajava L and Limonium wrightii, Okinawan medicinal plants, against ischemia-reperfusion injury in perfused rat hearts. Pharmacology 2003; 67(3): 128-35.
[http://dx.doi.org/10.1159/000067799] [PMID: 12571408]

[43]   Céspedes CL, El-Hafidi M, Pavon N, Alarcon J. Antioxidant and cardioprotective activities of phenolic extracts from fruits of Chilean blackberry *Aristotelia chilensis* (Elaeocarpaceae), Maqui. Food Chem 2008; 107(2): 820-9.
[http://dx.doi.org/10.1016/j.foodchem.2007.08.092]

[44]   Ashour OM, Abdel-Naim AB, Abdallah HM, Nagy AA, Mohamadin AM, Abdel-Sattar EA. Evaluation of the potential cardioprotective activity of some Saudi plants against doxorubicin toxicity. Z Naturforsch C J Biosci 2012; 67(5-6): 297-307.
[http://dx.doi.org/10.1515/znc-2012-5-609] [PMID: 22888535]

[45]   Alpsoy S, Aktas C, Uygur R, *et al.* Antioxidant and anti-apoptotic effects of onion (*Allium cepa*) extract on doxorubicin-induced cardiotoxicity in rats. J Appl Toxicol 2013; 33(3): 202-8.
[http://dx.doi.org/10.1002/jat.1738] [PMID: 21996788]

[46]   Patel KJ, Panchasara AK, Barvaliya MJ, *et al.* Evaluation of cardioprotective effect of aqueous extract of *Garcinia indica* Linn. fruit rinds on isoprenaline-induced myocardial injury in Wistar albino rats Res Pharm Sci 2015; 10(5): 388-96.
[PMID: 26752987]

[47]   Shanmugarajan T, Arunsundar M, Somasundaram I, Krishnakumar E, Sivaraman D, Ravichandiran V. Cardioprotective effect of *Ficus hispida* Linn on cyclophosphamide provoked oxidative myocardial injury in a rat model. Int J Pharmacol 2008; 1: 1-10.

[48]   Mehdizadeh R, Parizadeh MR, Khooei AR, Mehri S, Hosseinzadeh H. Cardioprotective effect of saffron extract and safranal in isoproterenol-induced myocardial infarction in wistar rats. Iran J Basic Med Sci 2013; 16(1): 56-63.
[PMID: 23638293]

[49]   Fung SY, Sim SM, Kandiah , *et al.* Prophylactic effect of Mucuna pruriens Linn (velvet bean) seed extract against experimental Naja sputatrix envenomation: gene expression studies. Indian J Exp Biol 2014; 52(9): 849-59.

[PMID: 25241584]

[50]   Oza MJ, Kulkarni YA. Traditional uses, phytochemistry and pharmacology of the medicinal species of the genus *Cordia* (Boraginaceae). J Pharm Pharmacol 2017; 69(7): 755-89.
[http://dx.doi.org/10.1111/jphp.12715] [PMID: 28266011]

[51]   Ramesh T, Mahesh R, Sureka C, Begum VH. Cardioprotective effects of *Sesbania grandiflora* in cigarette smoke-exposed rats. J Cardiovasc Pharmacol 2008; 52(4): 338-43.
[http://dx.doi.org/10.1097/FJC.0b013e3181888383] [PMID: 18791462]

[52]   Yashin A, Yashin Y, Xia X, Nemzer B. Antioxidant activity of spices and their impact on human health: A review. Antioxidants 2017; 6(3): 70.
[http://dx.doi.org/10.3390/antiox6030070] [PMID: 28914764]

[53]   Tsui PF, Lin CS, Ho LJ, Lai JH. Spices and Atherosclerosis. Nutrients 2018; 10(11): 1724.
[http://dx.doi.org/10.3390/nu10111724] [PMID: 30423840]

[54]   e J, R V, T JZ. Quality of dry ginger (*Zingiber officinale*) by different drying methods. J Food Sci Technol 2014; 51(11): 3190-8.
[http://dx.doi.org/10.1007/s13197-012-0823-8] [PMID: 26396311]

[55]   Otunola GA, Oloyede OB, Oladiji AT, Afolayan AJ. Comparative analysis of the chemical composition of three spices-*Allium sativum* L. *Zingiber officinale* Rosc. and *Capsicum frutescens* L. commonly consumed in Nigeria. Afr J Biotechnol 2010; 9(41): 6927-31.

[56]   Mao QQ, Xu XY, Cao SY, *et al.* Bioactive compounds and bioactivities of ginger (*Zingiber officinale* Roscoe). Foods 2019; 8(6): 185.
[http://dx.doi.org/10.3390/foods8060185] [PMID: 31151279]

[57]   Ghayur MN, Gilani AH, Afridi MB, Houghton PJ. Cardiovascular effects of ginger aqueous extract and its phenolic constituents are mediated through multiple pathways. Vascul Pharmacol 2005; 43(4): 234-41.
[http://dx.doi.org/10.1016/j.vph.2005.07.003] [PMID: 16157513]

[58]   Han X, Zhang Y, Liang Y, *et al.* 6-Gingerol, an active pungent component of ginger, inhibits L-type Ca^{2+} current, contractility, and Ca^{2+} transients in isolated rat ventricular myocytes. Food Sci Nutr 2019; 7(4): 1344-52.
[http://dx.doi.org/10.1002/fsn3.968] [PMID: 31024707]

[59]   Hatcher H, Planalp R, Cho J, Torti FM, Torti SV. Curcumin: From ancient medicine to current clinical trials. Cell Mol Life Sci 2008; 65(11): 1631-52.
[http://dx.doi.org/10.1007/s00018-008-7452-4] [PMID: 18324353]

[60]   Xu XY, Meng X, Li S, Gan RY, Li Y, Li HB. Bioactivity, health benefits, and related molecular mechanisms of curcumin: Current progress, challenges, and perspectives. Nutrients 2018; 10(10): 1553.
[http://dx.doi.org/10.3390/nu10101553] [PMID: 30347782]

[61]   Ahmad N, Fazal H, Abbasi BH, Farooq S, Ali M, Khan MA. Biological role of *Piper nigrum* L. (Black pepper): A review. Asian Pac J Trop Biomed 2012; 2(3): S1945-53.
[http://dx.doi.org/10.1016/S2221-1691(12)60524-3]

[62]   Dosoky NS, Satyal P, Barata LM, da Silva JKR, Setzer WN. Volatiles of black pepper fruits (*Piper nigrum* L.). Molecules 2019; 24(23): 4244.
[http://dx.doi.org/10.3390/molecules24234244] [PMID: 31766491]

[63]   El Hamss R, Idaomar M, Alonso-Moraga A, Muñoz Serrano A. Antimutagenic properties of bell and black peppers. Food Chem Toxicol 2003; 41(1): 41-7.
[http://dx.doi.org/10.1016/S0278-6915(02)00216-8] [PMID: 12453727]

[64]   Hirata N, Tokunaga M, Naruto S, Iinuma M, Matsuda H. Testosterone 5α-reductase inhibitory active constituents of Piper nigrum leaf. Biol Pharm Bull 2007; 30(12): 2402-5.
[http://dx.doi.org/10.1248/bpb.30.2402] [PMID: 18057734]

[65]   Meriga B, Parim B, Chunduri VR, *et al.* Antiobesity potential of Piperonal: promising modulation of body composition, lipid profiles and obesogenic marker expression in HFD-induced obese rats. Nutr Metab (Lond) 2017; 14(1): 72.
[http://dx.doi.org/10.1186/s12986-017-0228-9] [PMID: 29176994]

[66]   Nadeem M, Muhammad Anjum F, Issa Khan M, Tehseen S, El-Ghorab A, Iqbal Sultan J. Nutritional and medicinal aspects of coriander (*Coriandrum sativum* L.). Br Food J 2013; 115(5): 743-55.
[http://dx.doi.org/10.1108/00070701311331526]

[67]   Liang Y, Li Y, Sun A, Liu X. Chemical compound identification and antibacterial activity evaluation of cinnamon extracts obtained by subcritical n-butane and ethanol extraction. Food Sci Nutr 2019; 7(6): 2186-93.
[http://dx.doi.org/10.1002/fsn3.1065] [PMID: 31289667]

[68]   Gupta Jain S, Puri S, Misra A, Gulati S, Mani K. Effect of oral cinnamon intervention on metabolic profile and body composition of Asian Indians with metabolic syndrome: a randomized double -blind control trial. Lipids Health Dis 2017; 16(1): 113.
[http://dx.doi.org/10.1186/s12944-017-0504-8] [PMID: 28606084]

[69]   Jarvill-Taylor KJ, Anderson RA, Graves DJ. A hydroxychalcone derived from cinnamon functions as a mimetic for insulin in 3T3-L1 adipocytes. J Am Coll Nutr 2001; 20(4): 327-36.
[http://dx.doi.org/10.1080/07315724.2001.10719053] [PMID: 11506060]

[70]   Mang B, Wolters M, Schmitt B, *et al.* Effects of a cinnamon extract on plasma glucose, HbA1c, and serum lipids in diabetes mellitus type 2. Eur J Clin Invest 2006; 36(5): 340-4.
[http://dx.doi.org/10.1111/j.1365-2362.2006.01629.x] [PMID: 16634838]

[71]   Petrovska B, Cekovska S. Extracts from the history and medical properties of garlic. Pharmacogn Rev 2010; 4(7): 106-10.
[http://dx.doi.org/10.4103/0973-7847.65321] [PMID: 22228949]

[72]   Omar SH, Al-Wabel NA. Organosulfur compounds and possible mechanism of garlic in cancer. Saudi Pharm J 2010; 18(1): 51-8.
[http://dx.doi.org/10.1016/j.jsps.2009.12.007] [PMID: 23960721]

[73]   Farooqui A. Phytochemicals, signal transduction, and neurological disorders. Springer-Verlag New York 2012.
[http://dx.doi.org/10.1007/978-1-4614-3804-5]

[74]   El-Saber Batiha G, Magdy Beshbishy A, G Wasef L, Elewa Y, A Al-Sagan A, Abd El-Hack ME, *et al.* Chemical Constituents and Pharmacological Activities of *Garlic Allium sativum* L. A Review: Nutrients 2020; 12(3): 872.
[http://dx.doi.org/10.3390/nu12030872]

[75]   Zheng J, Zhou Y, Li Y, Xu DP, Li S, Li HB. Spices for prevention and treatment of cancers. Nutrients 2016; 8(8): 495.
[http://dx.doi.org/10.3390/nu8080495] [PMID: 27529277]

[76]   Srivastava SK, Nagpure NS, Kushwaha B, Ponniah AG. Efficacy of clove oil as an anaesthetic agent in fishes. Indian J Anim Sci 2003; 73: 466-7.

[77]   Kim HM, Lee EH, Hong SH, *et al.* Effect of *Syzygium aromaticum* extract on immediate hypersensitivity in rats. J Ethnopharmacol 1998; 60(2): 125-31.
[http://dx.doi.org/10.1016/S0378-8741(97)00143-8] [PMID: 9582002]

[78]   Zheng GQ, Kenney PM, Lam LKT. Sesquiterpenes from clove (*Eugenia caryophyllata*) as potential anticarcinogenic agents. J Nat Prod 1992; 55(7): 999-1003.
[http://dx.doi.org/10.1021/np50085a029] [PMID: 1402962]

[79]   Miyazawa M, Hisama M. Antimutagenic activity of phenylpropanoids from clove (*Syzygium aromaticum*). J Agric Food Chem 2003; 51(22): 6413-22.
[http://dx.doi.org/10.1021/jf030247q] [PMID: 14558756]

[80] Birari R, Javia V, Bhutani KK. Antiobesity and lipid lowering effects of *Murraya koenigii* (L.) Spreng leaves extracts and mahanimbine on high fat diet induced obese rats. Fitoterapia 2010; 81(8): 1129-33.
[http://dx.doi.org/10.1016/j.fitote.2010.07.013] [PMID: 20655993]

[81] Lee JJ, Kim HA, Lee J. The effects of *Brassica juncea* L. leaf extract on obesity and lipid profiles of rats fed a high-fat/high-cholesterol diet. Nutr Res Pract 2018; 12(4): 298-306.
[http://dx.doi.org/10.4162/nrp.2018.12.4.298] [PMID: 30090167]

[82] Verma SK, Jain V, Katewa SS. Blood pressure lowering, fibrinolysis enhancing and antioxidant activities of cardamom (*Elettaria cardamomum*). Indian J Biochem Biophys 2009; 46(6): 503-6.
[PMID: 20361714]

[83] Abourashed EA, El-Alfy AT. Chemical diversity and pharmacological significance of the secondary metabolites of nutmeg (*Myristica fragrans* Houtt.). Phytochem Rev 2016; 15(6): 1035-56.
[http://dx.doi.org/10.1007/s11101-016-9469-x] [PMID: 28082856]

[84] Vergara-Jimenez M, Almatrafi M, Fernandez M. Bioactive components in *Moringa oleifera* Leaves protect against chronic disease. Antioxidants 2017; 6(4): 91.
[http://dx.doi.org/10.3390/antiox6040091] [PMID: 29144438]

[85] Muni Swamy G, Ramesh G, Devi Prasad R, Meriga B. Astragalin, (3-O-glucoside of kaempferol), isolated from *Moringa oleifera* leaves modulates leptin, adiponectin secretion and inhibits adipogenesis in 3T3-L1 adipocytes. Arch Physiol Biochem 2020; 27: 1-7.
[http://dx.doi.org/10.1080/13813455.2020.1740742] [PMID: 32216601]

[86] Imran M, Butt MS, Suleria HAR. *Capsicum annuum* bioactive compounds: Health Promotion perspectives. In: Mérillon JM, Ramawat K, Eds. Bioactive molecules in food Reference series in phytochemistry. 2018.
[http://dx.doi.org/10.1007/978-3-319-54528-8_47-1]

[87] Mohd Yusof YA. Gingerol and its role in chronic diseases. Adv Exp Med Biol 2016; 929: 177-207.
[http://dx.doi.org/10.1007/978-3-319-41342-6_8] [PMID: 27771925]

[88] Gupta SC, Sung B, Kim JH, Prasad S, Li S, Aggarwal BB. Multitargeting by turmeric, the golden spice: From kitchen to clinic. Mol Nutr Food Res 2013; 57(9): 1510-28.
[http://dx.doi.org/10.1002/mnfr.201100741] [PMID: 22887802]

[89] Zikaki K, Aggeli IK, Gaitanaki C, Beis I. Curcumin induces the apoptotic intrinsic pathway *via* upregulation of reactive oxygen species and JNKs in H9c2 cardiac myoblasts. Apoptosis 2014; 19(6): 958-74.
[http://dx.doi.org/10.1007/s10495-014-0979-y] [PMID: 24668280]

[90] Agbor GA, Akinfiresoye L, Sortino J, Johnson R, Vinson JA. Piper species protect cardiac, hepatic and renal antioxidant status of atherogenic diet fed hamsters. Food Chem 2012; 134(3): 1354-9.
[http://dx.doi.org/10.1016/j.foodchem.2012.03.030] [PMID: 25005953]

[91] Sahib NG, Anwar F, Gilani AH, Hamid AA, Saari N, Alkharfy KM. Coriander (*Coriandrum sativum* L.): a potential source of high-value components for functional foods and nutraceuticals--a review. Phytother Res 2013; 27(10): 1439-56.
[http://dx.doi.org/10.1002/ptr.4897] [PMID: 23281145]

[92] Prachayasittikul V, Prachayasittikul S, Ruchirawat S, Prachayasittikul V. Coriander (*Coriandrum sativum*): A promising functional food toward the well-being. Food Res Int 2018; 105: 305-23.
[http://dx.doi.org/10.1016/j.foodres.2017.11.019] [PMID: 29433220]

[93] Akilen R, Tsiami A, Devendra D, Robinson N. Glycated haemoglobin and blood pressure-lowering effect of cinnamon in multi-ethnic Type 2 diabetic patients in the UK: a randomized, placebo-controlled, double-blind clinical trial. Diabet Med 2010; 27(10): 1159-67.
[http://dx.doi.org/10.1111/j.1464-5491.2010.03079.x] [PMID: 20854384]

[94] Rana SV, Pal R, Vaiphei K, Sharma SK, Ola RP. Garlic in health and disease. Nutr Res Rev 2011; 24(1): 60-71.

[http://dx.doi.org/10.1017/S0954422410000338] [PMID: 24725925]

[95] Stabler SN, Tejani AM, Huynh F, Fowkes C. Garlic for the prevention of cardiovascular morbidity and mortality in hypertensive patients. Cochrane Libr 2012; 8(8): CD007653.
[http://dx.doi.org/10.1002/14651858.CD007653.pub2] [PMID: 22895963]

[96] Adefegha SA, Oboh G, Adefegha OM, Boligon AA, Athayde ML. Antihyperglycemic, hypolipidemic, hepatoprotective and antioxidative effects of dietary clove (*Syzgium aromaticum*) bud powder in a high-fat diet/streptozotocin-induced diabetes rat model. J Sci Food Agric 2014; 94(13): 2726-37.
[http://dx.doi.org/10.1002/jsfa.6617] [PMID: 24532325]

CHAPTER 8

Ameliorative Potential of Biochanin-A against Dexamethasone Induced Hypertension through Modulation of Relative mRNA and Protein Expressions in Experimental Rats

V. V. Sathibabu Uddandrao[1,*], P. P. Sethumathi[2], Parim Brahma Naidu[3], S. Vadivukkarasi[1], Mustapha Sabana Begum[4] and G. Saravanan[1,*]

[1] *Centre for Biological Sciences, Department of Biochemistry, K.S. Rangasamy College of Arts and Science (Autonomous), Tiruchengode, Namakkal District, Tamilnadu, 637215, India*

[2] *Department of Pharmacology, Nandha College of Pharmacy, Erode, Tamil Nadu, 638052, India*

[3] *Animal Physiology and Biochemistry Laboratory, ICMR-National Animal Resource Facility for Biomedical Research (ICMR-NARFBR), Hyderabad, 500078, India*

[4] *Department of Biochemistry, Muthayammal College of Arts and Science, Rasipuram, Namakkal, Tamil Nadu 637408, India*

Abstract: In this study, we made an attempt to attenuate the dexamethasone induced hypertension through Biochanin-A (BCA) in experimental rats. Hypertension was induced in male albino Wistar rats by subcutaneous administration of dexamethasone (10µg/kg body weight). The rats were orally treated with BCA (10mg/kg body weight) once daily for 45 days and Nicorandil-treated group (6mg/kg body weight) included for comparison. We evaluated the changes in mean arterial pressure, heart rate, blood pressure, vascular function, oxidative stress markers, and gene expression of histone deacetylases (HDAC)-1, HDAC-2, and HDAC-8. Administration of BCA or Nicorandil showed noteworthy improvement in vascular function in experimental rats. Moreover, aortic eNOS expression was down regulated, and NADPH oxidase subunit p47^{phox} was up regulated in hypertensive rats. The antihypertensive effects of BCA were connected with concomitant downregulation of p47^{phox} expression and upregulation of eNOS expression. Dexamethasone exposure led to increased mRNA expression of HDACs expression in the kidneys and these were restored after BCA administration. In conclusion, our results are, therefore, BCA reduces hypertension in experimental rats and suggests that BCA might be used against the hypertension.

Keywords: Biochanin-A, Hypertension, Natural products, Vascular dysfunction.

---

[*] **Corresponding authors V. V. Sathibabu Uddandrao & G. Saravanan:** Centre for Biological Sciences, Department of Biochemistry, K.S. Rangasamy College of Arts and Science (Autonomous), Tiruchengode, Namakkal District, Tamilnadu, 637215-India; E-mails: sarabioc@gmail.com & sathibabu.u@gmail.com

1. INTRODUCTION

Hypertension is a disorder provoked by several factors, which belong to the foremost threat factors dependable for renal dysfunction, cardiovascular and metabolic diseases [1]. There are numerous substantial researches presenting the significance of vascular tone rise through the sympathetic nervous system and the renin angiotensin pathway in vital hypertension. Vascular tone is mostly reliant on the intracellular Ca^{2+} levels in vascular smooth muscle cells, which are synchronized by the endothelium, an essential module of the blood pressure and vascular wall [2]. The endothelium liberates vasodilators, together with prostaglandin I2, endothelium-derived hyperpolarizing factor, and nitric oxide (NO), as well as vasoconstrictors, such as endothelin, angiotensin-2 and thromboxane-A2, an extremely strong vasoconstrictor [3]. In normal states, the vascular quality is maintained by constrictor signals and vasodilator [4]. Nevertheless, in disease conditions, an increase in the endothelium-derived and a reduction in the endothelium-attained vasodilators or inflamed tissue-derived vasoconstrictors subsequently raise blood pressure and vascular tone, and leads to hypertension. In fundamental hypertension, systolic and diastolic blood pressures elevation is reassured by the combination therapy of angiotensin converting - adrenergic receptor blockers, diuretics, and β-enzyme inhibitors, angiotensin receptor blockers [5, 6]. On the other hand, the effectiveness of conventional antihypertensive agents cannot be expected in salt sensitive hypertension, reasonable to brutal hypertension, and metabolic disease induced hypertension to go together with endothelial damage [6]. For that reason, novel anti hypertension medications are necessary to combat against relentless and convoluted hypertension.

Biochanin-A (BCA) is a natural compound that is predominantly found in soy, chickpea, peanuts, alfalfa sprouts, and red clover. It is chemically known as Omethylated isoflavonoid and has several benefits against myocardial infarction [7], antiobesity [8] and obesity cardiomyopathy [9]. However, there was no scientific literature available to point out the antihypertensive efficacy of BCA. Hence, the present study is to evaluate the antihypertensive potential of BCA in dexamethasone (DMS)-induced hypertension in experimental rats.

2. MATERIALS AND METHODS

2.1. Chemicals

BCA was purchased from Sigma-Aldrich (St. Louis, Missouri, USA). All the reagents used in the experiments were analytic grade and had the highest purity.

2.2. Animals

Male Wistar rats were obtained from the Department of Biochemistry, Muthyammal College of Arts and Science, Rasipuram, Namakkal District, Tamilnadu, India. Experimental animals were kept under standard laboratory conditions (temperature; $22 \pm 2°C$: moistness; 40-60%), and permitted food and water *ad libitum*. Rats, at first weighing 180-200g, were separated into four groups of six each (n=6). All procedures involving laboratory animals were in accordance with the institutional animal ethical committee of Muthyammal College of Arts and Science (Approval number: IAEC/MCAS/07/2019).

2.3. Induction of Hypertension

In the experimental rats, hypertension was induced by subcutaneous injection of DMS ($10\mu g/kg/d$) in the evening [10].

2.4. Experimental Design

Group I: Normal control

Group II: Hypertensive control

Group III: Hypertensive + AA (20mg/kg body weight)

Group IV: Hypertensive + Nicorandil (6mg/kg body weight)

2.5. Measurement of Body Weight

The body weight of each rat was measured. At the end of the experiment, blood was collected from overnight fasted animals under inhalation of anaesthesia by retro-orbital puncture method. Blood was collected in anticoagulant coated vials and permitted for 15 minutes at room temperature. Plasma was separated by centrifugation at 2500 rpm for 15 minutes.

2.6. Indirect Measurement of Blood Pressure in Conscious Rats

Systolic blood pressure (SBP) of rats was determined every week end by non-invasive tail-cuff plethysmography (IITC/Life Science Instrument, USA). In short, awakened rats were positioned in a restrainer when quiet just before measurement. The rat tail was positioned within the tail cuff, and the cuff was mechanically exaggerated and released. Blood pressure was recorded in each rat as the mean value from the three measurements with 15 min gaps.

2.7. Hemodynamic and Vascular Responsiveness Measurements

At the end of the experiment, the rats were insensible by peritoneal injection of pentobarbital sodium (60mg/kg body weight). Temperature of the body was observed throughout the study using a heating pad by a rectal probe and maintained at $37\pm2°C$. A femoral artery was recognized, cleaned of a connective tissue and cannulated with a polyethylene tube. Baseline values of SBP, diastolic blood pressure (DBP), mean arterial pressure (MAP) and heart rate (HR) were constantly checked for 20 min by a way of a pressure transducer and recorded using Acknowledge Data Acquisition software (Biopac Systems Inc., USA). Hind limb blood flow (HBF) was incessantly recorded by an electromagnetic flow meter (Carolina Medical Electronics, USA) attached to an electromagnetic flow probe placed around the abdominal aorta. Hind limb vascular resistance (HVR) was calculated from baseline MAP and mean HBF.

2.8. Assay of Nitric Oxide Metabolites

The concentration of plasma NOx was measured using an enzymatic conversion method with some modifications [11].

2.9. Assay of Superoxide Production

Vascular O_2^- production was measured using a lucigenin-enhanced chemiluminescence method [12]. The carotid arteries were quickly cut apart and the supporter fat and connective tissue were cleaned on ice. The vessel segments (3-5mm) were located in Krebs-KCl buffer and authorized to equilibrate at $37°C$ for 30 min. Lucigenin was added to the test sample tube and positioned in a luminometer (Turner Biosystems, USA). The photon counts were included, each 30 s for 5 min and averaged. The vessels were desiccated at $45°C$ for 24 h to determine dry weight. O_2^- production in vascular tissue was demonstrated as relative light unit counts per minute per milligram of dry tissue weight.

2.10. RT-PCR Analysis

Kidney tissues were homogenized under standard conditions and then total RNA was extracted with the help of a Trizol reagent. The synthesis of cDNA was performed according to the manufacturer's protocol. The specifically designed primer pairs of histone deacetylase (HDAC)-1, HDAC-2, and HDAC-8 used for analysis are shown in Table **1**, and these were synthesized by Applied Biosystems, Foster City, USA. The amplification reaction was conducted in a 25μL capillary which contained 2μL of cDNA, 0.5μL each of the forward and reverse primers (final concentration of each, 0.5 μM), 12.5μL 2×SYBR green and sufficient nuclease free water for a final volume of 25μL for each reaction. The following thermal profile for RT-PCR, assays were used for all primer sets: 95°C for 1 min followed by 40 cycles of denaturation at 95°C for 10 s, annealing at 55°C and elongation at 64°C for 25 s with the acquisition of fluorescent data.

Table 1. Primer sequences.

Gene	Primer Sequence	Product Size (bp)
HDAC-1	F: 5'-GGAAATCTATCGCCCTCACA-3' R: 5'-AACAGGCCATCGAATACTGG-3'	89
HDAC-2	F: 5'-TAAATCCAAGGACAACAGTGG-3' R: 5'-GGTGAGACTGTCAAATTCAGG-3'	120
HDAC-8	F: 5'-AGATATTGGCCTGGGGAAAG-3' R: 5'-CCAGTCAAGTACGTCCAGCA-3'	175
β-actin	F: 5'GGCACCACACTTTCTACAAT3' R: 5'AGGTCTCAAACATGATCTGG3'	259

2.11. Western Blot Analysis

Protein eNOS and p47^{phox} expression levels were determined in aortic homogenates following an earlier described western blot method [13], with some modifications. Homogenates were electrophoresed on an SDS polyacrylamide gel electrophoresis system. The proteins were electrotransferred onto a polyvinylidene difluoride membrane, blocked with 5% skimmed milk in tris-buffered saline (TBS) with 0.1% tween 20 for 2 h at room temperature before overnight incubation at 4°C with mouse monoclonal antibodies to eNOS (BD Biosciences, CA, USA) and p47^{phox} (Santa Cruz Biotechnology, Indian Gulch, CA, USA). The membranes were washed with TBS and then incubated for 2 h at room temperature with horseradish peroxidase conjugated goat anti-mouse IgG (Santa Cruz Biotechnology). The blots were developed in Amersham™ ECL™ Prime solution (Amersham BiosciencesCorp., Piscataway, NJ, USA), and densitometric analysis was performed using an ImageQuant™ 400 imager (GE Healthcare Life Sciences, Piscataway, NJ, USA). The β-actin (Santa Cruz, USA) was used as the loading control.

2.12. Statistical Analysis

All statistical analyses were done using the SPSS software (Version 13.0). All data were shown as mean ± SD. One-way analysis of variance was used to detect significant differences between the control and treatment groups. Values of $p<0.05$ were deemed to be statistically considerable.

3. RESULTS

Fig. (1) depicts the changes in body weight in the control and DMS-induced hypertensive group of animals during the experiment. Administration of DMS showed a significant ($p<0.05$) decrease in body weight compared to the normal control group. Oral administration with BCA (10mg/kg body weight) or Nicorandil (6mg/kg body weight) significantly ($p<0.05$) increased the body weight when compared to the DMS control group.

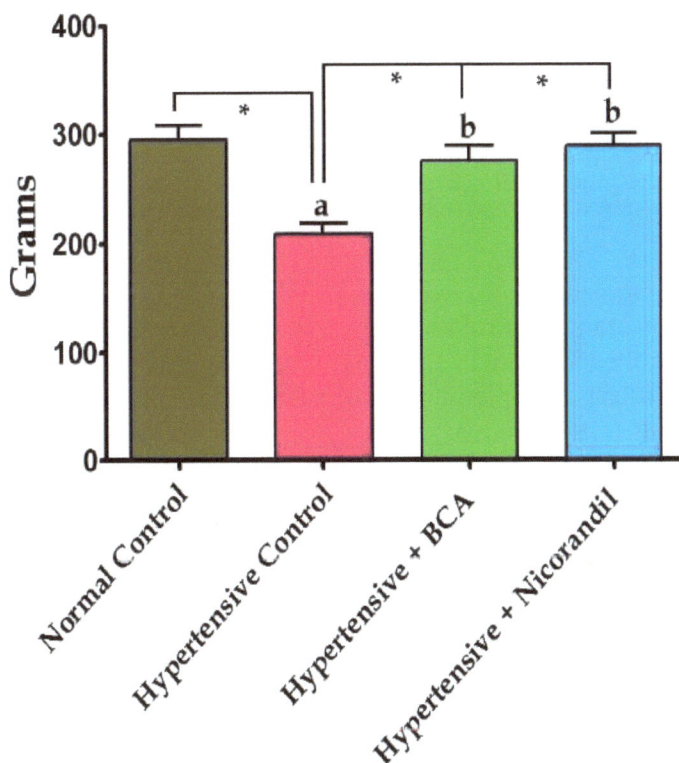

Fig. (1). Effect of BCA on body weight in control and experimental rats. Values are expressed as mean±SD for 6 animals in each group, [a]Significantly different from normal control, [b]Significantly different from hypertensive control, values are statistically significant at *$p<0.05$.

Fig. (**2**) shows the effect of BCA on SBP in control and hypertensive rats. There was no noteworthy dissimilarity in mean baseline values of SBP between all groups of rats at the beginning of the experiment. Administration of DMS caused a progressive increase in SBP compared with the normal control group ($p<0.05$). Treatment with BCA or Nicorandil considerably reduced SBP in hypertensive rats ($p<0.05$).

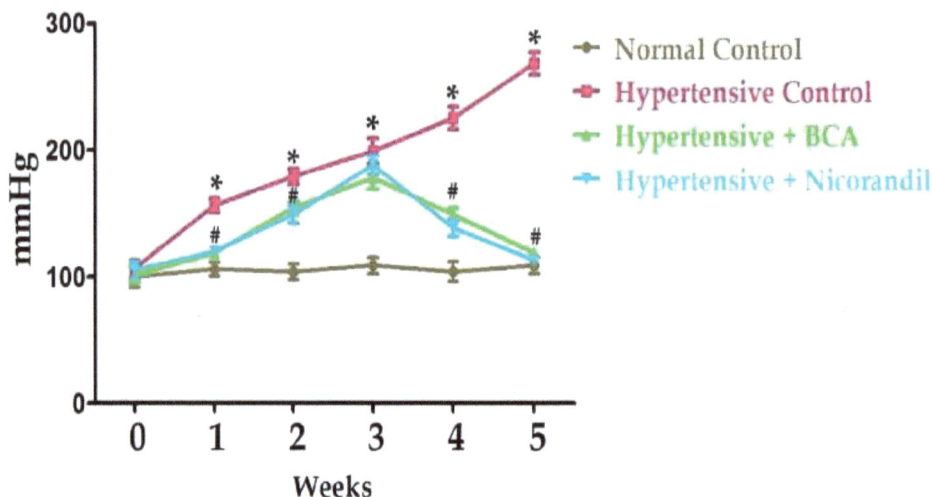

Fig. (2). Effect of BCA on SBP in control and hypertensive rats, values are expressed as mean ± SD for 6 animals in each group, *$p<0.05$ *versus* normal control, #$p<0.05$ *versus* hypertensive control.

Table **2** demonstrates the effects of BCA on hemodynamic and vascular responsiveness are in control and experimental hypertensive rats. SBP, DBP, and MAP all notably elevated in the DMS-administered groups when evaluated in group 1 ($p<0.05$). Supplementation with BCA or Nicorandil considerably decreased SBP, DBP, and MAP in DMS-induced hypertensive rats ($p<0.05$). There was also a momentous rise in HR noticed in DMS-induced hypertensive rats ($p<0.05$), which was considerably reduced by subsequent oral treatment with BCA or Nicorandil ($p<0.05$). The HBF of hypertensive rats was also identified to be lower than that of normal rats, reliable with a significant increase in HVR ($p<0.05$). BCA or Nicorandil administration noticeably enhanced both HVR and HBF in hypertensive rats ($p<0.05$).

Fig. (**3**) depicts the plasma NOx levels in the control and experimental groups. In DMS-induced hypertensive rats, plasma NOx concentrations were extensively ($p<0.05$) reduced when compared to those in the normal control group. Oral supplementation with BCA or Nicorandil significantly ($p<0.05$) enhanced the concentration of plasma NOx. On the other hand, DMS-induced hypertensive rats showed significant ($p<0.05$) increase in vascular O2$^-$ production when compared to normal control (Fig. **4**). But the rats administered with BCA significantly ameliorated the production of vascular O_2^- when compared to untreated hypertensive rats.

Table 2. Effect of BCA on hemodynamic and vascular responsiveness in control and experimental hypertensive rats.

-	Control	Hypertensive Control	Hypertensive + BCA	Hypertensive + Nicorandil
SBP (mmHg)	121.56±3.21	236.12±4.38[a*]	145.67±2.16[b*]	139.60±3.11[b*]
DBP (mmHg)	81.90±1.90	145.26±2.90[a*]	97.38±3.12[b*]	89.99±4.12[b*]
MAP (mmHg)	95.28±2.48	169.99±4.19[a*]	118.27±3.18[b*]	105.27±3.19[b*]
HR (beat/min)	340.37±9.09	453.28±8.69[a*]	364.81±5.85[b*]	354.64±5.91[b*]
HBF (mL/100 g tissue/min)	7.94±0.78	3.98±0.18[a*]	6.89±0.71[b*]	6.45±0.49[b*]
HVR (mmHg/min/100 g/mL)	13.64±3.12	47.14±3.10[a*]	17.59±1.89[b*]	19.56±1.01[b*]

Values are expressed as Mean ± SD for 6 animals in each group. Values are statistically significant at * $p<0.05$ [a]Significantly different from the control [b]Significantly different from hypertensive control.

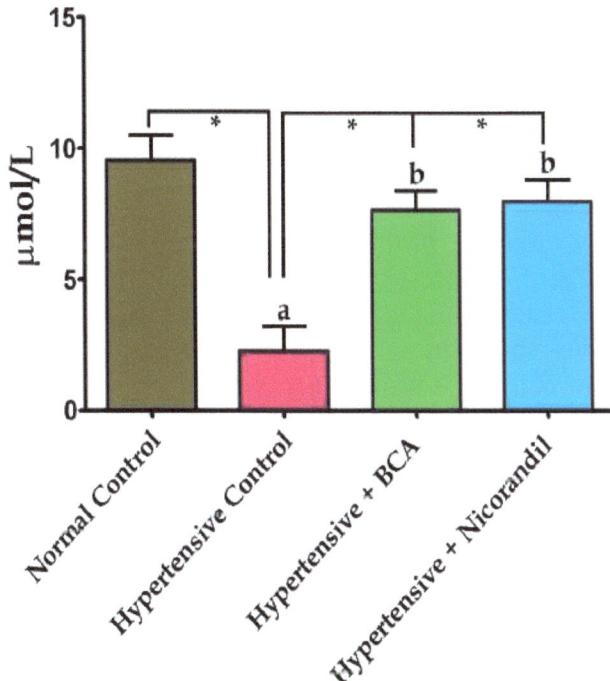

Fig. (3). Effect of BCA on plasma NOx levels in control and experimental rats. Values are expressed as mean±SD for 6 animals in each group, [a]Significantly different from normal control, [b]Significantly different from hypertensive control, values are statistically significant at *$p<0.05$.

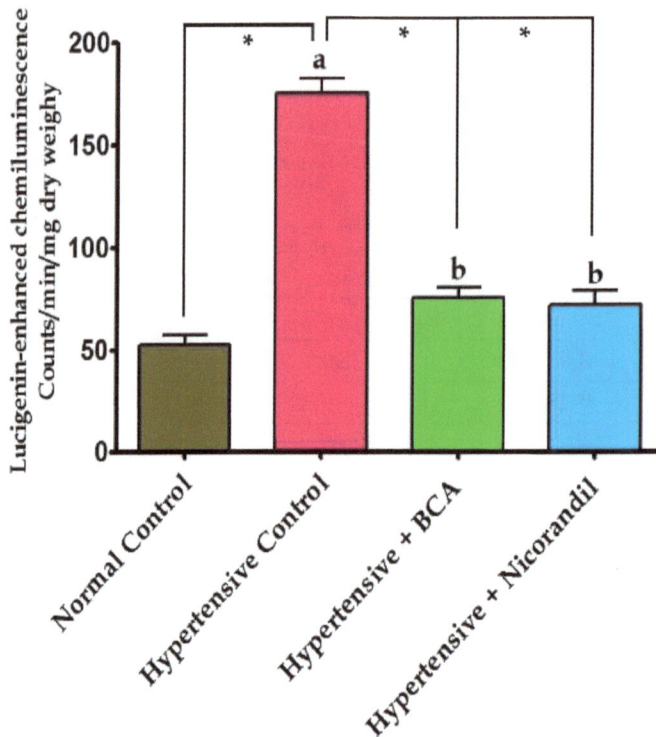

Fig. (4). Effect of BCA on vascular O_2^- production in control and experimental rats. Values are expressed as mean±SD for 6 animals in each group, [a]Significantly different from normal control, [b]Significantly different from hypertensive control, values are statistically significant at *$p<0.05$.

Fig. (**5**) demonstrates the effect of BCA or Nicorandil on the gene expressions (HDAC-1, HDAC-2, and HDAC-8) in control and experimental hypertensive rats. We observed significant up-regulations in the expressions of HDACs in DMS induced hypertensive rats when compared to the normal control rats. We found that supplementation with BCA or Nicorandil down-regulated mRNA expression of HDAC-1 (Fig. **5a**), HDAC-2 (Fig. **5b**), and HDAC-8 (Fig. **5c**) in experimental hypertensive rats.

Fig. (**6**) explains the expressions of eNOS and p47^{phox} proteins in control and hypertensive rats. Significant down regulation of eNOS protein expression was noticed in hypertensive rats (Fig. **6a**). Oral supplementation with BCA or Nicorandil completely restored aortic eNOS protein expression. The expression of p47^{phox} protein in aortic tissue from DMS-administered rats was considerably up-regulated when contrasted with that from group 1. Administration with BCA or Nicorandil inhibited the p47^{phox} protein over expression in hypertensive rats (Fig. **6b**).

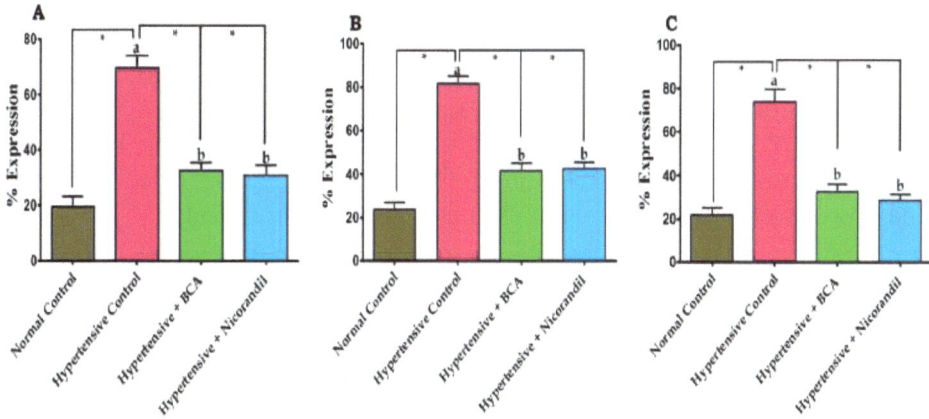

Fig. (5). Effect of BCA on mRNA expressions of **(A)** HDAC-1, **(B)** HDAC-2 and **(C)** HDAC-8 in control and experimental rats. Values are expressed as mean±SD for 6 animals in each group, [a]Significantly different from normal control, [b]Significantly different from hypertensive control, values are statistically significant at *$p<0.05$.

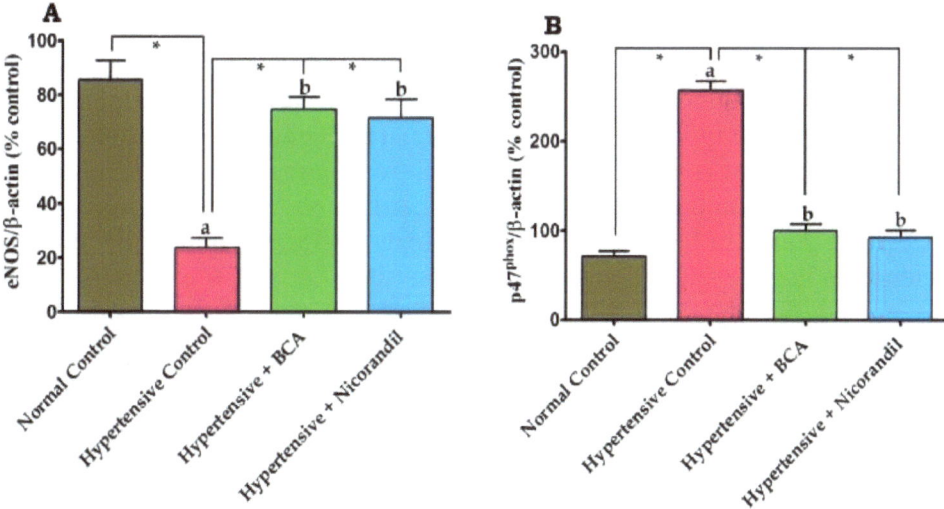

Fig. (6). Effect of BCA on protein expressions of **(A)** eNOS and **(B)** p47[phox] in control and experimental rats. Values are expressed as mean±SD for 6 animals in each group, [a]Significantly different from normal control, [b]Significantly different from hypertensive control, values are statistically significant at *$p<0.05$.

4. DISCUSSION

Hypertension is a well-documented impediment of surplus glucocorticoids, both synthetic and naturally-occurring. DMS is a powerful synthetic glucocorticoid, which has extensive clinical uses. As DMS has glucocorticoid activity entirely with insignificant mineralocorticoid effects, DMS-induced hypertension models have been considered for studying the mechanisms of glucocorticoid-induced hypertension [14]. In the current study, we were used the DMS to induce experimental hypertension to evaluate the anti hypertensive potential of BCA. We observed that administration of DMS to rats raised arterial blood pressure, HR, and HVR and takes place in damaged vascular response to the Phe and ACh vasoactive agents. These hemodynamic alterations were connected with reduced plasma NOx levels and enhanced oxidative stress markers levels [15].

DMS has efficiently induced nuclear translocation of both mineralocorticoid and glucocorticoid receptors but stimulates mineralocorticoid receptor-mediated transactivation at a much lower capacity than aldosterone [16]. Even though it can attach to mineralocorticoid receptors, DMS increases blood pressure in man without mineralocorticoid effects as substantiation by the lack of urinary sodium retention [17]. In the rat, DMS reduces body weight and enhances hematocrit [18]. Our results are in line with these findings; decreased body weights were found in hypertensive rats than in control and treatment with BCA or Nicorandil effectively increased the body weights in experimental rats.

SBP is resolute by both total peripheral resistance and cardiac output. By suppressing NO production, DMS may possibly influence both determinants. First of all, there is a support that NO acts to restrain central sympathetic nervous flood; so, condensed neuronal NO manufacture might lead to sympathetic over activity [19]. This outcome might improve cardiac output. In addition, the lofty HVR that we found in hypertensive rats has been documented to be linked to NO-deficiency induced systemic vasoconstriction [20]. Further, the rounded reaction to ACh, and the standard response to the NO donor SNP in DMS-induced hypertensive rats, point out a function for NO in endothelium-dependent vaso-relaxation. This extends and confirms earlier findings that the complications of the heart linked with experimental hypertension induced by DMS are connected with endothelial dysfunction [21]. Supplementation of BCA to hypertensive rats decreased blood pressure, HVR and augmented HBF representing that BCA could lower vascular resistance. Further, administration with BCA to hypertensive rats brought back normal vascular response to ACh, signifying that BCA might improve vascular endothelial function. Thus, it is expected that BCA ameliorates the hemodynamic alterations caused by DMS suppression of NO synthesis by improving NO bioavailability.

We observed discrepancy in mRNA and protein levels that were expected as a result of programming at the transcriptional and post-transcriptional levels [22]. Type I HDACs are vital for kidney homeostasis [23]. Numerous RAS components, including renin, AGT, AT1R, and ACE have been documented to be epigenetically controlled *via* HDACs [24]. Our results recommend that DMS led to programmed expression of specific genes in the RAS *via* HDACs, and that this was deprogrammed by BCA or Nicorandi administration. Class I HDACs, in particular HDAC-1, HDAC-2, and HDAC-3 are considered to reside principally in the nucleus, where they provide canonical roles in the control of gene expression through histone tails deacetylation. These HDACs are present in huge multi protein complexes such as Sin3, NuRD, CoREST, and NCoR/SMRT, which are employed as gene regulatory elements by sequence specific DNA binding transcription factors [25]. In general, HDAC-1 and HDAC-2 are instituted together in Sin3, NuRD, and CoREST complexes, whereas HDAC-3 is a component of the NCoR/SMRT complex. HDAC-8 has been revealed to cooperate with the estrogen-related receptor α [26] and cyclic adenosine monophosphate response element-binding protein [27] transcription factors, signifying a responsibility for this HDAC in the regulation of gene expression. Numerous small molecule inhibitors of HDAC enzymes have been revealed to be successful in experimental *in vivo* models of vascular breakdown, fibrosis and jamming pathological cardiac hypertrophy and recuperating ventricular function [28]. Induction of hypertension through DMS significantly increased the mRNA expressions of HDACs and, after treatment with BCA or Nicorandil, effectively suppressed the expressions of HDACs in experimental hypertensive rats.

The NO occurs in blood vessels produced in endothelial cells where L-arginine is transformed to NO by eNOS [29]. We noticed that administration of DMS notably decreased plasma NOx levels in rats and that this was connected with down-regulation of eNOS protein expression [24]. We found that supplementation with BCA to hypertensive rats elevated plasma NOx level and utterly re-established eNOS protein expression. These findings are in with earlier reports of betulinic acid and ursolic acid (triterpinoid compounds) up-regulated eNOS protein expression in human being endothelial cells [30]. The less concentration of plasma NO noticed in hypertensive rats might not only be the consequence of a malfunction to produce sufficient NO *via* eNOS, there could furthermore be improved inactivation of NO ensuing from improved oxidation of NO to $ONOO^-$ by $O2^-$ [31]. Up-regulation of $p47^{phox}$ protein expression, overproduction of $O2^-$, and reduced plasma NOx have all been found in hypertensive rats [32]. In the current study, we noticed up-regulated protein expressions of $p47^{phox}$ in aortic tissues accompanied by enhancement in vascular $O2^-$. NO may perhaps also proceed to reduce $O2^-$ formation directly by restraining a membrane constituent of NADPH oxidase and sinking NADPH oxidase 5 activity [33]. We recognized that oral administration with BCA was efficient in decreasing vascular $O2^-$, and expression of $p47^{phox}$ in DMS-induced hypertensive rats. BCA also demonstrates direct antioxidant activity [9] interceded by numerous hydroxyl groups.

CONCLUSION

In conclusion, BCA is able to progress hemodynamic status and restore vascular function in hypertensive rats induced by DMS. These antihypertensive potential of BCA are associated with the simultaneous up-regulation of eNOS and down-regulation of p47^{phox} expression foremost to increase NO bioavailability. Its advantageous effect may be endorsed by its capability to revise the expression of HDACs. This strongly recommends that BCA has ameliorative capability for the control of hypertension.

CONSENT FOR PUBLICATION

Not applicable.

CONFLICT OF INTEREST

The author declares no conflict of interest, financial or otherwise.

ACKNOWLEDGEMENTS

The authors thank the management of K.S. Rangasamy College of Arts and Science (Autonomous) for providing laboratory facilities and Muthyammal College of Arts and Science for providing ananimal house facility.

REFERENCES

[1]   Harrison DG, Coffman TM, Wilcox CS. Pathophysiology of Hypertension. Circ Res 2021; 128(7): 847-63.
[http://dx.doi.org/10.1161/CIRCRESAHA.121.318082] [PMID: 33793328]

[2]   Khalil RA. Modulators of the vascular endothelin receptor in blood pressure regulation and hypertension. Curr Mol Pharmacol 2011; 4(3): 176-86.
[http://dx.doi.org/10.2174/1874467211104030176] [PMID: 21222646]

[3]   Napoli C, Ignarro LJ. Nitric oxide and pathogenic mechanisms involved in the development of vascular diseases. Arch Pharm Res 2009; 32(8): 1103-8.
[http://dx.doi.org/10.1007/s12272-009-1801-1] [PMID: 19727602]

[4]   Félétou M, Vanhoutte PM. Endothelium-derived hyperpolarizing factor: where are we now? Arterioscler Thromb Vasc Biol 2006; 26(6): 1215-25.
[http://dx.doi.org/10.1161/01.ATV.0000217611.81085.c5] [PMID: 16543495]

[5]   Vogel RA. Optimal vascular protection: a case for combination antihypertensive therapy. Prev Cardiol 2006; 9(1): 35-41.
[http://dx.doi.org/10.1111/j.1520-037X.2006.4473.x] [PMID: 16407701]

[6]   Park BG, Shin WS, Oh S, Park GM, Kim NI, Lee S. A novel antihypertension agent, sargachromenol D from marine brown algae, Sargassum siliquastrum, exerts dual action as an L-type Ca^{2+} channel blocker and endothelin A/B$_2$ receptor antagonist. Bioorg Med Chem 2017; 25(17): 4649-55.
[http://dx.doi.org/10.1016/j.bmc.2017.07.002] [PMID: 28720331]

[7]   Sangeethadevi G, v v SU, Jansy Isabella RAR, *et al.* Attenuation of lipid metabolic abnormalities, proinflammatory cytokines, and matrix metalloproteinase expression by biochanin-A in isoproterenol-

induced myocardial infarction in rats. Drug Chem Toxicol 2021; 1-12.
[http://dx.doi.org/10.1080/01480545.2021.1894707] [PMID: 33719799]

[8]   Antony Rathinasamy JIR, Uddandrao VVS, Raveendran N, Sasikumar V. Antiobesity Effect of Biochanin-A: Effect on Trace Element Metabolism in High Fat Diet-Induced Obesity in Rats. Cardiovasc Hematol Agents Med Chem 2020; 18(1): 21-30.
[http://dx.doi.org/10.2174/1871524920666200207101920] [PMID: 32031077]

[9]   A JIR, Uddandrao VVS, G S, *et al.* Biochanin A attenuates obesity cardiomyopathy in rats by inhibiting oxidative stress and inflammation through the Nrf-2 pathway. Arch Physiol Biochem 2021; 1-16.
[http://dx.doi.org/10.1080/13813455.2021.1874017] [PMID: 33471570]

[10]   Ong SLH, Vickers JJ, Zhang Y, McKenzie KUS, Walsh CE, Whitworth JA. Role of xanthine oxidase in dexamethasone-induced hypertension in rats. Clin Exp Pharmacol Physiol 2007; 34(5-6): 517-9.
[http://dx.doi.org/10.1111/j.1440-1681.2007.04605.x] [PMID: 17439425]

[11]   Luangaram S, Kukongviriyapan U, Pakdeechote P, Kukongviriyapan V, Pannangpetch P. Protective effects of quercetin against phenylhydrazine-induced vascular dysfunction and oxidative stress in rats. Food Chem Toxicol 2007; 45(3): 448-55.
[http://dx.doi.org/10.1016/j.fct.2006.09.008] [PMID: 17084956]

[12]   Yamazaki T, Kawai C, Yamauchi A, Kuribayashi F. A highly sensitive chemiluminescence assay for superoxide detection and chronic granulomatous disease diagnosis. Trop Med Health 2011; 39(2): 41-5.
[http://dx.doi.org/10.2149/tmh.2011-08] [PMID: 22028609]

[13]   Sathibabu Uddandrao VV, Brahmanaidu P, Ravindarnaik R, Suresh P, Vadivukkarasi S, Saravanan G. Restorative potentiality of S-allylcysteine against diabetic nephropathy through attenuation of oxidative stress and inflammation in streptozotocin–nicotinamide-induced diabetic rats. Eur J Nutr 2019; 58(6): 2425-37.
[http://dx.doi.org/10.1007/s00394-018-1795-x] [PMID: 30062492]

[14]   Ong S, Zhang Y, Whitworth J. Mechanisms of Dexamethasone-Induced Hypertension. Curr Hypertens Rev 2009; 5(1): 61-74.
[http://dx.doi.org/10.2174/157340209787314315]

[15]   Bunbupha S, Pakdeechote P, Kukongviriyapan U, Prachaney P, Kukongviriyapan V. Asiatic acid reduces blood pressure by enhancing nitric oxide bioavailability with modulation of eNOS and p47phox expression in L-NAME-induced hypertensive rats. Phytother Res 2014; 28(10): 1506-12.
[http://dx.doi.org/10.1002/ptr.5156] [PMID: 24723332]

[16]   Rebuffat AG, Tam S, Nawrocki AR, *et al.* The 11-ketosteroid 11-ketodexamethasone is a glucocorticoid receptor agonist. Mol Cell Endocrinol 2004; 214(1-2): 27-37.
[http://dx.doi.org/10.1016/j.mce.2003.11.027] [PMID: 15062542]

[17]   Whitworth JA, Gordon D, Andrews J, Scoggins BA. The hypertensive effect of synthetic glucocorticoids in man: role of sodium and volume. J Hypertens 1989; 7(7): 537-49.
[http://dx.doi.org/10.1097/00004872-198907000-00005] [PMID: 2760458]

[18]   Hu L, Zhang Y, Lim P, *et al.* Apocynin but not L-arginine prevents and reverses dexamethasone-induced hypertension in the rat. Am J Hypertens 2006; 19(4): 413-8.
[http://dx.doi.org/10.1016/j.amjhyper.2005.09.023] [PMID: 16580579]

[19]   Cunha RS, Cabral AM, Vasquez EC. Evidence that the autonomic nervous system plays a major role in the L-NAME-induced hypertension in conscious rats. Am J Hypertens 1993; 6(9): 806-9.
[http://dx.doi.org/10.1093/ajh/6.9.806] [PMID: 7906520]

[20]   Baylis C, Mitruka B, Deng A. Chronic blockade of nitric oxide synthesis in the rat produces systemic hypertension and glomerular damage. J Clin Invest 1992; 90(1): 278-81.
[http://dx.doi.org/10.1172/JCI115849] [PMID: 1634615]

[21] Nakmareong S, Kukongviriyapan U, Pakdeechote P, *et al.* Antioxidant and vascular protective effects of curcumin and tetrahydrocurcumin in rats with l-NAME-induced hypertension. Naunyn Schmiedebergs Arch Pharmacol 2011; 383(5): 519-29.
[http://dx.doi.org/10.1007/s00210-011-0624-z] [PMID: 21448566]

[22] Tain YL, Chen CC, Sheen JM, *et al.* Melatonin attenuates prenatal dexamethasone-induced blood pressure increase in a rat model. J Am Soc Hypertens 2014; 8(4): 216-26.
[http://dx.doi.org/10.1016/j.jash.2014.01.009] [PMID: 24731552]

[23] Chen S, Bellew C, Yao X, *et al.* Histone deacetylase (HDAC) activity is critical for embryonic kidney gene expression, growth, and differentiation. J Biol Chem 2011; 286(37): 32775-89.
[http://dx.doi.org/10.1074/jbc.M111.248278] [PMID: 21778236]

[24] Song R, Van Buren T, Yosypiv IV. Histone deacetylases are critical regulators of the renin-angiotensin system during ureteric bud branching morphogenesis. Pediatr Res 2010; 67(6): 573-8.
[http://dx.doi.org/10.1203/PDR.0b013e3181da477c] [PMID: 20496471]

[25] Cunliffe VT. Eloquent silence: developmental functions of Class I histone deacetylases. Curr Opin Genet Dev 2008; 18(5): 404-10.
[http://dx.doi.org/10.1016/j.gde.2008.10.001] [PMID: 18929655]

[26] Wilson BJ, Tremblay AM, Deblois G, Sylvain-Drolet G, Giguère V. An acetylation switch modulates the transcriptional activity of estrogen-related receptor alpha. Mol Endocrinol 2010; 24(7): 1349-58.
[http://dx.doi.org/10.1210/me.2009-0441] [PMID: 20484414]

[27] Gao J, Siddoway B, Huang Q, Xia H. Inactivation of CREB mediated gene transcription by HDAC8 bound protein phosphatase. Biochem Biophys Res Commun 2009; 379(1): 1-5.
[http://dx.doi.org/10.1016/j.bbrc.2008.11.135] [PMID: 19070599]

[28] McKinsey TA. Therapeutic potential for HDAC inhibitors in the heart. Annu Rev Pharmacol Toxicol 2012; 52(1): 303-19.
[http://dx.doi.org/10.1146/annurev-pharmtox-010611-134712] [PMID: 21942627]

[29] Moncada S. Nitric oxide gas: mediator, modulator, and pathophysiologic entity. J Lab Clin Med 1992; 120(2): 187-91.
[PMID: 1500817]

[30] Steinkamp-Fenske K, Bollinger L, Völler N, *et al.* Ursolic acid from the Chinese herb Danshen (*Salvia miltiorrhiza* L.) upregulates eNOS and downregulates Nox4 expression in human endothelial cells. Atherosclerosis 2007; 195(1): e104-11.
[http://dx.doi.org/10.1016/j.atherosclerosis.2007.03.028] [PMID: 17481637]

[31] Pryor WA, Squadrito GL. The chemistry of peroxynitrite: a product from the reaction of nitric oxide with superoxide. Am J Physiol 1995; 268(5 Pt 1): L699-722.
[PMID: 7762673]

[32] Litterio MC, Jaggers G, Sagdicoglu Celep G, *et al.* Blood pressure-lowering effect of dietary (−)-epicatechin administration in L-NAME-treated rats is associated with restored nitric oxide levels. Free Radic Biol Med 2012; 53(10): 1894-902.
[http://dx.doi.org/10.1016/j.freeradbiomed.2012.08.585] [PMID: 22985936]

[33] Qian J, Chen F, Kovalenkov Y, *et al.* Nitric oxide reduces NADPH oxidase 5 (Nox5) activity by reversible S-nitrosylation. Free Radic Biol Med 2012; 52(9): 1806-19.
[http://dx.doi.org/10.1016/j.freeradbiomed.2012.02.029] [PMID: 22387196]

CHAPTER 9

Zingiberene, an Active Constituent from *Zingiber officinale* Ameliorated High-Fat Diet-Induced Obesity Cardiomyopathy in Rats

S. Jaikumar[1], G. Somasundaram[1] and S. Sengottuvelu[2,*]

[1] *Department of Pharmacology, Sri Lakshmi Narayana Institute of Medical Sciences, Puducherry, 605502, India*

[2] *Department of Pharmacology, Nandha College of Pharmacy, Erode, Tamilnadu, India*

Abstract: In the current study, we evaluated the effect of Zingiberene (ZB) is, a monocyclic sesquiterpene that is the principal constituent of ginger (*Zingiber officinale*), against high-fat-diet (HFD)-induced obesity cardiomyopathy (OC) in rats. ZB (50mg/kg/BW) was supplemented on obese rats for the period of 45 days and assessed its effect of body weight, anthropometrical and morphological parameters along with hyperglycemic markers. We also evaluated the effect of ZB on cardiac lipotoxicity and oxidative stress in cardiac tissue. The current study demonstrated that HFD supplementation significantly increased body weight, anthropometrical and morphological parameters, together developed hyperglycemia in rats. On the other hand, ZB supplementation in obese rats attenuated these altered parameters and ameliorated cardiac lipotoxicity as well as oxidative stress by decreasing lipid profiles of heart and enhancing the activities of endogenous antioxidant enzymes in the heart. Therefore, this study suggest that ZB might ameliorate the diet induced OC through the restoration of antioxidant system of the heart and attenuation of dyslipidemia in the cardiac.

Keywords: Nutraceuticals, Obesity cardiomyopathy, Oxidative stress, Zingiberene.

1. INTRODUCTION

Obesity cardiomyopathy (OC) is a multifaceted relationship of indirect and direct pathophysiologic factors connected to obesity. Obesity is an autonomous risk factor for coronary artery disease (CAD) and is robustly linked with diabetes mellitus (DM) and hypertension, which circuitously lead to the development of

*** Corresponding author S. Sengottuvelu:** Department of Pharmacology, Nandha College of Pharmacy, Erode, Tamilnadu, 638052, India; E-mail: sehejan@gmail.com

Dr. V. V. Sathibabu Uddandrao & Dr. Parim Brahma Naidu (Eds.)

hypertensive, ischemic and cardiomyopathy correspondingly [1]. There are definite structural changes related to OC and body weight and heart weight display a linear bond. Particularly, left ventricular remodelling with augmented wall width and mass, as well as ventricular dilatation are well-established consequences of obesity, even after controlling for age and hypertension [2]. Extreme fatty acids may direct prejudiced myocardial presentation due to the gathering of toxic long-chain non-esterified fatty acids and their by-products such as ceramides and diacylglycerols. This state is referred to as lipotoxic heart disease [3]. Insulin resistance (IR), one of many obesity-associated metabolic derangements, may also arbitrate the progress of cardiomyopathy through mutilation of myocardial oxygen utilization, myocardial fatty acid uptake and oxidation. Prominent myocardial triglyceride levels may also alter myocardial function and structure [4].

On the other hand, elevated oxidative stress in the cardiomyocytes arises through numerous mechanisms, including mitochondrial uncoupling and dysfunction, increased fatty acid oxidation, superior NADPH oxidase activity, and abridged antioxidant capacity [5]. It has been documented that obesity may persuade systemic oxidative stress. Biomarkers of oxidative stress are elevated in patients with obesity and correlate in a straight line with body mass index and the proportion of body fat; on the contrary, an opposite association between central adiposity, body fat and antioxidant capacity has been recommended. A number of processes are concerned with obesity-related oxidative stress, caused by a high intake of fat and carbohydrate meals [6, 7]. These observations point out that the modulation of oxidative stress by antioxidants appears to have an optimistic outcome in the avoidance of OC.

Several attempts have been made to spot the metabolic inconsistency of obesity state, producing a number of drugs like sibutramine, fibrates and orlistat, but they experience from substantial side effects [8]. Therapeutical approaches to obesity devoid of any side effects are still a dispute in the medical system of human beings. There is a mounting demand by individuals to use natural products with antiobesity nature because oral antiobesity drugs have numerous side effects [9]. In the same way, Zingiberene (ZB) is a monocyclic sesquiterpene that is the principal constituent of *Zingiber officinale* and in addition, previous reports indicated that ZB has various therapeutic effects [10]. On the other hand, there was no scientific evidence available on the antiobesity activity of ZB in animal models or any other clinical models. Therefore, the current study intended to find out the therapeutic efficacy of ZB against high-fat diet (HFD)-induced obesity and OC in rats.

2. MATERIALS AND METHODS

2.1. Chemicals

ZB was purchased from Sigma-Aldrich, India.

2.2. Animals

We procured male Wistar rats (weighing 120-140g) from the Nandha College of Pharmacy, Erode, Tamilnadu, India and rats were initially acclimatized for the period of one week with a 12 h day/night cycle, in a temperature of $22 \pm 2^\circ C$, and humidity of 45-64%. The protocol of this study was approved by the Institutional Animal Ethical Committee (IAEC), Nandha College of Pharmacy (Approval No: 688/PO/Re/S/02/CPCSEA).

2.3. HFD Composition

HFD was commercially obtained (National Institute of Nutrition, Hyderabad, India) and composed of corn starch (15%), sugar (27.5%), lard oil (17.6%), vitamin mixture (1%), mineral mixture (3.5%), casein (20%), cellulose powder (5%), corn oil (9.9%) and choline bitartrate (0.2%).

2.4. Experimental Design

Obesity was induced by the supplementation of HFD for the period of 15 weeks and treatment with respective drugs was initiated. At the same time, normal control rats were fed with a normal pellet diet. The rats were divided into four groups and each group contained six animals. All the respective drugs were administered orally by using intragastric tube for the period of 45 days once a day.

Group 1: Normal control

Group 2: HFD-induced obese control

Group 3: Obese + ZB (50mg/kg body weight)

Group 4: Obese + Lorcascrin (10mg/kg body weight)

At the end of the 45 days treatment period with respective drugs, all the rats were overnight fasted and blood was collected by retro orbital sinus puncture method with mild anaesthesia. Then, the rats were sacrificed by the cervical decapitation and vital organs were collected immediately and stored at -80°C until further use.

2.5. Measurement of Body Weight, Anthropometrical and Morphological Parameters

Body weight of all the animals were recorded at the end of the experimental period. At the end of the experimental period, rats were overnight fasted and their AC (abdominal circumference), TC (thoracic circumference), and body mass index (BMI) was measured by considering body length and body weight. On the other hand, morphological parameters such as WHR (waist-hip ratio), adiposity index = (sum of the weights of white adipose tissue (WAT) of perirenal, retroperitoneal WAT, and epididymal WAT divided by body weight X 100), obesity index = (body weight of rat/ nasoanal length (mm) X 104) were measured by the method of Singh and Krishan [11].

2.6. Estimation of Biochemical Markers

The biochemical markers such as glucose and insulin were measured with commercially available kits (Stanbio Laboratory, Boerne, TX, USA). IR was measured using the homeostasis model assessment.

2.7. Determination of Cardiac Lipid Profile

In brief, heart tissues were homogenised in lipid extraction buffer prepared with 5 volume isopropanol, 2 volume of water and 2 volumes of Triton X-100. After forcefully vortexing, the homogenates were centrifuged for 5 min at 14,000 rpm. Supernatants were obtained to inspect the levels of cholesterol, free fatty acids (FFA), triglycerides (TG) and phospholipids (PL) (BioAssay Systems).

2.8. Assessment of Oxidative Stress Markers in Heart

The oxidative stress markers, namely lipid peroxidation [12], glutathione (GSH), glutathione peroxidase (GPx), glutathione reductase (GR), glutathione--transferase (GST), superoxide dismutase (SOD) and catalase (CAT) were measured as described by Saravanan *et al.* [13].

2.9. Statistical Analysis

The results of the study were expressed as the mean ± SD and n=6. All the data in the group were evaluated statistically with SPSS\10.0 software. Statistical analysis was performed by one-way analysis of variance and the least-significant difference test. P values <0.05 were considered significant.

3. RESULTS

3.1. Effect of ZB on Anthropometrical and Morphological Parameters

Fig. (**1**) depicts the anthropometrical parameters in control and experimental obese rats. There was a noteworthy (*P*<0.05) elevation in the body weight (Fig. **1A**), AC (Fig. **1B**), TC (Fig. **1C**) and BMI (Fig. **1D**) in the obese control group when compared to the normal control group. At the same time, obese rats treated with ZB considerably (*P*<0.05) reduced their body weight, AC, TC and BMI.

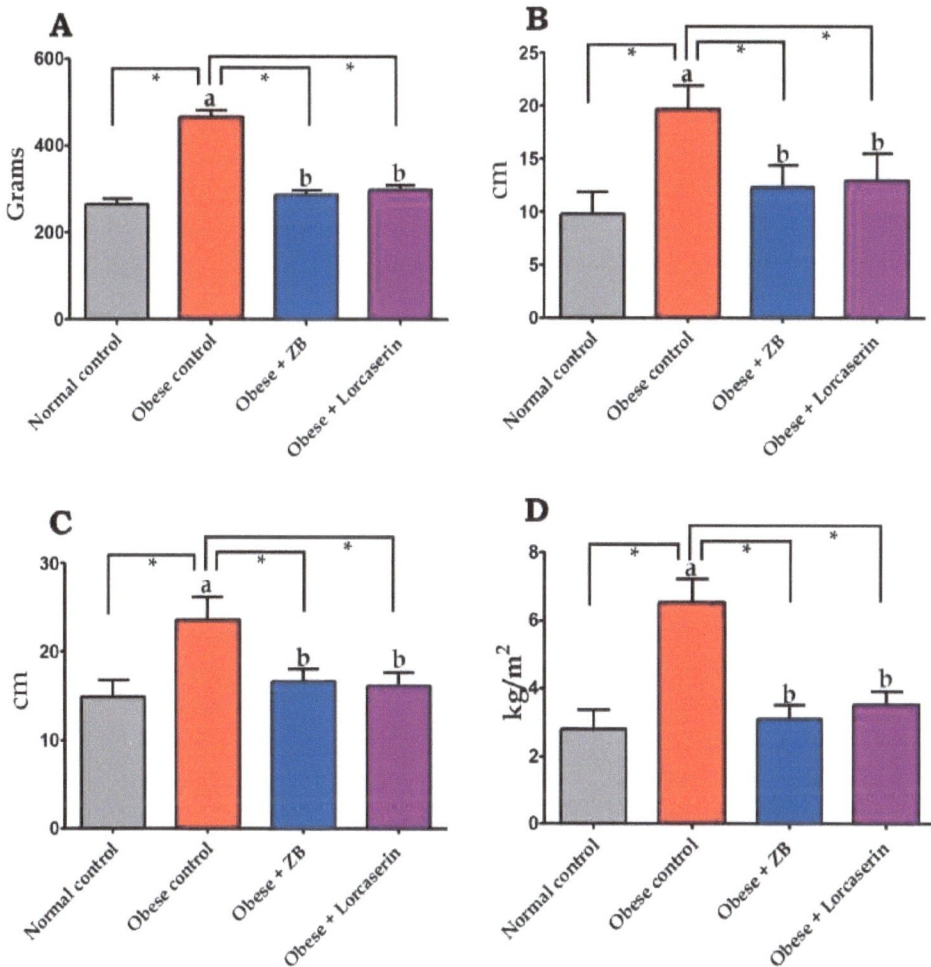

Fig. (1). Effect of ZB on (**A**) body weight, (**B**) AC, (**C**) TC and (**D**) BMI in control and experimental obese rats. All the values were expressed in mean ± SD, n=6, [a]Significantly different from the normal control, [b]Significantly different from the obese control, *P*<0.05.

Fig. (**2**) depicts that there was a significant increase in the WHR, adiposity index and obesity index in the obese control group when contrasted to normal rats. On the other hand, ZB treatment to obese rats for 45 days successfully ameliorated WHR (Fig. **2A**), adiposity index (Fig. **2B**) and obesity index (Fig. **2C**).

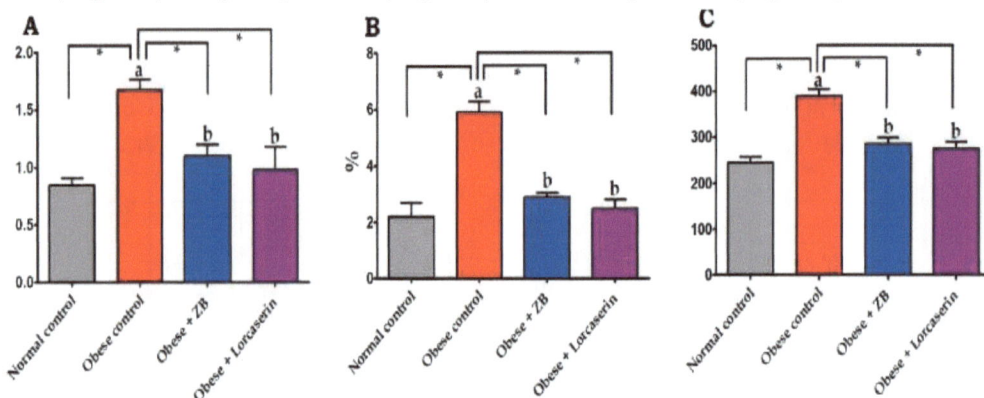

Fig. (2). Effect of ZB on (**A**) WHR, (**B**) adiposity index and (**C**) obesity index in control and experimental obese rats. All the values were expressed in mean ± SD, n=6, [a]Significantly different from the normal control, [b]Significantly different from the obese control, *$P<0.05$.

3.2. Influence of ZB on Diabetic Markers

Fig. (**3**) demonstrated that HFD supplementation caused diabetes in obese rats, which were confirmed by the elevated levels of blood glucose (Fig. **3A**), insulin (Fig. **3B**) and IR (Fig. **3C**). Conversely, supplementation of ZB to obese rats successfully ($P<0.05$) ameliorated the above altered parameters and restored them to near normal.

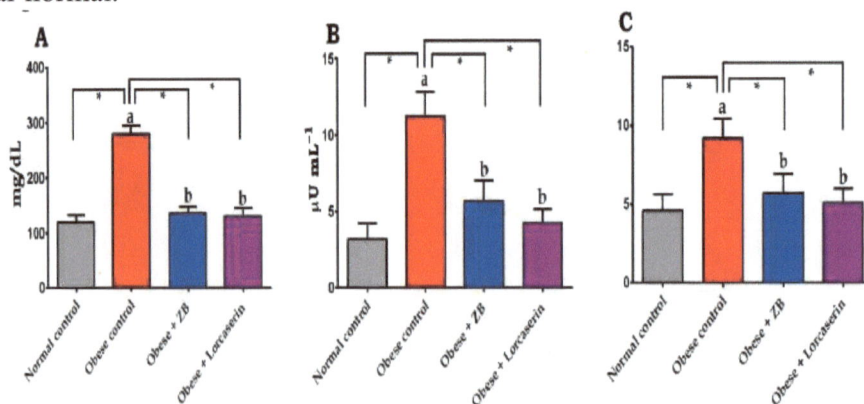

Fig. (3). Effect of ZB on diabetic markers (**A**) blood glucose, (**B**) insulin and (**C**) IR in control and experimental obese rats. All the values were expressed in mean ± SD, n=6, [a]Significantly different from the normal control, [b]Significantly different from the obese control, *$P<0.05$.

3.3. Effect of ZB on Cardiac Lipid Profiles

Fig. (**4**) explains the lipid profile of the heart in control and experimental obese rats. There was a significant ($P<0.05$) elevation of total cholesterol, TG and FFA and a simultaneous reduction in the levels of PL in obese control group. Interestingly, obese rats treated with ZB considerably attenuated the elevated levels of total cholesterol (Fig. **4a**), TG (Fig. **4b**) and FFA (Fig. **4c**) and restored PL levels (Fig. **4d**) to near normal as compared to untreated obese rats.

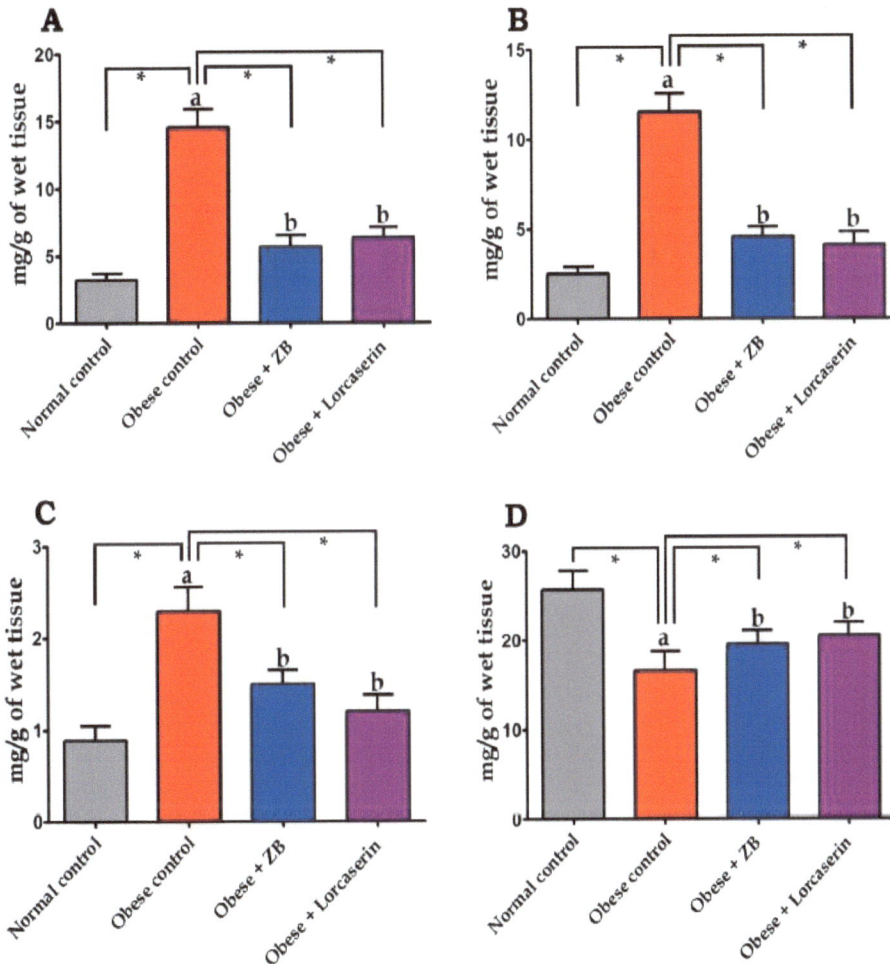

Fig. (4). Effect of ZB on cardiac lipid profiles **(A)** total cholesterol, **(B)** TG, **(C)** FFA and **(D)** PL in control and experimental obese rats. All the values were expressed in mean ± SD, n=6, [a]Significantly different from the normal control, [b]Significantly different from the obese control, *$P<0.05$.

3.4. ZB Ameliorated Oxidative Stress in Heart

Fig. (**5 and 6**) demonstrates the effect of ZB against oxidative stress in the heart of control and experimental obese rats. In the obese control group, there was a predominant ($P<0.05$) increase in lipid peroxidation (Fig. **5**) but the treatment with ZB in obese rats greatly attenuated the lipid peroxidation. On the other hand, there was a significant reduction in the levels of GSH (Fig. **6A**), GPX (Fig. **6B**), GR (Fig. **6C**), GST (Fig. **6D**), SOD (Fig. **6E**) and CAT (Fig. **6F**) in HFD-induced obese rats when compared to the normal control group. At the same time, obese rats treated with ZB for the period of 45 days successfully restored these markers to near normal, which emphasizes the antioxidant potentiality of ZB.

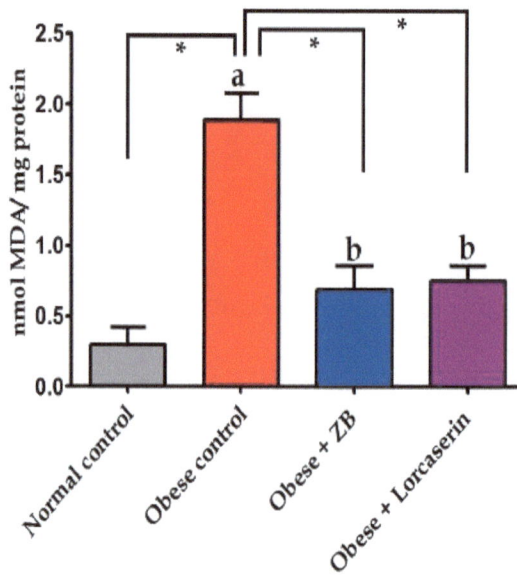

Fig. (5). Effect of ZB on cardiac lipid peroxidation in control and experimental obese rats. All the values were expressed in mean ± SD, n=6, [a]Significantly different from the normal control, [b]Significantly different from the obese control, *$P<0.05$.

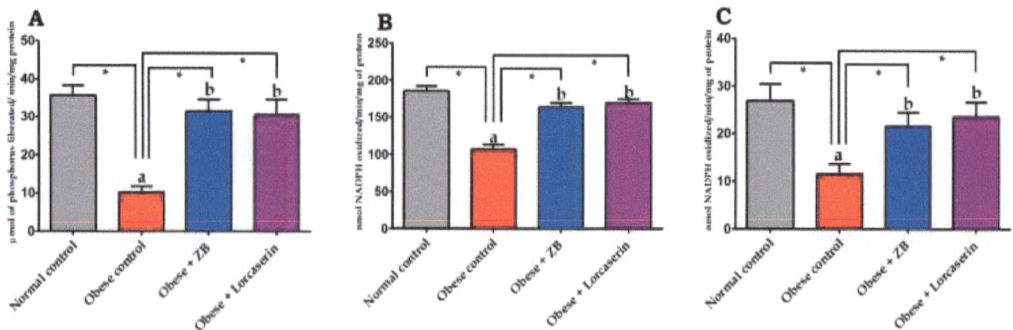

(Fig. 6) contd.....

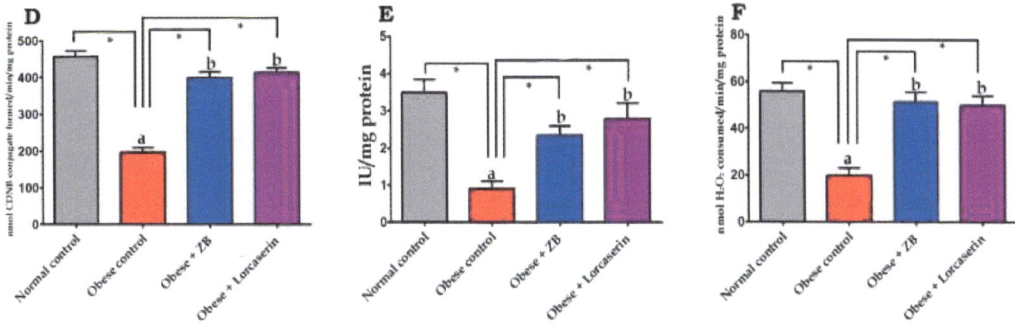

Fig. (6). Effect of ZB on oxidative stress markers **(A)** GSH content, **(B)** GPX, **(C)** GR, **(D)** GST, **(E)** SOD and **(F)** CAT in control and experimental obese rats. All the values were expressed in mean ± SD, n=6, [a]Significantly different from the normal control, [b]Significantly different from the obese control, *$P<0.05$.

4. DISCUSSION

Although the number of obese and chunky individuals globally continues to climb progressively, with obesity being linked with an augmented risk for cardiovascular disease and death, the categorization of an OC is a more recent development [2]. In the current study, we made an attempt to develop an OC model by using HFD supplementation and evaluated the therapeutic efficacy of ZB against OC. The current study demonstrated that HFD supplementation to the rats successfully developed obesity and OC, which was confirmed by the altered morphological and anthropometrical parameters and elevated body weight, lipid profiles and oxidative stress in rats.

Abundant wide-ranging studies have pointed out that HFD notably increases the accumulation of adipose tissue, due to their lofty energy solidity, leading to mounting body weight [14 - 16]. It might be due to the expenditure of a food rich in calories in the form of saturated fats and its deposition in different body fat pads [17], which leads to unnecessary growth of adipose tissue consequential in obesity, including two growth mechanisms: hypertrophic and hyperplastic of adipose tissue [16]. The present study established that HFD supplementation in rats is associated with increased body weight, BMI, TC, AC, adiposity index, and obesity index. The HFD-induced obese control rats weighed more than the normal controls because HFD is one of the risk factors for obesity [16]. These results are simultaneous with the findings of Jansy Isabella Rani *et al.* [14], who reported that the HFD induces the gathering of fat in the abdominal and thoracic regions. These findings substantiate that the noticed increase in body weight, WHR, adiposity index, and obesity index is due to the utilization of excessive food and adipose tissue accumulation. Rodrigues *et al.* [18] confirmed the association of the BMI with every day lipid eating and fat deposition. On the other hand, the observed diminished anthropometric measures in the obese rats subsequent ZB supplementation may be due to the reserve of dietetic lipid expenditure. Several researchers are documented that the adding together of medicinal plant extracts or their isolated compounds is connected with condensed energy mandatory for lipid and protein biosynthesis leading to inferior growth performance and nutrient utilization [19 - 21]. Therefore, ZB may have the potential of deteriorating body lipid and subsequently retaining energy. So, we hypothesised that the anthropometrical index may recognize obesity and may forecast its adverse effects on lipid profile and oxidative stress in rats.

Prolonged HFD supplementation is linked with dysregulated glucose and lipid metabolism and, therefore, overall deregulated energy homeostasis. Irregular in the energy balance is the chief cause of IR, obesity and type 2 DM. The combination of obesity and T2DM contributes considerably to the climb in cardiovascular diseases [22]. In the current study, the supplementation of HFD caused hyperglycemia, as revealed by the increased levels of plasma glucose, plasma insulin, and IR. HFD supplemented rats may be vulnerable to IR because the receptor cells are blocked by fat deposits; subsequently, DM becomes obvious. In the present study, we found that the HFD supplementation to rats clearly exhibited hyperglycemia and this consequence might be due to high HFD intake [15]. An unnecessary adipose tissue gathering was recognized to connect with metabolic alterations, which could be the threat issue for the increase of IR. In the body, adipose tissue is a very important place of energy storage and is vital for energy balance [19]. Enduring expenditure of HFD is one of the reasons for obesity and has been exposed to direct IR by plummeting the interaction between insulin receptor substrate-1 and insulin *via* diacylglycerol signalling [23]. Therefore, HFD may play a momentous function in the augmented incidence of obesity and can be a provoking factor in the development of hyperinsulinemia and hyperglycemia. Furthermore, an HFD not only holdback glucose uptake but also poorly suppresses hepatic glucose production enthused by insulin leading to IR as well as hyperglycemia [19, 24]. In the current study, HFD-induced obese rats have developed IR as selected by augmented plasma glucose, plasma insulin which maybe connected with the mutilation in the regulation of insulin-mediated glucose uptake caused by IR in skeletal muscle [25]. ZB endorses insulin sensitivity, subsequently declining IR, diminishing glucose level in obese rats, possibly by falling FFAs or regulating the cell energy metabolism.

Dyslipidemia is a conventional risk factor for cardiovascular disease, and many proofs exist regarding cardiac lipid metabolism that is openly linked to heart failure [14, 26]. Lipids are momentous controllers of cardiac function because of their function in cell membrane structure, cell signalling and transport. They also provide a substrate for β-oxidation and energy to the mitochondria [27]. Cardiac lipotoxicity involves not only a surplus deposition of intramyocellular TG in the cardiac but also the changes in lipid classes and the FFA profile. Therefore, the development of active lipid mediators enhances the heart metabolism and function to a certain extent by allowing the development of cardiac fibrosis, a very important provider of cardiac muscle dysfunction [28]. In addition, the HFD-provoked cardiac cholesterol levels point out that HFD may cause myocardial damage through extreme cholesterol deposition within cardiac tissues. Normal cells are confined from unnecessary cholesterol accumulation through diverse processes such as cholesterol synthesis, efflux and deluge [29], which might be destabilized by different pathophysiological circumstances. FFAs are accountable for the production of physiologically imperative substrates through oxidation. On the other hand, elevated levels of FFAs have been established to be a risk factor for heart failure [14]. Cardiomyocytes manufacture up to 70% of their essential requirements through the β-oxidation of FFAs [30]. Increased cardiac FFA levels are injurious to the heart in numerous ways [31]. Due to their cleanser-like and amphiphilic properties, FFAs can interrupt ion channels and membrane integrity and disengage mitochondrial enzymes, as a result diminishing the output of the respiratory cycle and the contractile capacity of the heart [14]. PLs are decisive for the precise localisation, capacity of the key mitochondrial enzymes, and myocardial suitability and contractility at the same time [28]. In the current study, we found that there was a significant elevation in the levels of total cholesterol, TG and FFA and concomitant decrease in the PL in heart. The changed heart lipid profiles were re-established to normal after treatment with ZB for 45 days, signifying the antihyperlipidimic potential of ZB and may attenuate cardio lipotoxicity caused by consumption of HFD.

Tissue damage provoked by free radicals is attention to be a significant feature in the pathogenesis of obesity and OC. Measuring the antioxidant defence system in the heart is a persuasive forecaster of cardiovascular damage, especially in metabolic disorders [32]. In the numerous models of cardiovascular disease models, including congestive heart failure, the tissue antioxidant system be unsuccessful to function and as a result, oxygen derived free radicals are augmented 4-fold and their levels in the cardiac tissue predicts the brutality of heart failure [33, 34]. Altitude of oxidative stress markers and reactive oxygen species products in the heart leads to straight oxidative damage of cellular machinery [35]. Similarly, in the current study, we establish a noteworthy rise in heart lipid peroxidation and concomitant reduction in the antioxidant enzymes (GPX, GR, GST, SOD and CAT) along with GSH content. Oxidative stress is one of the contributing factors that connect hypercholesterolemia with atherogenesis and myocardial infarction. Lipid peroxidation is a procession event that increases Malondialdehyde production [36]. There is also a relationship between hypercholesterolemia and lipid peroxidation. Our results confirmed an enhanced lipid peroxidation, in that way inducing free radical production in obese rats.

In addition, oxidative stress is infuriated by the decline in antioxidant enzymes activities such as SOD, CAT, GST, GR and GPx in cardiac tissue, which acts as free radical scavengers in conditions linked with oxidative stress [37]. It has been shown that animal body has an effectual mechanism to put off the free radical induced tissue cell damage, this is consummated by a set of inbuilt antioxidant enzymes and proteins such as GST, SOD, CAT, GPX, GR and GSH. When the balance between antioxidant defense and ROS production is vanished oxidative stress occurs; which through severe events deregulate the cellular functions, leading to heart failure [38]. GST, CAT and GPX constituted a reciprocally compassionate team of defence against reactive oxygen species. In the present study, SOD, GST, CAT, GPX, GR and GSH protein were measured in cardiac tissue and the data revealed that a significant decrease in the activities of these antioxidant enzymes in obese rats. On the other hand, ZB administration to obese rats restored the cardiac antioxidant system by uplifting the GSH content and increasing the activities of GPx, GR, GST, SOD and CAT. Earlier report suggests that antioxidants can make improvements in cholesterol absorption and antioxidant status [39]. Subsequently, we hypothesise the possible elucidation for the anti-obesity efficacy of ZB and its outcome on OC through the prevention of oxidative stress in the heart of obese rats.

CONCLUSION

In conclusion, this study exposed that treatment with ZB to obese rats for the period of 45 days might ameliorate obesity and its associated cardiomyopathy through reduction of cardiac lipotoxicity and oxidative stress. Hence, these results recommend that ZB may be used to treat OC and might develop as a pharmaceutical ingredient to combat cardiovascular disorders associated with obesity. However, a further detailed study is necessary to elucidate the mode of action against OC in the molecular level.

CONSENT FOR PUBLICATION

Not applicable.

CONFLICT OF INTEREST

The author declares no conflict of interest, financial or otherwise.

ACKNOWLEDGEMENTS

Declared none.

REFERENCES

[1]   Bhatheja S, Panchal HB, Ventura H, Paul TK. Obesity Cardiomyopathy: Pathophysiologic Factors and Nosologic Reevaluation. Am J Med Sci 2016; 352(2): 219-22.
       [http://dx.doi.org/10.1016/j.amjms.2016.05.014] [PMID: 27524223]

[2]   Newmarch W, Weiler M, Casserly B. Obesity cardiomyopathy: the role of obstructive sleep apnea and obesity hypoventilation syndrome. Ir J Med Sci 2019; 188(3): 783-90.
       [http://dx.doi.org/10.1007/s11845-018-01959-5] [PMID: 30645718]

[3]   Dela Cruz CS, Matthay RA. Role of obesity in cardiomyopathy and pulmonary hypertension. Clin Chest Med 2009; 30(3): 509-523, ix.
       [http://dx.doi.org/10.1016/j.ccm.2009.06.001] [PMID: 19700049]

[4]   Timoh T, Bloom ME, Siegel RR, Wagman G, Lanier GM, Vittorio TJ. A perspective on obesity cardiomyopathy. Obes Res Clin Pract 2012; 6(3): e181-8.
       [http://dx.doi.org/10.1016/j.orcp.2012.02.011] [PMID: 24331520]

[5]   Niemann B, Rohrbach S, Miller MR, Newby DE, Fuster V, Kovacic JC. Oxidative Stress and Cardiovascular Risk: Obesity, Diabetes, Smoking, and Pollution. J Am Coll Cardiol 2017; 70(2): 230-51.
       [http://dx.doi.org/10.1016/j.jacc.2017.05.043] [PMID: 28683970]

[6]   Kalaivani A, Vadivukkarasi S, Sathibabu Uddandrao VV, Saravanan G. Attenuation of Obesity-Associated Oxidative Stress by Cucurbita maxima Seed Oil in High Fat Diet-Induced Obese Rats. Pathophysiology of Obesity-Induced Health Complications Advances in Biochemistry in Health and Disease. Springer, Cham 2020.
       [http://dx.doi.org/10.1007/978-3-030-35358-2_18]

[7]   De Marchi E, Baldassari F, Bononi A, Wieckowski MR, Pinton P. Oxidative stress in cardiovascular diseases and obesity: role of p66Shc and protein kinase C. Oxid Med Cell Longev 2013; 2013: 1-11.
       [http://dx.doi.org/10.1155/2013/564961] [PMID: 23606925]

[8]   Kang JG, Park CY. Anti-Obesity Drugs: A Review about Their Effects and Safety. Diabetes Metab J 2012; 36(1): 13-25.
       [http://dx.doi.org/10.4093/dmj.2012.36.1.13] [PMID: 22363917]

[9]   Balaji M, Ganjayi MS, Hanuma Kumar GEN, Parim BN, Mopuri R, Dasari S. A review on possible therapeutic targets to contain obesity: The role of phytochemicals. Obes Res Clin Pract 2016; 10(4): 363-80.
       [http://dx.doi.org/10.1016/j.orcp.2015.12.004] [PMID: 26740473]

[10]   Togar B, Turkez H, Tatar A, Hacimuftuoglu A, Geyikoglu F. Cytotoxicity and genotoxicity of zingiberene on different neuron cell lines *in vitro*. Cytotechnology 2015; 67(6): 939-46.
       [http://dx.doi.org/10.1007/s10616-014-9729-9] [PMID: 24801579]

[11]   Singh R, Krishan P. Modulation of impact of high fat diet in pathological and physiological left ventricular cardiac hypertrophy by fluvastatin. Biomed Pharmacother 2010; 64(3): 147-53.
       [http://dx.doi.org/10.1016/j.biopha.2009.06.016] [PMID: 20053524]

[12]   Ohkawa H, Ohishi N, Yagi K. Assay for lipid peroxides in animal tissues by thiobarbituric acid reaction. Anal Biochem 1979; 95(2): 351-8.
       [http://dx.doi.org/10.1016/0003-2697(79)90738-3] [PMID: 36810]

[13]   Saravanan G, Ponmurugan P, Sathiyavathi M, Vadivukkarasi S, Sengottuvelu S. Cardioprotective activity of *Amaranthus viridis* Linn: Effect on serum marker enzymes, cardiac troponin and antioxidant system in experimental myocardial infarcted rats. Int J Cardiol 2013; 165(3): 494-8.

[http://dx.doi.org/10.1016/j.ijcard.2011.09.005] [PMID: 21962802]

[14]   A JIR, Uddandrao VVS, G S, *et al.* Biochanin A attenuates obesity cardiomyopathy in rats by inhibiting oxidative stress and inflammation through the Nrf-2 pathway. Arch Physiol Biochem 2021; 1-16.
[http://dx.doi.org/10.1080/13813455.2021.1874017] [PMID: 33471570]

[15]   Rameshreddy P, Uddandrao VVS, Brahmanaidu P, *et al.* Obesity-alleviating potential of asiatic acid and its effects on ACC1, UCP2, and CPT1 mRNA expression in high fat diet-induced obese Sprague–Dawley rats. Mol Cell Biochem 2018; 442(1-2): 143-54.
[http://dx.doi.org/10.1007/s11010-017-3199-2] [PMID: 28993954]

[16]   Brahma Naidu P, Uddandrao VVS, Ravindar Naik R, *et al.* Ameliorative potential of gingerol: Promising modulation of inflammatory factors and lipid marker enzymes expressions in HFD induced obesity in rats. Mol Cell Endocrinol 2016; 419: 139-47.
[http://dx.doi.org/10.1016/j.mce.2015.10.007] [PMID: 26493465]

[17]   A K, Uddandrao VVS, Parim B, *et al.* Reversal of high fat diet-induced obesity through modulating lipid metabolic enzymes and inflammatory markers expressions in rats. Arch Physiol Biochem 2019; 125(3): 228-34.
[http://dx.doi.org/10.1080/13813455.2018.1452036] [PMID: 29553847]

[18]   Rodrigues A, Paula CP, Ana FV, Jose AB, Maria A. Food Intake, Body Mass Index and Body Fat Mass in Elderly. Asia J Clin Nutr 2012; 4: 107-15.
[http://dx.doi.org/10.3923/ajcn.2012.107.115]

[19]   Uddandrao VVS, Rameshreddy P, Brahmanaidu P, *et al.* Antiobesity efficacy of asiatic acid: down-regulation of adipogenic and inflammatory processes in high fat diet induced obese rats. Arch Physiol Biochem 2020; 126(5): 453-62.
[http://dx.doi.org/10.1080/13813455.2018.1555668] [PMID: 30739501]

[20]   Antony Rathinasamy JIR, Uddandrao VVS, Raveendran N, Sasikumar V. Antiobesity Effect of Biochanin-A: Effect on Trace Element Metabolism in High Fat Diet-Induced Obesity in Rats. Cardiovasc Hematol Agents Med Chem 2020; 18(1): 21-30.
[http://dx.doi.org/10.2174/1871524920666200207101920] [PMID: 32031077]

[21]   Kalaivani A, Sathibabu Uddandrao VV, Brahmanaidu P, *et al.* Anti obese potential of *Cucurbita maxima* seeds oil: effect on lipid profile and histoarchitecture in high fat diet induced obese rats. Nat Prod Res 2018; 32(24): 2950-3.
[http://dx.doi.org/10.1080/14786419.2017.1389939] [PMID: 29047298]

[22]   Sikder K, Shukla SK, Patel N, Singh H, Rafiq K. High Fat Diet Upregulates Fatty Acid Oxidation and Ketogenesis *via* Intervention of PPAR-γ. Cell Physiol Biochem 2018; 48(3): 1317-31.
[http://dx.doi.org/10.1159/000492091] [PMID: 30048968]

[23]   Meriga B, Parim B, Chunduri VR, *et al.* Antiobesity potential of Piperonal: promising modulation of body composition, lipid profiles and obesogenic marker expression in HFD-induced obese rats. Nutr Metab (Lond) 2017; 14(1): 72.
[http://dx.doi.org/10.1186/s12986-017-0228-9] [PMID: 29176994]

[24]   Sathibabu Uddandrao VV, Brahmanaidu P, Ravindarnaik R, Suresh P, Vadivukkarasi S, Saravanan G. Restorative potentiality of S-allylcysteine against diabetic nephropathy through attenuation of oxidative stress and inflammation in streptozotocin–nicotinamide-induced diabetic rats. Eur J Nutr 2019; 58(6): 2425-37.
[http://dx.doi.org/10.1007/s00394-018-1795-x] [PMID: 30062492]

[25]   Brahmanaidu P, Uddandrao VVS, Sasikumar V, *et al.* Reversal of endothelial dysfunction in aorta of streptozotocin-nicotinamide-induced type-2 diabetic rats by S-Allylcysteine. Mol Cell Biochem 2017; 432(1-2): 25-32.
[http://dx.doi.org/10.1007/s11010-017-2994-0] [PMID: 28258439]

[26]   Han Q, Yeung SC, Ip MSM, Mak JCW. Dysregulation of cardiac lipid parameters in high-fat high-

cholesterol diet-induced rat model. Lipids Health Dis 2018; 17(1): 255.
[http://dx.doi.org/10.1186/s12944-018-0905-3] [PMID: 30428911]

[27]   Schulze PC, Drosatos K, Goldberg IJ. Lipid Use and Misuse by the Heart. Circ Res 2016; 118(11): 1736-51.
[http://dx.doi.org/10.1161/CIRCRESAHA.116.306842] [PMID: 27230639]

[28]   Marín-Royo G, Ortega-Hernández A, Martínez-Martínez E, *et al.* The Impact of Cardiac Lipotoxicity on Cardiac Function and Mirnas Signature in Obese and Non-Obese Rats with Myocardial Infarction. Sci Rep 2019; 9(1): 444.
[http://dx.doi.org/10.1038/s41598-018-36914-y] [PMID: 30679580]

[29]   Li C, Gong D, Chen L, *et al.* Puerarin promotes ABCA1-mediated cholesterol efflux and decreases cellular lipid accumulation in THP-1 macrophages. Eur J Pharmacol 2017; 811: 74-86.
[http://dx.doi.org/10.1016/j.ejphar.2017.05.055] [PMID: 28576406]

[30]   Nagoshi T, Yoshimura M, Rosano GM, Lopaschuk GD, Mochizuki S. Optimization of cardiac metabolism in heart failure. Curr Pharm Des 2011; 17(35): 3846-53.
[http://dx.doi.org/10.2174/138161211798357773] [PMID: 21933140]

[31]   Seo WK, Jung JM, Kim JH, Koh SB, Bang OY, Oh K. Free Fatty Acid Is Associated with Thrombogenicity in Cardioembolic Stroke. Cerebrovasc Dis 2017; 44(3-4): 160-8.
[http://dx.doi.org/10.1159/000478895] [PMID: 28715812]

[32]   Farhangi MA, Nameni G, Hajiluian G, Mesgari-Abbasi M, Bang OY, Oh K. Cardiac tissue oxidative stress and inflammation after vitamin D administrations in high fat- diet induced obese rats. BMC Cardiovasc Disord 2017; 17(1): 161.
[http://dx.doi.org/10.1186/s12872-017-0597-z] [PMID: 28629326]

[33]   Parim B, Sathibabu Uddandrao VV, Saravanan G. Diabetic cardiomyopathy: molecular mechanisms, detrimental effects of conventional treatment, and beneficial effects of natural therapy. Heart Fail Rev 2019; 24(2): 279-99.
[http://dx.doi.org/10.1007/s10741-018-9749-1] [PMID: 30349977]

[34]   Sathibabu Uddandrao VV, Brahmanaidu P, Nivedha PR, Vadivukkarasi S, Saravanan G. Beneficial Role of Some Natural Products to Attenuate the Diabetic Cardiomyopathy Through Nrf2 Pathway in Cell Culture and Animal Models. Cardiovasc Toxicol 2018; 18(3): 199-205.
[http://dx.doi.org/10.1007/s12012-017-9430-2] [PMID: 29080123]

[35]   Skibska B, Goraca A. The protective effect of lipoic acid on selected cardiovascular diseases caused by age-related oxidative stress. Oxid Med Cell Longev 2015; 2015: 1-11.
[http://dx.doi.org/10.1155/2015/313021] [PMID: 25949771]

[36]   Naidu PB, Sathibabu Uddandrao VV, Naik RR, *et al.* Effects of S-Allylcysteine on Biomarkers of the Polyol Pathway in Rats with Type 2 Diabetes. Can J Diabetes 2016; 40(5): 442-8.
[http://dx.doi.org/10.1016/j.jcjd.2016.03.006] [PMID: 27373435]

[37]   Noeman SA, Hamooda HE, Baalash AA. Biochemical study of oxidative stress markers in the liver, kidney and heart of high fat diet induced obesity in rats. Diabetol Metab Syndr 2011; 3(1): 17.
[http://dx.doi.org/10.1186/1758-5996-3-17] [PMID: 21812977]

[38]   Pavithra K, Sathibabu Uddandrao VV, Chandrasekaran P, *et al.* Phenolic fraction extracted from *Kedrostis foetidissima* leaves ameliorated isoproterenol-induced cardiotoxicity in rats through restoration of cardiac antioxidant status. J Food Biochem 2020; 44(11): e13450.
[http://dx.doi.org/10.1111/jfbc.13450] [PMID: 32839989]

[39]   Kalaivani A, Vadivukkarasi S, Sathibabu Uddandrao VV, Saravanan G. Attenuation of Obesity-Associated Oxidative Stress by Cucurbita maxima Seed Oil in High Fat Diet-Induced Obese Rats. Pathophysiology of Obesity-Induced Health Complications Advances in Biochemistry in Health and Disease. 2020.
[http://dx.doi.org/10.1007/978-3-030-35358-2_18]

CHAPTER 10

Betaine, a Nutraceutical Ameliorated Myocardial Infarction by Attenuation of Pro-Inflammatory Cytokines and Matrix Metalloproteinase Production in Rats

G. Somasundaram[1,*], S. Jaikumar[1] and S. Sengottuvelu[2]

[1] *Department of Pharmacology, Sri Lakshmi Narayana Institute of Medical Sciences, Puducherry, 605502, India*

[2] *Department of Pharmacology, Nandha College of Pharmacy, Erode, Tamilnadu, 638052, India*

Abstract: Cardiovascular disease is a key community health challenge and presently the condition with the utmost deaths around the globe, even though enormous development has been made in its management but there are still many difficulties. In the current study, we made an attempt to evaluate the therapeutic action of betaine, an active nutraceutical against isoproterenol-induced myocardial infarction (MI) in rats. The rats were pre-treated with betaine (250mg/Kg BW) for the period of 30 days and on the 31st and 32nd days, they were administered with isoproterenol (20mg/Kg BW) to produce MI in rats. Then we evaluated the effects of betaine on the ratio of heart weight to the body weight. Cardiac diagnostic markers and the production of pro-inflammatory cytokines and matrix metallopreoteinases along with their mRNA expressions were also studied in the heart by RT-PCR. We found that there was a significant elevation in the heart size, levels of LDH, CK-MB, CRP, homocysteine and serum pro-inflammatory cytokines (TNF-α, IL-1α, IL-1β, IL-6, MCP-1 and RANTES) and matrix metallopreoteinases (MMP-2 and MMP-9) in MI rats. On the other hand, pre-treatment of MI rats with betaine revealed a noteworthy reduction in the pro-inflammatory cytokines and matrix metallopreoteinases in the serum. RT-PCR study revealed that betaine successfully down-regulated the mRNA expressions of NF-κB, TNF-α, IL-6, MMP-2 and MMP-9 in MI rats. In conclusion, this study revealed that betaine is able to ameliorate MI by restraining the production of pro-inflammatory cytokines and matrix metallopreoteinases. Hence, betaine might be used as a dietary supplement as an alternative for cardio-protection.

Keywords: Betaine, Cardiovascular disease, Myocardial infarction, Natural products, Nutraceuticals.

---

* **Corresponding author G. Somasundaram:** Department of Pharmacology, Sri Lakshmi Narayana Institute of Medical Sciences, Puducherry, 605502-India; E-mail: umeshkumar82@gmail.com

Dr. V. V. Sathibabu Uddandrao & Dr. Parim Brahma Naidu (Eds.)

1. INTRODUCTION

Cardiovascular disease (CVD) is the main reason for morbidity and mortality both in developing and urbanized countries. A foremost form of CVD is myocardial infarction (MI), which usually comes across as a quiet infarction due to its late diagnosis in the disease development. When the equilibrium between the blood supply to the heart vessels and the necessity of the cardiac tissue is affected, the cardiomyocytes are subjected to a long-lasting ischemic damage ensuing in necrosis, frequently well-known as acute MI [1]. In recent decades, with changes in the way of life and predilection to co-morbidities, the frequency of MI has been found in the adolescent to be mounting with age in the middle and elder age groups, affecting both women and men [2]. The condensed blood supply to the heart results in the deficiency of oxygen to cardiac muscles, which if left untreated, results in permanent necrotic harm to the myocardium. In most cases, the cardiac arrest is sudden with no noticeable symptoms of ache and a severe impulsivity [3].

MI is an extremely multifaceted disorder with multistep progression in which numerous physiological systems contribute. Wide-ranging investigational data exposed that MI is intricately connected with the commencement of an inflammatory reaction [4]. Inflammatory mediators are openly implicated in the pathogenesis of the susceptible plaque, foremost to occlusion of the coronary vessel and consequent necrosis of the myocardial region served by the vessel [5]. Scientific studies have identified critical molecular signals mediating the inflammatory response following MI. Therapeutic interventions in experimental animal models recommended that the balanced reserve of particular inflammatory signals may protect the infarcted heart from acute damage and delay unwanted remodelling following MI [6]. On the other hand, matrix metalloproteases (MMPs) play a vital role in post-MI cardiac remodelling and in the increase of unpleasant outcomes. MMPs synchronize key life activities, along with inflammation and developmen. The changes in MMPs may direct to unwanted circumstances, resulting in the progress of a variety of possible complications, including sudden cardiac arrest, left ventricular rupture, or the increase of congestive heart failure. The potential roles of MMPs as a therapeutic target for MI setting, thus, are warranted. Simultaneously, lots of currently used medications to treat MI encourage MMPs activity. Identifying specific MMPs inhibition approaches for the post-MI patient; predominantly treatments that limit the development of heart failure, remains a greatly needed target [7].

For acute conditions, such as MI, modern drugs have been alleged as the only available therapeutic approach. On the other hand, an understanding pertaining to conventional medicine for MI has been rising. Therapeutic plants have been mostly used for healthcare around the globe even before the arrival of modern medicine [8], and the consumption of diets rich in plant foods is connected with an abridged CVD risk [9, 10]. Betaine is circulated widely in plants, animals and rich dietary sources which include seafood, spinach and wheat bran [11]. Betaine has several therapeutic effects which include antioxidants [12], antiobesity, antidiabetic [13] and hepatoprotective [14]. However, the protective effect of betaine on myocardial inflammation and the MMP system in experimentally induced MI conditions has not yet been previously explored. Hence, the current study was designed to evaluate the effect of betaine on pro-inflammatory cytokines and MMPs production in isoproterenol (ISO)-induced MI in rats.

2. MATERIALS AND METHODS

Betaine ($(CH_3)_3N^+CH_2COO^-$) and ISO were purchased from the Sigma-Aldrich, India.

2.1. Animals

The Wistar rats (weighing 120-140g) were utilized for this study and obtained from the Nandha College of Pharmacy, Erode, Tamilnadu, India. The animals were maintained at a 12 h day/night cycle, at a temperature of $22 \pm 2°C$, and humidity of 45-64%. The protocol of this study was approved by the Institutional Animal Ethical Committee, Nandha College of Pharmacy (Approval No: 688/PO/Re/S/02/CPCSEA).

2.2. Experimental Design

Group 1: Normal control

Group 2: ISO-induced MI untreated control

Group 3: Rats were pre-treated with betaine (250mg/kg BW) orally for 30 days and ISO (20mg/kg BW) administered once a day subcutaneously on the 31st and 32nd days.

Group 4: Rats were pre-treated with α-tocopherol (60mg/kg BW) orally for 30 days and ISO (20mg/kg BW) administered once a day subcutaneously on the 31st and 32nd days.

2.3. Measurement of Heart Weight and the Ratio of Heart Weight to Body Weight

After completion of the treatment period and ISO induction, the rats were anaesthetized by injecting pentobarbital sodium (40mg/kg/BW, i.p). Then rats were sacrificed by cervical decapitation and then straight away harvested hearts were weighed, and the ratio of the heart weight to the body weight was measured.

2.4. Assessment of Cardiac Diagnostic Markers

The cardiac diagnostic markers such as lactate dehydrogenase (LDH), creatine kinase-MB isoenzyme (CK-MB), cardiac troponin and homocysteine were determined by the commercially available kits procured from the Roche Diagnostics, Switzerland.

2.5. Estimation of Serum Inflammatory Markers

The serum levels of inflammatory cytokines such as C-reactive protein (CRP), tumour necrosis factor-alpha (TNF-α), interleukin (IL)-1α, IL-1β, IL-6, monocyte chemoattractant protein-1 (MCP-1), and regulated upon activation, normal T cell expressed and secreted (RANTES) were estimated as per the standard protocols described by the manufacturer (Thermo Fisher Scientific, India).

2.6. Determination of Serum Matrix Metalloproteinases

The levels of MMP-2 and MMP-9 in serum were determined by using the ELISA method (Stat Fax 303 Plus Microstrip Reader, Minneapolis, MN, USA).

2.7. RT-PCR Analysis

The total RNA was extracted from the cardiac tissue using Trizol reagent (Thermo Fisher Scientific, India) and reverse transcribed to accomplish cDNA using a DNA synthesis kit (Thermo Fisher Scientific, India). 20ng of cDNA was collected for semi-quantitative PCR. The PCR amplification was performed for 38 cycles using the following cycling conditions: 30 sec of denaturation at 94°C, 30 sec of annealing at 59°C and 1 min of extension at 72°C, with the primers (Table 1) and β-actin gene was used as housekeeping gene for normalization.

Table 1. Primer sequences for RT-PCR.

Gene	Primer
NF-κB	F 5'- ACCTTTGCTGGAAACACACC-3' R 5'-ATGGCCTCGGAAGTTTCTTT-3'
TNF-α	F: 5'-ATGTGGAACTGGCAGAGGAG-3' R: 5'-AGAAGAGGCTGAGGCACAGA-3'
IL-6	F: 5'-ATGTTGTTGACAGCCACTGC-3' R: 5'-GTCTCCTCTCCGGACTTGTG-3'
MMP-2	F5'-GTGCTGAAGGACACCCTCAAGAAGA-3' R: 5'-TTGCCGTCCTTCTCAAAGTTGTACG-3':
MMP-9	F: 5'-ACGGCAAGGATGGTCTACTG-3' R: 5'-AGTTGCCCCCAGTTACAGTG-3'
β-actin	F: 5'-CCTGCTTGCTGATCCACA-3' R: 5'-CTGACCGAGCGTGGCTAC-3'

2.8. Statistical Analysis

All the results were expressed as the mean ± S.D, n=6 and all the grouped data were statistically analysed with SPSS\10.0 software. Hypothesis testing methods ANOVA followed by the LSD test, with significance level at $P<0.05$ were considered to indicate statistical significance.

3. RESULTS

Fig. (**1**) represents that the ISO-induced MI rats demonstrated a significant ($P<0.05$) increase in the size of the heart which was confirmed by the elevated heart weight (Fig. **1A**) and heart/body weight index (Fig. **1B**). But, the MI rats pre-treated with betaine displayed a normal heart/body weight index similar to the normal control group.

Fig. (**2**) demonstrates the cardiac diagnostic markers in control and experimental MI rats. There was a significant ($P<0.05$) elevation in the levels of LDH (Fig. **2A**), CK-MB (Fig. **2B**), cardiac troponin (Fig. **2C**) and homocysteine (Fig. **2D**) in the serum of the ISO-induced MI rats. On the other hand, rats pre-treated with betaine successfully ameliorated the alterations of the cardiac markers in ISO-induced MI rats when compared to untreated MI rats.

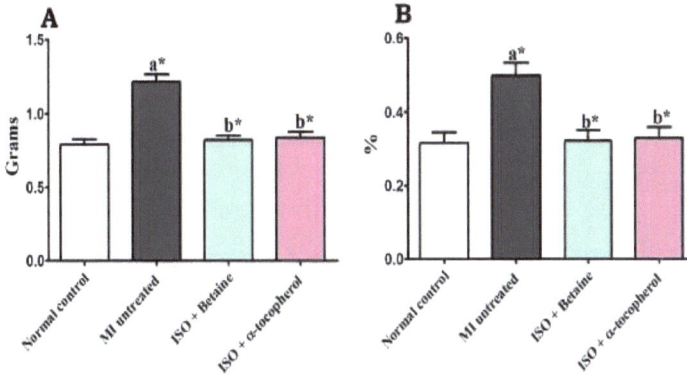

Fig. (1). Influence of betaine on **(A)** heart weight and **(B)** heart/body weight index. Values are expressed in mean±SD, n=6, [a]Significantly different from the normal control, [b]Significantly different from the MI control, *$P<0.05$.

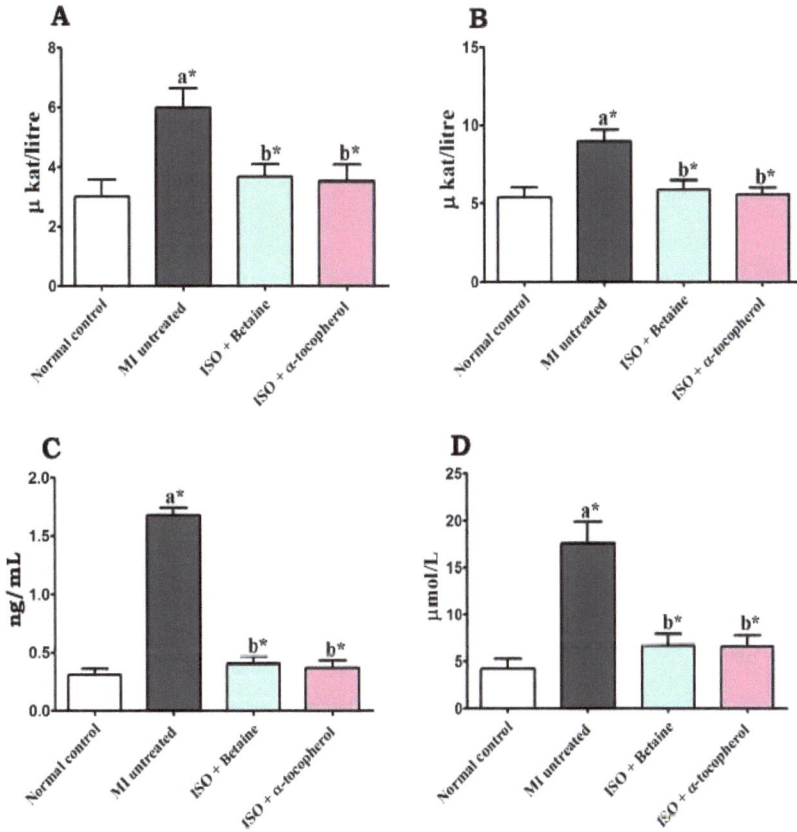

Fig. (2). Effect of betaine on cardiac diagnostic markers **(A)** LDH, **(B)** CK-MB, **(C)** cardiac troponin and **(D)** homocysteine. Values are expressed in mean±SD, n=6, [a]Significantly different from the normal control, [b]Significantly different from the MI control, *$P<0.05$.

Figs. (**3** and **4**) illustrate the effect of betaine on serum inflammatory markers production in control and experimental MI rats. The inflammatory markers such as CRP (Fig. **3A**), TNF-α (Fig. **3B**), IL-1α (Fig. **3C**), IL-1β (Fig. **3D**), IL-6 (Fig. **4A**), MCP-1 (Fig. **4B**) and RANTES (Fig. **4C**) were notably ($P<0.05$) elevated in MI rats when compared to group 1. Interestingly, the MI rats pre-treated with betaine did not show any alterations in these markers in the serum and were shown as near normal as group 1.

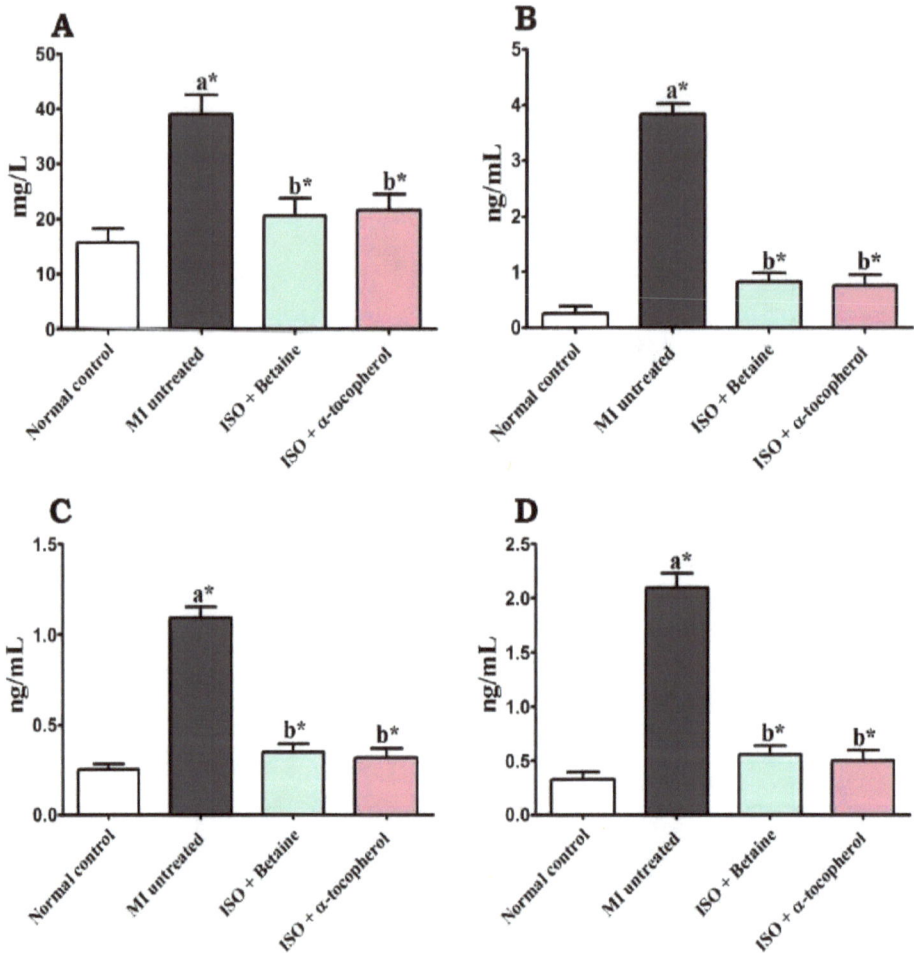

Fig. (3). Effect of betaine on serum **(A)** CRP, **(B)** TNF-α, **(C)** IL-1α and **(D)** IL-1β. Values are expressed in mean±SD, n=6, [a]Significantly different from the normal control, [b]Significantly different from the MI control, *$P<0.05$.

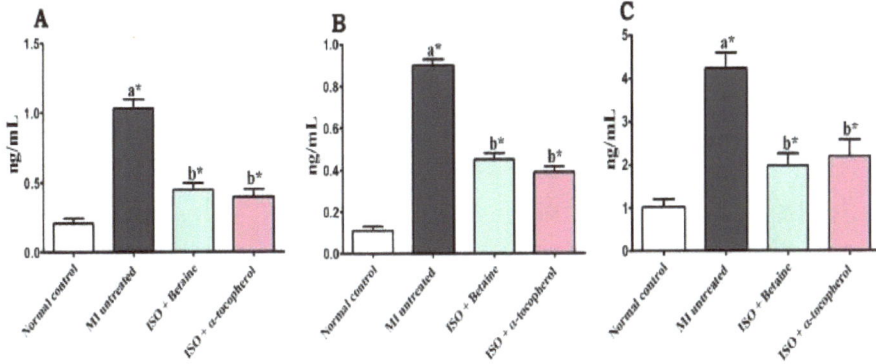

Fig. (4). Effect of betaine on serum **(A)** IL-6, **(B)** MCP-1 and **(C)** RANTES. Values are expressed in mean±SD, n=6, [a]Significantly different from the normal control, [b]Significantly different from the MI control, *$P<0.05$.

Fig. (**5**) displays the effect of betaine on the MMPs production in control and experimental MI rats. In this study, we found a momentous ($P<0.05$) increase in the levels of MMP-2 (Fig. **5A**) and MMP-9 (Fig. **5B**) in the serum of the ISO-induced MI rats. At the same time, there was a noteworthy ($P<0.05$) reduction in the production of MMP-2 and MMP-9 when the MI rats were pre-treated with betaine.

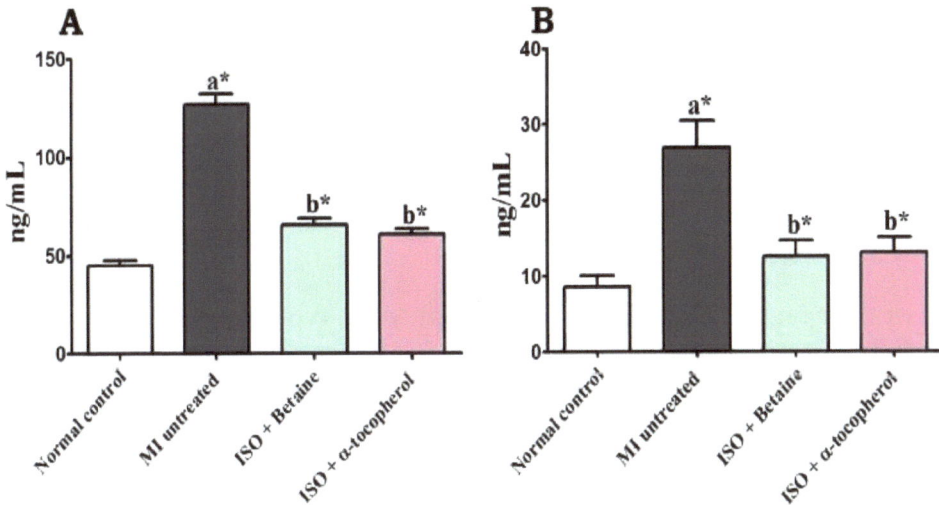

Fig. (5). Effect of betaine on **(A)** MMP-2 and **(B)** MMP-9. Values are expressed in mean±SD, n=6, [a]Significantly different from the normal control, [b]Significantly different from the MI control, *$P<0.05$.

We also studied the mRNA expressions of NF-κB, TNF-α, IL-6, MMP-2 and MMP-9 in the control and experimental MI rats by RT-PCR which revealed that there was a significant ($P<0.05$) up-regulation of these genes when compared to the normal control group (Fig. **6**). At the same time, when MI rats pre-treated with betaine, it effectively down-regulated the mRNA expressions of NF-κB (Fig. **6A**), TNF-α (Fig. **6B**), IL-6 (Fig. **6C**), MMP-2 (Fig. **6D**) and MMP-9 (Fig. **6E**) when compared to untreated MI rats.

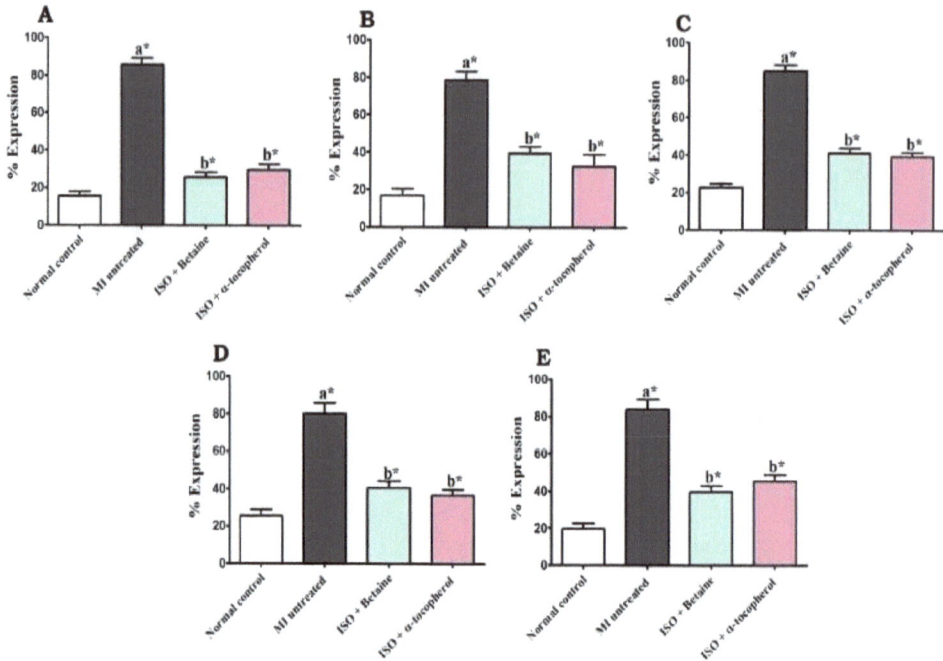

Fig. (6). Effect of betaine on cardiac mRNA expressions of **(A)** NF-κB, **(B)** TNF-α, **(C)** IL-6, **(D)** MMP-2 and **(E)** MMP-9. Values are expressed in mean±SD, n=6, [a]Significantly different from the normal control, [b]Significantly different from the MI control, *$P<0.05$.

4. DISCUSSION

Modern therapeutics have been used to treat MI, a type of CVD, and have been comparatively successful but not without side effects. Therefore, this concern has moved attention to the exploitation of natural products, which may be similarly effective and better tolerated [15]. Several studies have found the cardioprotective effect of natural products, such as plant-derived phytoconstituents, against ISO-induced MI; these have demonstrated promising results at the root of their anti-atherosclerotic, anti-apoptotic, antioxidant and anti-inflammatory activities [16, 17]. Therefore, in the current study, we evaluated the effect of betaine against ISO-induced MI in rats and its influence on the production of pro-inflammatory cytokines and MMPs. We supplemented the rats with betaine for a period of 30 days prior to the administration of ISO to evaluate its therapeutic action against MI and we found a significant cardioprotective effect with betaine supplementation.

ISO is a β-Adrenergic agonist that has been recognized to make use of both chronotropic and inotropic cardiac effects that ultimately lead to cell infiltration, necrosis induced by inflammation, fibrosis and myocardial hypertrophy [18]. ISO in high doses induces functional and morphological changes in the cardiac condition leading to subendocardial myocardial hypoxia, necrosis, ischemia and finally fibroblastic hyperplasia with reduced myocardial compliance and inhibition of systolic and diastolic tasks, which directly resemble local MI-like pathological alterations seen in human MI [19]. In the present study, we have observed a significant increase in the heart weight and the ratio of heart weight to body weight in ISO-induced rats. Patel *et al.* [20] observed an increase in the heart weight in ISO-induced MI rats which might be due to the increased water content, oedematous intramuscular space and wide-ranging necrosis of the heart muscle fibres followed by the incursion of damaged tissues by the inflammatory cells. Pre-treatment with betaine significantly decreased the heart weight and heart weight to body weight index in ISO-induced rats which may be due to the cardioprotective activity of betaine by preventing inflammation and necrosis.

CK-MB and LDH are cytosolic enzymes which give an insightful index to measure the severity of MI. Elevated activities of these marker enzymes in the serum are indications of cellular damage and failure of functional integrity and/or permeability of cell membrane [17, 19]. Furthermore, most recent data have indicated an assessment of cardiac troponin, a contractile and low molecular weight protein which is generally not found in serum, but discharged when myocardial scar occurs. It may be even further noteworthy in diagnosing cardiac damage and for risk prediction in subsequent MI [16]. At the same time, homocysteine could be considered a marker for the diagnosis of CVD or a pathologic metabolite causing inflammation and oxidative stress [21]. In the present study, a significant increase observed in the activities of CK-MB and LDH and the levels of cardiac troponin and homocysteine in the serum of ISO-induced MI rats may due to their leakage from the cardiac attack as a result of necrosis induced by ISO. To be exact, the cardiac membrane becomes porous or may shatter, due to lacking glucose and/or oxygen supply [17], thus resulting in the leakage of enzymes and/or cardiac troponin and homocysteine. Betaine is likely to protect the functional and structural integrity and/or permeability of the heart membrane and thus restricting the leak of these marker enzymes and cardiac troponin and homocysteine from the myocardium, as evident from the noticeably decreased levels of these markers in betaine + ISO group when compared to untreated groups, thereby establishing the cardioprotective effect of betaine.

Subsequent to MI, different mechanisms activate the immune system, causing inflammation [22]. In the access of inflammatory cells, high amounts of cytokines are produced that are involved in the inflammatory response after MI, including cell death, cell infiltration and extracellular remodelling stimulated by cell factors. Inflammation plays a role in the whole process of MI pathogenesis [22]. The altitude of inflammatory cytokines in serum is connected to the severity level and length; determining the levels of inflammatory cytokines in serum is of enormous value for correct diagnosis of patients with severe MI. Proper inflammation can endorse the renovation of cardiac tissue and angiogenesis, but overreaction will guide the configuration of a set of scar tissue and fibrosis, causing ventricular remodelling, and eventually distressing cardiac function [23].

TNF-α and IL-6 are proinflammatory cytokines linked with the synthesis of collagen and scar arrangement after acute MI [24]. Serum levels of IL-6 increase after MI, and because high IL-6 and CRP levels correspond to peak cardiac troponin, these could confirm the relationship between inflammation and infarct range [25]. In MI, serum levels of IL-1β are explained and they produce myofibroblasts engaged with cardiac rebuilding and adjustment of systolic capability after MI [26]. IL-1α, leaked from necrotic cardiomyocytes, may serve as an indication of the ratification of post-MI inflammatory reaction that adds to the detrimental effects on the heart. It has been projected that the discharge of constitutive IL-1α may enlarge ischemic myocardial damage by mounting apoptosis of cardiomyocytes [27]. On the other hand, in individuals with MI, a remarkable rise in the serum level of RANTES was documented [28]. Similarly, in this study, we found a significant increase in pro-inflammatory cytokines such as TNF-α, IL-1α, IL-1β, IL-6, MCP-1, and RANTES in ISO-induced MI rats. At the same time, MI rats pre-treated with betaine hold back the production of these pro-inflammatory cytokines and this could be because betaine may diminish the constant reperfusion injury arbitrated during inflammatory reactions by interfering with NF-κB authorization; this pathway is fundamental in the control of translation of proinflammatory-associated genes [29]. This was supported by our RT-PCR analysis, which revealed that there was a significant up-regulation of the mRNA expressions of NF-κB, TNF-α, and IL-6 in ISO-induced MI rats. In addition to that, MI rats pre-treated with betaine down-regulated these inflammatory gene mRNA expressions. This could emphasize the anti-inflammatory efficacy of betaine.

MMPs have been extensively researched as potential markers to predict the prognosis of CVD, predominantly in post-MI remodeling and cardiac failure. MMP-2 is expressed by cardiomyocytes, vascular smooth muscle cells, macrophages, endothelial cells and fibroblasts [30]. Because of its high constitutive activity, MMP-2 is well thought-out an MMP maintenance gene that helps to control typical tissue turnover [31]. Post-MI, MMP-2 levels rise both in plasma and within the infarct due to stimulation of the cardiac fibroblast and cardiomyocyte [32]. In MI rats, MMP-2 mRNA expressions increase within 24 hours post-MI and reach at peak around day 14 of post-MI [17]. In MI, MMP-9 within the infarcted tissue is substantial from neutrophils and may probably function reasonably on the ventricular tissue as a protease, yet it might encourage neutrophil degranulation and diffusion and fuel the ischemic insult [33]. MMP-9 reserve prompts a lower episode of myocardial apoptosis after MI and lowers left ventricular swelling due to a reduced amount of collagen redeployment in the infarcted region [34]. In the current study, we found that there was a significant elevation in the levels of MMP-2 and MMP-9 in serum and also the mRNA expressions were up-regulated in cardiac tissue. At the same time, MI rats pre-treated with betaine effectively restrain the production of MMPs and this established that betaine can be proficient to restrain the production of MMP-2 and MMP-9, thereby this may ameliorate MI and maintain the characteristic cardiac function.

CONCLUSION

In conclusion, this study revealed that betaine, an active nutraceutical present in various animals and plants, can able to ameliorate the ISO-induced MI in rats. Betaine can able to hold back the production of pro-inflammatory cytokines and MMPs, thereby maintaining the normal function of the heart. Hence, this study recommended that supplementation of betaine might be able to protect from heart failure.

CONSENT FOR PUBLICATION

Not applicable.

CONFLICT OF INTEREST

The author declares no conflict of interest, financial or otherwise.

ACKNOWLEDGEMENTS

Declared none.

REFERENCES

[1]   Boarescu PM, Chirilă I, Bulboacă AE, *et al.* Effects of Curcumin Nanoparticles in Isoproterenol-Induced Myocardial Infarction. Oxid Med Cell Longev 2019; 2019: 1-13.
       [http://dx.doi.org/10.1155/2019/7847142] [PMID: 31205590]

[2]   Bhushan A, Kulshreshtha M. A scientific update on myocardial infarction: A life-threatening issue.

Cardiology Plus 2019; 4(3): 71-80.
[http://dx.doi.org/10.4103/cp.cp_13_19]

[3]   Hoffman JIE, Buckberg GD. The myocardial oxygen supply:demand index revisited. J Am Heart Assoc 2014; 3(1): e000285.
[http://dx.doi.org/10.1161/JAHA.113.000285] [PMID: 24449802]

[4]   Frangogiannis NG. The inflammatory response in myocardial injury, repair, and remodelling. Nat Rev Cardiol 2014; 11(5): 255-65.
[http://dx.doi.org/10.1038/nrcardio.2014.28] [PMID: 24663091]

[5]   Huang S, Frangogiannis NG. Anti-inflammatory therapies in myocardial infarction: failures, hopes and challenges. Br J Pharmacol 2018; 175(9): 1377-400.
[http://dx.doi.org/10.1111/bph.14155] [PMID: 29394499]

[6]   Kleveland O, Kunszt G, Bratlie M, *et al.* Effect of a single dose of the interleukin-6 receptor antagonist tocilizumab on inflammation and troponin T release in patients with non-ST-elevation myocardial infarction: a double-blind, randomized, placebo-controlled phase 2 trial. Eur Heart J 2016; 37(30): 2406-13.
[http://dx.doi.org/10.1093/eurheartj/ehw171] [PMID: 27161611]

[7]   Yabluchanskiy A, Li Y, Chilton RJ, Lindsey ML. Matrix metalloproteinases: drug targets for myocardial infarction. Curr Drug Targets 2013; 14(3): 276-86.
[PMID: 23316962]

[8]   Wei H, Li H, Wan SP, *et al.* Cardioprotective Effects of Malvidin Against Isoproterenol-Induced Myocardial Infarction in Rats: A Mechanistic Study. Med Sci Monit 2017; 23: 2007-16.
[http://dx.doi.org/10.12659/MSM.902196] [PMID: 28445445]

[9]   Parim B, Sathibabu Uddandrao VV, Saravanan G. Diabetic cardiomyopathy: molecular mechanisms, detrimental effects of conventional treatment, and beneficial effects of natural therapy. Heart Fail Rev 2019; 24(2): 279-99.
[http://dx.doi.org/10.1007/s10741-018-9749-1] [PMID: 30349977]

[10]   Sathibabu Uddandrao VV, Brahmanaidu P, Nivedha PR, Vadivukkarasi S, Saravanan G. Beneficial Role of Some Natural Products to Attenuate the Diabetic Cardiomyopathy Through Nrf2 Pathway in Cell Culture and Animal Models. Cardiovasc Toxicol 2018; 18(3): 199-205.
[http://dx.doi.org/10.1007/s12012-017-9430-2] [PMID: 29080123]

[11]   Cholewa JM, Wyszczelska-Rokiel M, Glowacki R, *et al.* Effects of betaine on body composition, performance, and homocysteine thiolactone. J Int Soc Sports Nutr 2013; 10(1): 39.
[http://dx.doi.org/10.1186/1550-2783-10-39] [PMID: 23967897]

[12]   Ganesan B, Buddhan S, Anandan R, Sivakumar R, AnbinEzhilan R. Antioxidant defense of betaine against isoprenaline-induced myocardial infarction in rats. Mol Biol Rep 2010; 37(3): 1319-27.
[http://dx.doi.org/10.1007/s11033-009-9508-4] [PMID: 19288277]

[13]   Du J, Shen L, Tan Z, *et al.* Betaine Supplementation Enhances Lipid Metabolism and Improves Insulin Resistance in Mice Fed a High-Fat Diet. Nutrients 2018; 10(2): 131.
[http://dx.doi.org/10.3390/nu10020131] [PMID: 29373534]

[14]   Li Y, Xu S, Mihaylova MM, *et al.* AMPK phosphorylates and inhibits SREBP activity to attenuate hepatic steatosis and atherosclerosis in diet-induced insulin-resistant mice. Cell Metab 2011; 13(4): 376-88.
[http://dx.doi.org/10.1016/j.cmet.2011.03.009] [PMID: 21459323]

[15]   Wong ZW, Thanikachalam PV, Ramamurthy S. Molecular understanding of the protective role of natural products on isoproterenol-induced myocardial infarction: A review. Biomed Pharmacother 2017; 94: 1145-66.
[http://dx.doi.org/10.1016/j.biopha.2017.08.009] [PMID: 28826162]

[16]   Pavithra K, Sathibabu Uddandrao VV, Chandrasekaran P, *et al.* Phenolic fraction extracted from

Kedrostis foetidissima leaves ameliorated isoproterenol-induced cardiotoxicity in rats through restoration of cardiac antioxidant status. J Food Biochem 2020; 44(11): e13450.
[http://dx.doi.org/10.1111/jfbc.13450] [PMID: 32839989]

[17]   Sangeethadevi G, v v SU, Jansy Isabella RAR, *et al.* Attenuation of lipid metabolic abnormalities, proinflammatory cytokines, and matrix metalloproteinase expression by biochanin-A in isoproterenol-induced myocardial infarction in rats. Drug Chem Toxicol 2021; 1-12.
[http://dx.doi.org/10.1080/01480545.2021.1894707] [PMID: 33719799]

[18]   Tasatargil A, Kuscu N, Dalaklioglu S, *et al.* Cardioprotective effect of nesfatin-1 against isoproterenol-induced myocardial infarction in rats: Role of the Akt/GSK-3β pathway. Peptides 2017; 95: 1-9.
[http://dx.doi.org/10.1016/j.peptides.2017.07.003] [PMID: 28720397]

[19]   Li H, Xie YH, Yang Q, *et al.* Cardioprotective effect of paeonol and danshensu combination on isoproterenol-induced myocardial injury in rats. PLoS One 2012; 7(11): e48872.
[http://dx.doi.org/10.1371/journal.pone.0048872] [PMID: 23139821]

[20]   Patel V, Upaganlawar A, Zalawadia R, Balaraman R. Cardioprotective effect of melatonin against isoproterenol induced myocardial infarction in rats: A biochemical, electrocardiographic and histoarchitectural evaluation. Eur J Pharmacol 2010; 644(1-3): 160-8.
[http://dx.doi.org/10.1016/j.ejphar.2010.06.065] [PMID: 20624385]

[21]   Chaturvedi P, Kalani A, Givvimani S, Kamat PK, Familtseva A, Tyagi SC. Differential regulation of DNA methylation *versus* histone acetylation in cardiomyocytes during HHcy *in vitro* and *in vivo*: an epigenetic mechanism. Physiol Genomics 2014; 46(7): 245-55.
[http://dx.doi.org/10.1152/physiolgenomics.00168.2013] [PMID: 24495916]

[22]   Kain V, Ingle KA, Colas RA, *et al.* Resolvin D1 activates the inflammation resolving response at splenic and ventricular site following myocardial infarction leading to improved ventricular function. J Mol Cell Cardiol 2015; 84: 24-35.
[http://dx.doi.org/10.1016/j.yjmcc.2015.04.003] [PMID: 25870158]

[23]   Boufenzer A, Lemarié J, Simon T, *et al.* TREM-1 Mediates Inflammatory Injury and Cardiac Remodeling Following Myocardial Infarction. Circ Res 2015; 116(11): 1772-82.
[http://dx.doi.org/10.1161/CIRCRESAHA.116.305628] [PMID: 25840803]

[24]   Tian M, Yuan YC, Li JY, Gionfriddo MR, Huang RC. Tumor necrosis factor-α and its role as a mediator in myocardial infarction: A brief review. Chronic Dis Transl Med 2015; 1(1): 18-26.
[PMID: 29062983]

[25]   Govindasami S, Uddandrao VVS, Raveendran N, Sasikumar V. Therapeutic Potential of Biochanin-A Against Isoproterenol-Induced Myocardial Infarction in Rats. Cardiovasc Hematol Agents Med Chem 2020; 18(1): 31-6.
[http://dx.doi.org/10.2174/1871525718662200206114304] [PMID: 32026788]

[26]   Nagaraju CK, Dries E, Popovic N, *et al.* Global fibroblast activation throughout the left ventricle but localized fibrosis after myocardial infarction. Sci Rep 2017, 7(1). 10801.
[http://dx.doi.org/10.1038/s41598-017-09790-1] [PMID: 28883544]

[27]   Frangogiannis N. Interleukin-1 in cardiac injury, repair, and remodeling: pathophysiologic and translational concepts. Discoveries (Craiova) 2015; 3(1): e41.
[http://dx.doi.org/10.15190/d.2015.33] [PMID: 26273700]

[28]   Cavalera M, Frangogiannis N. Targeting the chemokines in cardiac repair. Curr Pharm Des 2014; 20(12): 1971-9.
[http://dx.doi.org/10.2174/13816128113199990449] [PMID: 23844733]

[29]   Mokhtari-Zaer A, Marefati N, Atkin SL, Butler AE, Sahebkar A. The protective role of curcumin in myocardial ischemia–reperfusion injury. J Cell Physiol 2019; 234(1): 214-22.
[http://dx.doi.org/10.1002/jcp.26848] [PMID: 29968913]

[30]   DeLeon-Pennell KY, Meschiari CA, Jung M, Lindsey ML. Matrix Metalloproteinases in Myocardial Infarction and Heart Failure. Prog Mol Biol Transl Sci 2017; 147: 75-100.
[http://dx.doi.org/10.1016/bs.pmbts.2017.02.001] [PMID: 28413032]

[31]   Vanhoutte D, Schellings M, Pinto Y, Heymans S. Relevance of matrix metalloproteinases and their inhibitors after myocardial infarction: A temporal and spatial window. Cardiovasc Res 2006; 69(3): 604-13.
[http://dx.doi.org/10.1016/j.cardiores.2005.10.002] [PMID: 16360129]

[32]   Baghirova S, Hughes BG, Poirier M, Kondo MY, Schulz R. Nuclear matrix metalloproteinase-2 in the cardiomyocyte and the ischemic-reperfused heart. J Mol Cell Cardiol 2016; 94: 153-61.
[http://dx.doi.org/10.1016/j.yjmcc.2016.04.004] [PMID: 27079252]

[33]   Walz W, Cayabyab FS. Neutrophil Infiltration and Matrix Metalloproteinase-9 in Lacunar Infarction. Neurochem Res 2017; 42(9): 2560-5.
[http://dx.doi.org/10.1007/s11064-017-2265-1] [PMID: 28417261]

[34]   Ducharme A, Frantz S, Aikawa M, *et al.* Targeted deletion of matrix metalloproteinase-9 attenuates left ventricular enlargement and collagen accumulation after experimental myocardial infarction. J Clin Invest 2000; 106(1): 55-62.
[http://dx.doi.org/10.1172/JCI8768] [PMID: 10880048]

SUBJECT INDEX

A

Abdomen 113
  bloated 113
Abdominal obesity 4, 126
Abnormal glucose tolerance 58
Absorption 7, 11, 34, 141
  intestinal 34
Acid(s) 6, 8, 13, 14, 15, 16, 39, 46, 82, 84,
    133, 135, 136, 137, 142, 145, 167, 174,
    177, 180, 181
  acetylsalicylic 8
  alpha-linolenic (ALA) 13
  amino 6, 84
  arachidonic 14
  arjunolic 137
  ascorbic 15
  betulinic 167
  docosahexaenoic 13
  eicosapentaenoic 13
  folic 39
  free fatty (FFAs) 174, 177, 180, 181
  gallotannic 145
  glutamic 84
  gymnemic 137
  hydroxycitric 135
  lactic 13
  linoleic 142
  nicotinic 133
  nucleic 82
  oleanolic 145
  oleic 16, 142
  palmitic 142
  petroselinic 142
  phenolic 135, 136
  thiobarbituric 46
  ursolic 167
Acquired coronary heart diseases 89
Actions 6, 7, 14, 116, 138, 139, 186, 195
  aldosterone-secreting 6
  anti-atherogenic 116
  anticlotting 138

cardiac 7
  electrical 7
  inhibitory 139
  lipid-lowering 14
  therapeutic 186, 195
Activities 31, 65, 104, 107, 112, 137, 138,
    139, 140, 142, 143, 165, 172, 194
  anthelmintic 142
  anticancer 139
  antihypercholesterolemic 143
  antihyperlipidemic 142
  antihypertensive 137
  anti-inflammatory 194
  antiobesity 172
  cardiac cell 31
  distorted 112
  glucocorticoid 165
  hypocholesterolemic 140
  metabolic 65, 138
  paracrine 104, 107
  superior NADPH oxidase 172
Adam stroke syndrome 115
Adaptive immune responses 43
Adeno-associated virus (AAVs) 67, 91, 94
Adipocytes 43, 142, 146
  mature 43
Adipogenesis 146
Aldosterone 166
Allium Sativum 12, 143
Alzheimer's disease 40
Amalgamations 90
Ameliorate 171, 197
Amplification reaction 160
Anaemia 30, 131
Anaesthesia 69, 158
Angina 2, 10, 116, 130, 134, 137
  pectoris 137
Angiogenesis 196
Angiography 69
Angiotensin-converting enzyme (ACE) 29,
    133, 166
  inhibitors 29

Anthocyanidins 135
Anthocyanins 14, 16, 135, 136, 139
Anthocynins 136
Anthropometrical index 180
Antiarrhythmics 6, 13, 129, 137
Anti-atherogenesis 147
Antiatherogenic agent 55
Anti-atherosclerotic effects 136
Anti-coagulants drugs 8
Anti-dyslipidemia 147
Anti-flatulent properties 145
Anti-hypercholesterolemic effects 45
Anti-inflammatory 11, 16, 39, 42, 43, 45
    action 16
    agents 11, 42, 43, 45
    effects 39
Antinuclear antibodies 131
Antioxidant(s) 11, 12, 13, 14, 16, 38, 45, 46,
        115, 118, 135, 136, 137, 138, 140, 142,
        143, 145, 147, 148, 181, 182
    activities 118, 136, 137
    capacity, non-enzymatic 46
    effects 11, 13
    endogenous 115
    enzymes 16, 138, 181, 182
    polyphenolic 12
    properties 13, 14, 118
    response 16
Antioxidant system 171, 182
    cardiac 182
Antioxidant vitamins 15, 18
    food-containing 18
Aortic constriction 52, 61, 71, 72
Apolipoprotein 17, 54, 55, 56, 88, 128
Apoprotein 54
Apoptosis 60, 88, 106, 115, 197
    myocardial 60, 197
Apoptotic process 88
Appendicitis 133
Applications, translational 52
Arrhythmias 10, 12, 13, 33, 52, 90, 91, 108,
        114, 116, 130, 131, 132
    cardiac 33, 52
Arrhythmogenic right ventricular
cardiomyopathy (ARVC) 27
Arteriosclerosis 128
Arthritis 45, 138
Atherogenesis 9, 42, 54, 55, 181
    vascular bed 9
Atherogenesis lesions 56

Atherosclerosis 2, 4, 5, 9, 42, 52, 53, 54, 55,
        56, 66, 67, 126, 127, 128, 129, 144
    aortic 67
    coronary 66
    lesions 9
    risk of 9, 129
Atherosclerotic 9, 54, 55, 56, 66, 67
    aortic 54
    lesions 54, 55, 56, 66, 67
Atherothrombosis 8
ATPase 31, 33, 34
    enzyme 31
ATPase pump 33
    sodium-potassium 33
Atrial 3, 25, 26, 30, 31, 34, 35, 115
    arrhythmia 31
    fibrillation 3, 25, 26, 30, 34, 35, 115
Autosomal disease 87

B

Bacteria 14, 82, 87
    health-promoting 14
Bacterial plasmids 82
Beta-adrenergic blocking 30
    agents 30
    drugs 30
Bioactive peptides 10, 14
BioAssay systems 174
Bioinformatics 2, 17
    application 17
    approach 2
Biological phenotypes 95
Biomarkers 2, 172
    novel therapeutic 2
    of oxidative stress 172
Blood 11, 15, 54, 57, 67, 106, 107, 108, 113,
        128, 129, 130, 132, 133, 134, 158, 176
    disorders 129, 130, 132
    glucose 57, 176
    lipids 15
Blood pressure 6, 8, 12, 13, 71, 115, 134, 137,
        138, 139, 156, 157, 158, 159
    diastolic 71, 159
    reduction 13
    systolic 71, 158
Body 172, 174, 175, 179, 180
    lipid 180
    mass index (BMI) 172, 174, 175, 179
Brachial neuralgia 117

Bradycardia 72
Bronchospasm 131
Bufodienolide poisoning 33

C

Calcium 33, 41, 42, 139, 146
   channels, voltage-dependent 139
   release 33
Cancer 2, 11, 14, 15, 40, 42, 44, 45, 46, 80,
     82, 87, 88, 141, 144
   human cervical 88
   surpassed 2
Capsicum annum 146
Carbohydrate(s) 10, 39, 40, 41, 42, 134, 138,
     140, 141, 143, 144, 145, 172
   diet 10
   high glycemic index 39
   meals 172
   refined 41
   restricting high glycemic index 41
Cardiac 2, 14, 27, 34, 52, 60, 61, 63, 64, 89,
     91, 105, 107, 114, 115, 180, 181, 187,
     189, 190, 191, 194, 195, 196, 197
   arrest 64, 187
   computed tomography 2
   diseases 27, 52, 89, 91
   events 114
   fibroblast 197
   fibrosis 60, 61, 181
   function responses 63
   functions 14, 34, 107, 115, 180, 196
   ischemia 61
   magnetic resonance imaging 2
   membrane 195
   MRI 114
   mRNA expressions 194
   muscle dysfunction 181
   toxicity 63
   troponin 189, 190, 191, 195, 196
Cardiac glycoside(s) 25, 31, 32, 33, 34, 35,
     134, 140
   biotransformation 34
   containing plants 34
Cardiac hypertrophy 52, 60, 167
   pathological 167
Cardiac lipid 174, 177, 178
   peroxidation 178
   profile 174, 177
Cardiac lipotoxicity 171, 182

ameliorated 171
Cardiomyocytes 12, 89, 90, 91, 115, 172, 187,
     196, 197
   infect 91
   necrotic 91, 196
Cardio-myopathic complication 71
Cardiomyopathy 2, 27, 79, 90
   hypertrophic 2, 27, 90
   inherited 79
   restrictive 27
Cardioprotective 12, 134, 135, 137, 146, 194,
     195
   activities 137, 146, 195
   effect 194, 195
Cardiotoxins 62
Cardiovascular diseases 18, 41, 131, 136
   developing 41
   prevention of 41, 131
   risk of 18, 41, 136
Cardiovascular 9, 38, 39, 53, 132
   diseases research 53
   events 9, 132
   inflammation 38, 39
Carminative agent 46
Carnitine 13
   content reductionis 13
Carolina medical electronics 159
Carotenoids 15, 16, 134, 135, 136
   lycopene antioxidant 16
Catalase 46, 174
Catastrophic health 4
   costs 4
   spending 4
Catechins 14, 15, 16, 136, 142
Cell 11, 93, 116, 180, 195, 196
   cycle arrest 11
   energy metabolism 180
   infiltration 195, 196
   metabolism 116
   penetrating peptides 93
Cellular adhesion 27
Cerebrovascular 2, 9, 126
   disease 2, 126
   events 9
Chemistry of cardiac glycosides 31
Chest 34, 62, 113, 127
   incision 62
   radiograph 34
Chinese 13, 45
   medicine 45

plant coptischinensis 13
Cholecystokinin 58
Cholesterol 4, 5, 9, 11, 13, 14, 15, 41, 42, 54, 55, 56, 60, 64, 66, 127, 133, 147, 181
  deposition 5
  developed elevated plasma 56
  diet 60, 66
  efflux 147
  high-density lipoprotein 127
  ingested 11
    lowering medications 133
    synthesis 13, 15, 181
Cholesterol absorption 11, 133, 182
  inhibitors 133
Cholinergic-mediated vascular effects 139
Chow diet 55
Chronic 31, 46, 56, 70, 71, 87, 136
  congestive heart failure 70
  dialysis 46
  diseases 136
  granulomatous disorders (CGD) 87
  obstructive pulmonary disease (COPD) 31, 56
  valvular disease 71
Chronic inflammations 42, 43, 87
  disease 42
Cinnamaldehyde 142
Cinnamon 142, 143, 147
  polyphenols 143
CIRSPR technology 92
Cleaves plasminogen 9
Clogging 108, 138
  preventing 138
CMD prognosis 105, 106, 119
Collagen redeployment 197
Combination therapy 157
Computed tomography (CT) 2
Concomitant reduction 181
Conditions 7, 26, 27, 29, 35, 40, 42, 52, 53, 67, 70, 83, 87, 138, 182, 186, 195
  atherosclerotic 42
  cardiac 7, 195
  rheumatological 138
Congestive heart failure (CHF) 10, 12, 25, 26, 27, 29, 31, 33, 34, 35, 64, 70, 181
Consumption 4, 14, 26, 41, 45, 125, 137, 181, 188
  excessive alcohol 4, 26
Contractile dysfunctions 108, 115
Contractility 108, 115, 181

cardiac 108
  myocardial 115
Contraction 7, 8, 25, 29, 33, 107, 115, 116
  cardiac myocyte 8
  force 29
  myocardial 25, 115
Control 16, 40, 41, 134, 158, 161, 162, 163, 164, 165, 166, 167, 168, 175, 176, 177, 178, 179, 192, 193
  anti-oxidative 16
  blood pressure 41
  glycemic 134
  hypertensive 158, 161, 162, 163, 164, 165
  lifelong weight 40
Coriandrum sativum 141
Corn starch 173
Coronary 2, 9, 11, 13, 14, 26, 52, 53, 62, 64, 67, 68, 89, 90, 91, 113, 138, 144, 146, 171
  artery disease (CAD) 2, 26, 52, 138, 171
  disease 90
  heart disease (CHD) 9, 11, 13, 14, 26, 53, 89, 90, 91, 144, 146
  occlusion 62
  vasculature 64
Creatine 114, 189
  kinase-MB isoenzyme 189
  Phospho-Kinase-MB (CPKMB) 114
CRISPR 79, 80, 81, 82, 83, 84, 85, 86, 88, 89, 92, 93, 94, 95, 96
  gene technology 89
  method 85
  nickase enzyme 94
  system 81, 86, 88
  techniques 84, 85, 86
  technologies 79, 80, 81, 82, 83, 84, 86, 92, 93, 94, 95, 96
Crocus sativus 135
Cryptoxanthin 141
Curcuma longa 139
Curcumin 12, 136, 140
Curcuminoids 46
CVD 2, 4, 9, 43, 126, 147, 195
  diagnosis 4, 195
  disorders 9
  morbidity 126
  mortality 2, 4
  promoting conditions 43
  protection 147
  related deaths 2

risk 9
Cyclic adenosine monophosphate 14
Cystic-fibrosis transmembrane 84
Cytokines 43, 44, 45, 55, 118, 189, 196
  inflammatory 43, 44, 118, 189, 196
  proatherogenic 43
  proinflammatory 196

D

Damage 12, 29, 45, 82, 119, 128, 157, 181,
    182, 195
  cardiac 195
  cardiovascular 181
  endothelial 157
  free radical induced tissue cell 182
  polyunsaturated LDL 12
  tissue 45, 181
Deaths 2, 3, 4, 11, 52, 53, 79, 87, 90, 126,
    179, 186
  proportionate 4
Defective phagocytes 87
Dehydrated garlic 143
Demands 61, 105, 107
  metabolic 105, 107
  perfusion 61
Demerits 89, 95
  heart lopping 89
Dendritic cells 140
Densitometric analysis 160
Deposition 12, 42, 113, 127, 179
  atheromatous 12
Detoxification genes 16
Dexamethasone 156, 157
  exposure 156
Diabetes mellitus (DM) 4, 56, 59, 66, 114,
    132, 143, 171, 180
Diabetic nephropathy 129, 130
Diacylglycerol signalling 180
Diastolic blood pressure (DBP) 71, 157, 159,
    162, 163
Diet 38, 39, 40, 44, 45, 55, 67
  atherogenic 55
  high-cholesterol 55, 67
  ketogenic 40, 44
  low carbohydrate 38, 40, 45
  low-cholesterol 67
  pro-inflammaotry 39
Dietary 39, 60, 137
  foods 137

inflammation 39
  Inflammatory Index (DII) 39
  manipulation 60
Diet-associated inflammation 39
Diet induced 38, 56
  inflammation 38
  steatohepatitis 56
Digitoxigenin 34
Digoxin medication 34
Dihydrocoriandrin 142
Dihydrodigoxin 34
Disease(s) 1, 2, 42, 43, 45, 46, 53, 54, 55, 56,
    71, 80, 88, 90, 96, 112, 114, 117, 129,
    157
  communicable 129
  etiology 96
  metabolic 157
  pathogenesis 53
  prognosis 112, 117
  skin 117
Disorders 4, 30, 44, 53, 54, 80, 81, 84, 86, 87,
    91, 105, 108, 116, 117, 126, 137, 142,
    144, 145, 181, 187
  alcohol use 30
  allergic 145
  autoimmune 44
  cardiac 91
  hereditary dyslipidemic 54
  metabolic 105, 108, 116, 137, 181
  multifaceted 187
  multifactorial 87
  neurodegenerative 44
  stomach 142
Dizziness 127, 129, 130, 131, 132
DNA 16, 80, 81, 82, 88, 93, 94, 95, 96, 167
  binding transcription factors 167
  cleavage 93, 96
  exogenous 80, 82
  splicing protein 96
  target locus 81
Doppler echocardiography 62
Double-strand breaks (DSB) 81, 82, 90, 96
Drugs 7, 25, 31, 54, 56, 60, 62, 64, 66, 68, 72,
    91, 129, 130, 134, 172
  anti-arrhythmia 91
  anti-diabetic 60
  atherosclerotic 54
  cytotoxic 62
  hypolipidemic 56
  immune-suppressive 72

oral antiobesity 172
Duchenne muscle dystrophy (DMD) 71, 86
Dysfunction 5, 26, 29, 127, 131, 132, 133,
    157, 166, 172
  diastolic 26
  endothelial 5, 127, 166
  hepatic 131, 132
  myocardial 29
  renal 157
  sexual 133
Dyslipidemia 4, 9, 40, 43, 56, 57, 58, 125,
    126, 127, 146, 171, 180
  diabetic 56, 57
  pro-atherogenic 43
Dyspepsia 131, 133
Dyspnea 25, 26, 30, 31, 34
Dyspnoea 132

E

Echocardiography 116
Edema 9, 30, 108, 117
  acute pulmonary 9
Effective nutraceuticals 138
Effect(s) 11, 141, 144, 146, 147, 156, 172,
    178, 188, 194, 195,
  antihyperlipidemic 141
  antihypertensive 156
  atheroprotective 147
  cardiac 195
  hallucinogenic 146
  of betaine on cardiac mRNA expressions
    194
  of ZB on cardiac lipid peroxidation 178
  on nutraceuticals on cardiovascular health
    11
  therapeutic 144, 172, 188
Efficacy 12, 29, 54, 57, 63, 68, 95, 118, 125,
    139, 157, 182, 196
  antihypertensive 157
  anti-inflammatory 196
  anti-obesity 182
  therapeutic 125, 139
Electrocardiograms 2, 90, 114
Electrophysiology 64
Elettaria cardamomum 146
ELISA method 189
Emboli coil implantation 70
Emerging CRISPR Technologies 95

Endocarditis 4
Endogenous retrovirus 92
Endothelial 13, 15, 16, 42, 115, 137
  functions 13, 15, 16, 115, 137
  integrity 42
Energy 25, 26, 34, 115, 117, 118, 180
  balance 180
  condensed 180
  depletion 115
  metabolism 118
  storage 180
Engineered mega nucleases 81
Enzymatic proteolysis 6
Enzyme 8, 13, 93, 114, 133, 141, 181, 195
  cardiac 114
  cytosolic 195
  gastro-intestinal 141
  mitochondrial 181
  reverse transcriptase 93
Epicatechins 136, 142
Equilibrium 106, 111, 112, 119, 187
  body's thermal 106
Erectile dysfunctions 56, 117
Escherichia coli 82
Euvolemic hyponatremia 30
Exercise tolerance 25, 29, 34
Expression 15, 18, 79, 84, 85, 107, 108, 111,
    115, 156, 164, 167, 168
  down-regulated mRNA 164
  genetic 79
  phenotypic 85

F

Factors 2, 5, 15, 30, 38, 39, 52, 53, 80, 96,
    105, 110, 111, 112, 114, 115, 117, 118,
    157, 181
  dietary 2
  endothelium-derived hyperpolarizing 157
  endothelium-derived relaxing 115
  environmental 53, 80
  etiological 112, 117
  genetic 5
  hepatic transcription 15
  tumor necrosis 114, 118
Fagonia Arabica 118
Failure 26, 30, 33, 55, 69, 70, 195, 196
  cardiac 26, 33, 69, 196
  myocardial infarction/heart 70
Fatal disease 61

Fat(s) 39, 40, 41, 42, 54, 55, 56, 113, 172, 179
  hydrogenated 39
  milk 55
    soluble lubrication 113
Fatty acid(s) 1, 10, 13, 15, 17, 18, 39, 40, 43,
    146, 148, 172
  polyunsaturated 18, 148
  bsynthase 17
  toxic long-chain non-esterified 172
  unsaturated 39, 40
Fever 114, 131, 142
  seasonal 142
Fiber 1, 15, 18, 38, 41, 90, 143
  dietary 1, 18
  smooth muscle 90
Fibroblasts, fetal 68
Fibrosis 29, 60, 61, 71, 80, 82, 83, 110, 113,
    115, 167, 195, 196
  cystic 80, 82, 83
  myocardial 115
Ficus hispida 135
Flavonoids 2, 12, 14, 134, 135, 136, 138, 140,
    142, 144, 145
Flow 104, 106, 108, 110, 113, 115, 133
  oscillatory 115
Food and drug administration (FDA) 30, 34,
    134
Foods 1, 10, 12, 18, 34, 40, 106, 111, 112,
    118, 141, 144, 146, 179
  excessive 179
  healthy fats-rich 40
  swallowing 106
  therapeutic 1
Free radical scavenging 147
Fruits 12, 14, 15, 39, 40, 41, 134, 135, 136,
    137, 142
  citrus 136
  low-glycemic 41
Functions 6, 12, 13, 26, 61, 79, 84, 85, 89, 91,
    104, 105, 106, 108, 109, 113, 119, 172,
    180, 181
  cardiovascular 61
  cognitive 85
  compromised 105
  contractile 104, 105, 119
  explicit gene 79
  myocardial 172
  neuroendocrine 26

G

Gallate 135, 136
  epicatechin 136
Garcinia indica 135
Garlic 1, 12, 18, 143, 144, 147
  therapeutic effects of 144
Gastritis 132
Gene(s) 6, 12, 13, 16, 17, 18, 57, 67, 71, 79,
    80, 81, 82, 83, 84, 85, 86, 87, 88, 89, 90,
    91, 92, 94, 95, 96, 119, 129, 156, 164,
    166, 167, 189, 190, 196
  adeno-associated virus-mediated 67
  alterations 95
  allele-dominant 85
  cytoprotective 16
  delivery 91
  duplication 6
  dystrophin 71, 86
  expression 12, 13, 88, 119, 156, 164, 167
  housekeeping 189
  hub 18
  hunting 85
  induced 80
  leptin 57
  leptin-receptor 57
  lipoprotein 129
  multi-factorial 96
  mutations 67, 86, 91
  proinflammatory-associated 196
  therapy 79, 81, 91
  therapy tools 81
Generations 12, 80, 93, 94
  mitochondrial energy 12
Genesis 31, 104, 115
  abnormal 115
Genetic(s) 41, 42, 54, 61, 79, 80, 81, 85, 86,
    90, 128
  alleles 86
  diseases 80
  disorders 80
  modifying human 81
  mutations 80
  tool kits 85
Genome editing 82, 83, 84
  natural 83
  tools 83
Genome-wide association studies (GWAS) 90
Genomic 16, 96
  databases 96
  processes 16

Glucose 14, 39, 40, 113, 143, 174, 180, 195
  dysregulated 180
  intake 39
  tolerance test (GTT) 113
Glucose uptake 142, 180
  insulin-mediated 180
Glucosinolates 146
Glutathione 46, 174, 178, 179, 181, 182
  peroxidase 46, 174
  reductase (GR) 174, 178, 179, 181, 182
Glycosides 14, 32, 33, 134, 135, 138, 141
  cardiotonic 33
  flavonoid 14
  steroid 32
Glycosuria 57, 59
Glycyrrhiza glabra 137
Growth 4, 89, 140, 179
  economic 4
  suppress tumor 140
GSH protein 182
Guanylyl cyclase 139

H

Haemophilia 82
Haemorrhage 131, 132
  intestinal 131
Haemorrhagic strokes 3
HDL cholesterol levels 136, 137
Headache 129, 130, 131, 132, 133, 138
Health 45, 104
  disorders 45
  restoring 104
Healthy eating index 39
Heart 2, 6, 7, 8, 25, 26, 27, 33, 34, 35, 60, 89,
    105, 106, 107, 108, 115, 119, 126, 134,
    144, 171, 178, 181, 187
  attacks 2, 8, 26, 126, 144
  contraction 33, 34
  infarcted 187
  lipid peroxidation 181
  metabolism 181
  tonics 34
  transplantation 27, 35
Heart diseases 2, 3, 12, 14, 26, 53, 63, 70, 71,
    89, 116, 126, 172
  adult congenital 26
  congenital 89, 126
  hypertensive 3, 12
  ischaemic 70

  ischemic 3, 12, 116
  lipotoxic 172
  rheumatic 2, 3, 53
Heart failure 26, 29, 30, 31, 61, 62, 72,
  nonischemic 29, 30
  stable chronic 72
  stimulus 61
  symptoms 26, 31
  syndromes 62
Heart muscle 7, 14, 29, 107, 195
  contractions 29
  fibres 195
Hemodynamic forces 108
Hemoglobin 84, 85, 114
  glycosylated 114
Hemophilia 86
Hemostasis 113
Hepatic 34, 130, 146
  biotransformation 34
  encephalopathy 130
  steatosis 146
Hepatoprotective 135, 145, 188
Herbaceous perennial plant 146
High-cholesterol content 54
High density lipoprotein (HDL) 9, 67, 127
High-fat-diet 171
High reproductive efficiency 58
High-risk papillomavirus 88
Histone deacetylases 156, 160
HMG CoA reductase inhibitors 9
Homeostasis 84, 107, 113, 166, 180
  deregulated energy 180
  electrolytic 84
  kidney 166
Homocysteine 15, 61, 186, 189, 190, 191, 195
  lowering blood 15
Homogenates 160, 174
  aortic 160
Homologous mending processes 87
Homology-directed repair (HDR) 81, 82, 83,
    90, 93, 94
Human 56, 57
  obesity 57
  vasculopathy 56
Huntington's 80, 85
  disease 80, 85
  protein 85
Hydronephrosis 58
Hypercholesterolemia 54, 58, 67
Hyperglycemia 58, 146, 148, 180

Hyperinsulinemia 56, 57, 58, 59, 180
Hyperleptinemia 60
Hyperlipidaemias 133
Hyperlipidemia 2, 10, 57, 58, 127, 148
Hyperphagia 59
Hyperplasia 58, 195
   fibroblastic 195
Hypertension 2, 4, 12, 13, 14, 57, 125, 129,
     130, 131, 132, 137, 156, 157, 158
   sensitive 157
Hyperthyroidism 131
Hypertriglyceridemia 13, 56, 59
Hypertrophic cardiomyopathy (HCM) 2, 27,
     90
Hypertrophy 12, 16, 27, 58, 60, 61, 113, 195
   adipocyte 58
   myocardial 195
Hyponatremia 30
Hypotension 129, 130, 132

I

Illnesses 12, 18, 26, 88
   cardiac 12
   cardiovascular 18
   monogenetic 88
   thyroid 26
Immune 14, 47
   boosting properties 47
   function 14
Immunoboosting 148
Immunological deficiencies 87
Impaired glucose tolerance (IGT) 57, 59
Impairment 25, 26, 59, 107, 108, 116, 118,
     126, 129
   cognitive 25, 26
   gestational metabolic 59
   renal 129
Induction of hypertension 158, 167
Infarction 4, 7, 8, 60, 64, 69, 72, 131, 186
   acute myocardial 4, 7, 60, 64, 131
   chronic myocardial 72
   developing Myocardial 69
   isoproterenol-induced myocardial 186
Infections 26, 82, 87, 132, 136
   pathogenic 136
   urinary tract 132
Inflammation 39, 43, 44, 45, 55, 56, 59, 111,
     113, 127, 128, 188, 195, 196
   myocardial 188

Inflammatory 13, 91, 137, 187, 196
   enzyme COX-2 13
   processes 137
   reaction 91, 187, 196
Inhibitors 6, 29, 92, 133
   angiotensin-converting enzyme 6, 29
   angiotensin receptor-neprilysin 133
   lipoprotein lipase 92
Injury 8, 11, 29, 114, 116, 118, 196
   cardiac 29
   constant reperfusion 196
   ischemia reperfusion 11
   myocardial 114, 116, 118
Insulin 143, 174, 176, 180
   sensitivity 180
Intermediate-density lipoprotein (IDL) 54,
     128
Ischemia 8, 36, 60, 113, 136, 195
   myocardial 136
Ischemic heart disease (IHD) 3, 12, 29, 116

K

Ketosis 40
Kidney disease 41

L

Lactate dehydrogenase 189
Lagenaria siceraria 135
Left ventricular 25, 26, 27
   ejection fraction (LVEF) 25, 26
   noncompaction (LVNC) 27
Lentivirus-mediated CRISPR technologies 94
Leptin 56, 57
   hormone 57
   mutation 57
Leucoanthocyanin 140
Lipid 14, 60, 61, 64, 116, 147, 174, 177, 178,
     179, 180, 181, 182
   homeostasis 116
   peroxidation 147, 174, 178, 181, 182
   profile 14, 64, 147, 177, 179, 180
   rich occlusion 60, 61
Lipid metabolism 52, 53, 56, 108, 180
   cardiac 180
Lipoproteins 9, 17, 54, 55
   high density 9
   lipase 17

Low-density lipoprotein(s) (LDL) 4, 5, 11, 12, 13, 46, 54, 67, 88, 127, 128, 129, 147
  cholesterol 88
  oxidized 46
Lowering 9, 18
  blood lipids 18
  LDL cholesterol 9

M

Macronutrients 39, 43
  eating 43
Macrophages 13, 44, 55, 137, 140, 196
  pro-inflammatory 44
Malfunction 167
Malignant tendencies 88
MAPKs activation 147
Matrix 186, 187
  metallopreoteinases 186
  metalloproteases 187
Mechanical cell deformations 93
Mechanism 6, 7, 8, 9, 15, 29, 31, 33, 45, 47, 79, 82, 83, 84, 93, 112, 137, 165, 196
  anti-inflammatory 45
  cholesterol-lowering 15
  homology-directed repair 83
  immunological 82
  of action of amiodarone 7
  of action of amlodipine 8
  of action of aspirin 8
  of action of candesartan 6
  of action of lidocaine 7
  of action of procainamide 7
  of action of trandolapril 6
  of action of urokinase 9
  of cardiac glycosides 33
  protein refolding 84
  thermoregulatory 112
Mediators, inflammatory 39, 44, 66, 187
Medications 6, 7, 8, 9, 34, 117, 118, 187
  anti-arrhythmic 7
  cardiac 8
  herbal 9
Medicines 6, 7, 8, 9, 10, 18, 33, 45, 79, 96, 139, 142, 144
  antiarrhythmic 7
  antithrombotic 9
  genomic 96
  traditional 139
Mediterranean dietary index 39

Metabolic 2, 18, 38, 43, 46, 53, 105, 114, 116, 126, 130
  alkalosis 130
  program 18
  syndrome 2, 38, 43, 46, 53
  syndrome disorders 126
  system (MS) 105, 114, 116
Metabolism 14, 17, 25, 54, 64, 137
  cardiac 54, 64, 137
  lipoprotein 54, 137
Metabolites 6, 17, 106, 119, 195
  pathologic 195
Methods 17, 55, 62, 79, 84, 87, 93, 159, 190
  ANOVA 190
  enzymatic conversion 159
  gene therapy 87
  gene therapy treatment 79
  homologous recombination 84
  hydrodynamic delivery 93
  imaging 55
  lucigenin-enhanced chemiluminescence 159
  reductionist 17
  surgical 62
  transduction 93
Microdeposits 131
Microembolisation 70
Microflora, intestinal 14
Micronutrients 39, 134
Milk 18, 146, 160
  protein peptides 18
  skimmed 160
Mineralocorticoid effects 166
Minneapolis 189
Monocyclic sesquiterpene 171, 172
Monogenic diseases 82
Morbidities 42, 53, 107, 110, 117, 125, 187
  cardiovascular 42
Moringa oleifera 134, 146
Mucuna pruriens 135
Multifactorial diseases 82, 87
Multiple 15, 60, 83
  diffuse lipid-rich stenosis 60
  organ dysfunctions 83
  sclerosis 15
Muscle cells 7, 8, 14, 33, 91, 115, 157, 196
  cardiac 7, 14, 33, 91
  smooth 91
  vascular smooth 8, 115, 157, 196
Muscle contraction 7, 8
  smooth 8

Muscle(s) 6, 8, 13, 14, 31, 62, 71, 107, 108,
    109, 112, 116, 119, 139, 187
  cardiac 8, 14, 107, 187
  metabolism 116
  progressive 71
  respiratory 31
  vascular smooth 6, 8, 139
Mutations, transcriptase-introduced 93
Myeloperoxidase 46
Myocardial 4, 5, 8, 13, 25, 26, 62, 68, 70, 72,
    79, 116, 186, 187, 195, 196, 197
  infarction (MI) 4, 5, 8, 13, 25, 26, 68, 70,
    72, 79, 186, 187, 195, 196, 197
  ischemia-induced heart failure 62
  stiffness 116
Myocardial damage 181, 196
  ischemic 196
Myocarditis 26
Myocytes 8, 13, 7, 33, 104, 115
  cardiac 8, 13
Myofibroblasts 196
Myosin filaments 29
Myristica fragrans 146
Myristicin 146

N

NADPH oxidase 167
Nausea 132, 133, 142
Necrosis 106, 111, 115, 131, 187, 195
Neomycin resistance gene 68
Nephropathy 128
Neprilysin 133
Nerium oleander plant 32
Neurohormonal 26, 29, 31
  dysregulation 31
  systems 29
Neuropathy 58, 131
  peripheral 131
Neurotransmission 116
Neutrophil(s) 140, 197
  degranulation 197
Nitric oxide metabolites 159
Non-alcoholic fatty liver disease 44
Non-communicable disease (NCDs) 3, 52,
    129
Nonenzymatic anti-oxidant systems 15
Non-homologous end joining (NHEJ) 81, 82,
    91, 94
Noninvasive tail-cuff plethysmography 158

Nourishing metabolite 107
Nuclear acetylation 12
Numerous surgical methods 62
Nutraceuticals modulate genetic expression 16
Nutrient utilization 180

O

Obesity 43, 44, 56, 57, 58, 114, 116, 125, 157,
    171, 172, 173, 174, 176, 179, 180, 181,
    182
  ameliorate 182
  associated metabolic derangements 172
  cardiomyopathy (OC) 157, 171, 172, 179,
    181, 182
  index 174, 176, 179
Occlusion 8, 60, 69, 70, 187
  temporary 70
  vascular 8
Oil(s) 11, 13, 16, 40, 41, 134, 138, 140, 142,
    143, 144, 145, 173
  canola 13
  corn 173
  essential 138, 140, 142, 145
  olive 16, 40, 41
  seeds 40
  vegetable 11, 13
Olea europaea 135
Oral supplementation 162, 164
Organ failure 115
Osmocytosis 94
Oxidation 12, 13, 15, 16, 172, 181
  reducing 13
Oxidative 12, 16, 45
  burst 45
  damage 12, 16
Oxidative stress 16, 45, 59, 115, 171, 172,
    178, 179, 180, 181, 182
  obesity-related 172
  systemic 172
  vanished 182

P

Pain 25, 26, 31, 109, 113, 127, 131, 132, 133
  abdominal 131, 133
Palpitations 114, 130
Pancreas 58, 59, 66, 83
  offspring 59

Pancreatitis 132, 133
Pathogenesis 25, 42, 44, 57, 89, 96, 106, 112,
    113, 116, 181, 187
  diabetic 44
  related issues 96
Pathological dryness 111. 112, 113
  promoting 111, 112
Pathologic thirst 113
Pathophysiology, diabetic 57
Pathways 16, 17, 62, 81, 82, 139, 157, 196
  disease progress 81
  renin angiotensin 157
  vasodilator 139
Periodontal disease 58
Peripheral 2, 4, 52, 116
    arterial disease 2
    vascular disease 4, 52, 116
Peroxisome-proliferator-activated receptors
    (PPARs) 17
Peroxynitrite inactivation 12
Phenotype 55, 56, 119
  plasma lipoprotein 56
Phenotypic constitution 111
Phenylpropanoids 146
Phospholipids 174
Phytochemicals 10, 11, 15, 134, 136, 137,
    138, 144, 145, 148
    Mahanimbine 145
Phyto-pharmacological interventions of
    antioxidants 114
Phytosterols 11, 140
Piper nigrum 140, 141
Plant(s) 1, 11, 18, 31, 32, 134, 136, 138, 142,
    143, 148, 188, 194, 197
  and herbs 134, 148
  derived phytoconstituents 194
  sterols 1, 11
Plaque 8, 12, 43, 53, 54, 55, 128
  aortic 55
  atheromatous 43
  atherosclerotic 8, 12, 128
Plaque 60, 66
  haemorrhage 66
  stenosis 60
Plasma 54, 55, 88, 158, 167, 180, 197
  insulin 180
  lipoprotein profile 54
Plasma glucose 180
  augmented 180
Plasmid-based delivery systems 94

Platelet aggregation 8, 13, 16, 18, 136, 137,
    147
  inhibiting 8
  preventing 18
Platelet-derived growth factor (PDGF) 12
Pneumonitis 131
Polydipsia 58, 59, 113
Polyphenolic anti-oxidants 141
Polyvinylidene difluoride membrane 160
Predisposition, genetic 67
Pressure 26, 62, 64
  pulmonary capillary wedge 26
  systolic 64
Preventive cardiology 104
Problems 3, 81, 92, 93, 125
  biomedical 81
  global health 125
Production 8, 12, 13, 17, 85, 89, 94, 159, 162,
    163, 164, 166, 180, 181, 186, 192
  hepatic glucose 180
  inflammatory markers 192
  lipid 17
  malondialdehyde 181
  mitochondrial 12
Prognosis 2, 27, 52, 64, 104, 105, 118, 196
Programming 59, 166
  epigenetic 59
Progression 5, 42, 43, 54, 58, 71
  atherosclerotic plaque 43
Pro-inflammatory 39, 43, 186, 188, 196
    cytokines 186, 188, 196
    effects 39
    lipoproteins 43
Properties 12, 33, 68, 105, 111, 115, 118, 119,
    137, 138, 139, 142, 143, 148, 181
  amphiphilic 181
  anti-apoptotic 12
  antiatherosclerotic 148
  anti-oxidant 105
  biomechanical 68
  cardio-suppressant 139
  intrinsic 105, 111, 119
  intrinsic oxidant 115
  metal chelating 137
  thrombolytic 118
  triacylglycerols lipase 142
Prostaglandins 8, 9, 13
  pain-inducing 8
Protease 9, 55, 197
  active fibrinolytic 9

secretion 55
serine 9
Protein(s) 14, 15, 16, 38, 40, 41, 42, 82, 84,
        86, 93, 119, 138, 141, 143, 146, 160,
        164, 165, 167, 180
    biosynthesis 180
    dystrophin 86
    expressions 119, 165, 167
    fusion 93
    inhibitory 16
    lupin 14
    regulatory element binding 15
Proteomics 119
Psidium guajava 135
Pulmonary 2, 89
    atresia 89
    embolism 2
Pumps 33, 105
    calcium ions 33
    sodium-potassium 33
Purpurea, thrombocytopenic 131

R

Reactive oxygen species (ROS) 11, 42, 87,
        136, 182
Recovery, myocardial 72
Reduction of hyperlipidemia and
        hyperglycemia 148
Regulation 15, 88, 91, 93, 164, 167, 180
    metabolic 91
Regulatory mechanisms, genetic 89
Rehabilitation 31
    breathlessness 31
Research, translational 52, 71
Respiratory cycle 181
Response, inflammatory 187, 196
Restrictive cardiomyopathy (RCM) 27
Reteplase 9
Retinopathy 128
Reverse 93, 119, 189
    transcription 93
Rheumatic heart disease (RHD) 2, 3, 53
Right ventricular diastolic pressure 65
Risk 1, 4, 5, 9, 10, 11, 12, 13, 18, 40, 41, 42,
        134, 136
    cardiovascular 5, 9, 134
    chronic disease 40
    socioeconomic 18

Risk factors 1, 4, 5, 9, 43, 125, 127, 128, 143,
        171, 179, 180, 181
    autonomous 171
    cardiovascular 1, 4
    for cardiovascular diseases 5
RNA 81, 82
    target-oriented 81
    trans-activating 82
RT-PCR Analysis 159, 189, 196

S

Secoiridoids 135
Sensitivity 25, 26
    therapeutic 26
Sheath 69
    arterial vascular 69
Sickle cell 80, 84
    anemia 80, 84
    disease 84
Signaling pathways 16, 116, 118
    inhibitory 118
Skin 62, 65, 69, 131, 137
    discoloration 131
    incision 62, 69
Sleep disturbances 130
Somatic cell 67, 93
    gene-editing 93
Source 12, 32, 65, 66, 85, 91
    of cardiac glycosides 32
SPSS software 161
Staphylococcus aureus 92
Stem cells 72, 79, 89
    human mesenchymal 72
    induced pluripotent 79, 89
Stenosis 64, 113
    aortic 64
Stents 63, 66, 68
    drug-eluting 66
Steptokinase 118
Steroids 135, 138, 139, 140, 141, 144, 145
Strategy 133, 137
    combinatorial treatment 133
Streptokinase 9
Stress 111, 179, 180
    lipid profiles and oxidative 179, 180
Stroke 2, 4, 8, 9, 52, 126, 128, 137, 146
    ischemic 8
Super oxide dismutase (SOD) 46, 115, 174,
        178, 179, 181, 182

Supra-ventricular arrhythmias 131
Surgeries 71, 72
  cardiac 72
  cardiovascular 71, 72
Surplus glucocorticoids 165
Syndrome 40, 91, 114, 118, 130, 131, 132
  acute coronary 118, 132
  cardiac 91
  polycystic ovary 40
  respiratory distress 131
Synthesis 9, 118, 142, 159, 165, 166, 196
  glycogen 142
Synthetic glucocorticoid 165
System 29, 35, 84, 105, 119, 127, 157, 181
  antioxidant defence 181
  dysfunctional endothelial 127
  gastrointestinal 35
  metabolic 105
  musculoskeletal 119
  organoid 84
  renin-angiotensin 29
  sympathetic nervous 157
Systolic 26, 27, 30, 71, 158, 159, 162, 163,
    166
  blood pressure (SBP) 71, 158, 159, 162,
    163, 166
  dysfunction 26, 30
  function 27

T

Techniques 63, 68, 81, 82, 83, 89, 93, 114,
    119
  gene-editing 89
  genome-editing 81
  homology-based base-pairing 83
  imaging 63, 114
Technology 66, 80, 81, 92
  emerging 66
  gene editing 80
  genome-editing 92
  target gene-editing 81
  technology-based editing 92
Terpene hydrocarbons 146
Thalassemia 80, 82, 85
Therapeutic activity 139, 142, 143, 145
  of cinnamon 143
  of cloves 145
  of coriander 142
Therapeutic(s) 18, 79, 83, 88, 95, 187

molecule RNA 79
plants 187
targets 18, 187
tools 83, 88, 95
Therapies 6, 9, 18, 25, 31, 33, 35, 84, 88, 117
  device 35
Thermoregulation 111, 112, 113
Thrombocytopenia 131
Thrombolytic treatment 8
Thrombosis 2, 126
  vein 2
Thrombotic events 132
Thyroid disease 30
Tissues 6, 8, 25, 26, 32, 44, 59, 61, 93, 108,
    111, 112, 113, 119, 164, 167, 195
  aortic 164, 167
  cardiac nodal 8
  damaged 195
  insulin target 59
  interstitial 111
  mammalian 32
  matured adipose 44
  metabolizing 108, 112, 119
  myocardial 61
  visceral adipose 44
TNF-sensitive regulatory factor 90
Transcription activator-like effector nucleases
    (TALENs) 80, 81, 84, 96
Transcription factors 16, 17, 81, 167
  octamer-binding 81
Transcriptomics approach 17
Transferring vehicles 91
Transmyocardial implantation 72
Transplantations 72, 92
  intramyocardial 72
Transport, metabolite 106, 115
Transporter 12, 89
  electron 12

U

Urokinase 9, 118

V

Valvular 26, 89
  heart disease (VHD) 26, 89
Vascular 38, 55, 104, 137, 156, 159
  diseases 104

dysfunction 156
inflammation 38
lumen morphology 55
reactivity 137
resistance 159
Vasoactive agents 166
Vasoconstriction 108, 112, 113, 115, 166
induced systemic 166
Vasoconstrictors 9, 157
inflamed tissue-derived 157
Vasodilation 9, 108, 115, 139
mediated 139
Vasodilators 133, 134, 139, 157
endothelium-independent 139
Vasopressin receptor antagonists 25, 30
Vasopressor ionotropes 30
Vata disorders 112
Vectors 68, 91, 92, 94
adenovirus 91
defective lentiviral 92
viral-based 94
Very-low-density lipoprotein (VLDL) 54,
        129, 146, 147
Viral vector systems 94
Vomiting 127, 131, 132, 133

W

World health organization 41

X

Xeno transplantations 92
X-linked 86, 87
degenerative disease 86
genetic illness 86
granulomatous disease 87

Z

Zinc-finger nucleases (ZFNs) 80, 81
Zingiber Officinale 138, 171, 172
Zucker 58
diabetic fatty (ZDF) 58
fatty rat for hyperglycemia 58

www.ingramcontent.com/pod-product-compliance
Lightning Source LLC
Chambersburg PA
CBHW050836220326
41598CB00006B/377